Advances in Preventing and Treating Violence and Aggression

Series Editor

Peter Sturmey
Queens College and The Graduate Center
City University of New York
Flushing, NY, USA

The series publishes books focused and developed across three domains. The first is understanding and explaining violence and aggression. Books in this domain address such subject matter as genetics, physiology, neurobiology, cultural evolution, biobehavioral, learning, cognitive, psychoanalytic, sociological and other explanations of violence. The second domain focuses on prevention and treatment for individuals and couples. Examples of books in this domain include cognitive behavioral, behavioral, counseling, psychopharmacological, psychosocial, couples, and family therapy approaches. They also explore extant treatment packages for individually focused treatments (e.g., mindfulness, cognitive analytic therapies). Within this domain, books focus on meeting the information needs of clinicians and professionals who work in youth facilities, emergency rooms, special education, criminal justice, and therapy settings. Finally, books in the third domain address prevention and treatment for groups and society, including topical focus on early intervention programs, school violence prevention programs, policing strategies, juvenile facility reform as well as socio-legal and ethical issues. Books in this series serve as must-have resources for researchers, academics, and upper-level undergraduate and graduate students in clinical child and school psychology, public health, criminology/criminal justice, developmental psychology, psychotherapy/counseling, psychiatry, social work, educational policy and politics, health psychology, nursing, and behavioral therapy/rehabilitation.

More information about this series at http://www.springer.com/series/15332

József Haller

Neurobiopsychosocial Perspectives on Aggression and Violence

From Biology to Law Enforcement

Springer

József Haller
Department of Behavioral Neurobiology
Institute of Experimental Medicine
Budapest, Hungary

Faculty of Law Enforcement, Department of Criminal Psychology
National University of Public Service
Budapest, Hungary

Advances in Preventing and Treating Violence and Aggression
ISBN 978-3-030-46330-4   ISBN 978-3-030-46331-1 (eBook)
https://doi.org/10.1007/978-3-030-46331-1

This Springer imprint is published by the registered company Springer Nature Switzerland AG
The registered company address is: Gewerbestrasse 11, 6330 Cham, Switzerland

Preface

About Aggression

Aggression and violence are and continues to be in the forefront of public attention because they result in so much damage to the society. It is easy to substantiate this claim by figures. For instance, "interpersonal violence" occupies a distinguished rank in the World Health Organization's list of "Disease burden and mortality estimates" [1]. Another aggression-related item specifically "Collective violence and legal intervention" is 32 places lower but still in the upper third of the list, alongside neighbors like "schizophrenia" and "exposure to mechanical forces." Although it is difficult to understand why violence was listed among diseases – this author has never understood it – it is telling that a measure of disease burden called "disability adjusted life years" (DALY) attributes interpersonal violence more weight than to various types of cancer (breast, colon, liver, and stomach cancer), drug abuse, alcohol use disorders, hypertensive heart disease, and osteoarthritis to name just a few of the 165 diseases responsible for fewer DALY than interpersonal violence. A regrettable statistics shows that about 10 million people were killed only between 1990 and 2016 (i.e., a medium-sized country over 26 years), with yearly rates varying from 300 to 400 thousand [2]. This compares very unfavorably with the deadly victims of terrorism which number only around 20,000 over a much larger period (1970–2017, i.e., 47 years) according to the Global Terrorism Database [3]. Although these figures are high enough, they may constitute just the tip of the iceberg if we consider non-lethal aggression and violence that are often missing from crime statistics. A study performed in the barrooms of Toronto for instance suggests that fights break out every third hour in these locations [4]. The authors of the study observed 108 pubs and bars for 3335 hours in total and recorded 1052 instances of violence, which were committed by 1754 perpetrators. It is unknown whether these figures are generalizable to cities located elsewhere; nevertheless, one can rather confidently assume that people readily frequent places where physical aggression is common, and where they fight on their own accord without being admonished too often by the police and without being recorded in criminal statistics. The problem grows even larger if we consider accepted forms of aggression, e.g., indirect, relational, and social aggression (see below), which are far more frequent than fistfights, and, although physically not damaging, they still inflict a heavy psychological strain and health risks on their victims [5].

About this Book

In this volume we address the mechanisms of aggression and violence, which are also risk factors for violent crime. This volume proposes a hierarchical stratification of the mechanisms of aggression and violence and integrates the findings from all those scientific fields where they are major issues, i.e., biology, psychology, psychiatry, and law enforcement.

Explanations of aggression and violence can be addressed from various viewpoints. For instance, a US Department of Justice document evaluated the risk factors of delinquency by corroborating the bio-psychological properties of the individual with social influences exerted by the family, school, peer group, and community [6], whereas the International Society for Research on Aggression arranged risk factors into two major groups: personal and environmental risk factors [7]. These and other systems of grouping risk factors and mechanisms into a coherent line of thought appear naturally valid. Here we chose, however, another approach, which takes into consideration the causal relationship and the temporal succession of various risk factors. We consider that at the bottom of all mechanisms and risk factors are the genes that the individual inherits. Gene function, however, is readily changed by the phenomenon called epigenetics, which is prompted by social influences mediated by the stress hormones glucocorticoids. As such, the social factors of biological change and stress hormones and their epigenetic consequences constitute the second and third levels of influences. Under their effect, development is altered, which brings about significant changes in brain structure and function (fourth level), which are consequential for altered psychological functions, the psychological being the last level to be discussed here. The selection of the topics and their order of presentation will follow the logic of this hierarchically stratified system of mechanisms and risk factors.

Within each level, the findings of animal, psychological, psychiatric, and law enforcement studies will be presented in conjunction, with the hope of synthesizing knowledge into a common system. The relationships between these areas of research, however, are not entirely clear. We will start our investigations by addressing this issue in the first chapter.

Budapest, Hungary József Haller

References

1. WHO. *Disease burden and mortality estimates*. WHO. http://www.who.int/healthinfo/global_burden_disease/estimates/en/
2. Roser, M. (2013). Homicides. *Our World Data*.
3. Global Terrorism Database. https://www.start.umd.edu/gtd/
4. Graham, K., et al. (2006). Harm, intent, and the nature of aggressive behavior: measuring naturally occurring aggression in barroom settings. *Assessment, 13*, 280–296.
5. Archer, J., & Coyne, S. M. (2005). An integrated review of indirect, relational, and social aggression. Personality and Social Psychology Review: An Official Journal of the Society for Personality and Social Psychology, Inc., 9, 212–230.
6. Shader, M. *Risk factors for delinquency: An overview*. https://www.ncjrs.gov/pdffiles1/ojjdp/frd030127.pdf. Retrieved 3 Feb 2020.
7. Youth Violence Commission, International Society for Research on Aggression. *Risk factors for youth violence*. https://static1.squarespace.com/static/57530523f850829dde1dc031/t/5ad202726d2a73331c4449c1/1523712626745/isra-youth-violence-statement-2018.pdf. Retrieved 3 Feb 2020.

Contents

About the Author

József Haller, Ph.D., D.Sc. studied the neurobiology of aggression for most of his scientific career. He published more than 150 articles in peer-reviewed scientific journals and authored three books on the subject. His last book was *Neurobiological Bases of Aggression and Violent Behavior* (Springer, 2014). As a leader of the Behavioral Neurobiology Department of the Institute of Experimental Medicine, Budapest, Hungary, he contributed to aggression research by initiating the concept of abnormal aggression in animals, developing two laboratory models of aggression-related psychopathologies, and differentiating the neurobiological bases of normal manifestations of aggression from those of its abnormal forms and violence. His scientific work is widely known and cited in the field. He was recently appointed the head of the Institute of Behavioral Sciences and Law Enforcement, University of Public Service, Budapest, Hungary, where he teaches criminal psychology and conducts research in this field.

Chapter 1
Dissecting the Concept of Aggression from Biology to Law Enforcement

Introduction

There are four main approaches to aggression: the biological, psychological, psychiatric, and law enforcement approaches. This chapter compares these four approaches to answer an essential question: Is knowledge achieved in one area usable by another? In many studies, a positive answer to this question is taken for granted. For instance, Allan Siegel, a pioneer of the studies into the neurobiology of aggression, who still has a great influence on current thinking, used his findings on electrically evoked defensive rage and quiet biting (i.e., emotionless bites on prey) in cats to suggest mechanistic explanations for human aggression [1]. Moreover, he and his coworkers proposed pharmacological treatments for aggression-related psychopathologies [2] and addressed philosophical-like issues related to criminal responsibility [3] based largely on electric stimulation and brain lesion studies performed in cats. Are such inferences warranted? The question is important because other researchers seem to avoid references to work performed in areas other than their own, creating the impression that they answered the above question negatively. Naturally, the final answer may be given after an overview of experimental findings; however, it seems worthwhile to start the systematic comparison of the four main approaches by having the basic question in mind: Do these four approaches address the same or different issues?

J. Haller, *Neurobiopsychosocial Perspectives on Aggression and Violence*, Advances in Preventing and Treating Violence and Aggression,
https://doi.org/10.1007/978-3-030-46331-1_1

1.1 Biology: Aggression as Competition

1.1.1 Definition and Implications

In biology, aggressive behavior is conceptualized as a form of competition for resources and opportunities for reproduction. Usually, definitions either do not identify the ways by which the competition is carried out because they do not refer to particular behaviors or just enumerate examples. One such definition reads as follows "Aggressive behaviors in animals, *for example, threat, attack, and defense*, are commonly related to competition over resources, competition over mating opportunities, or fights for survival" (see Abstract in Ref. [4]). Note that the behaviors are described in terms of their alleged purposes. For instance, the authors do not define what threat behaviorally means.

The concept of aggression as competition is generally attributed to Darwin and assumed to be formulated in two of his major works on the origin of species [5] and on sexual selection [6]. However, Darwin never used the term "aggression" in these books, where he preferred the term "fight" without meticulously defining it. The sentence closest to the biological definition discussed here reads as follows: "The males fight for the possession of the females" (Darwin on sexual selection, p. 246). As a mating partner is a resource for leaving offspring, this statement is in line with the biological approach to aggression, but neither this nor several other Darwinian sentences can be considered definitions, although all suggest that animals have purposes when they fight.

Historically speaking, an early and more explicit formulation of the concept comes from Wallace Craig, who wrote in 1918: "Fundamentally, among animals, fighting is not sought nor valued for its own sake; it is resorted to rather as an unwelcome necessity, a means of defending the agent's interests [...]" [7]. The term "defending interests" can easily be equated with competition for resources; consequently, the concept was ready for use by the beginning of the twentieth century although not yet articulated into a definition-like statement. The wordings of various definition-like statements may be different; the definition may be attributed to Darwin [8, 9, 10] or Craig [11], but for most biologists, aggression is a form of competition for resources. As such, biologists perceive aggression as having an important function.

The functional definition of aggression has several implications, which all are highly important from the point of view of the other three approaches. Specifically, these implications impact how aggression is conceptualized as a disorder or as violent crime and from a psychological point of view. The main implications of the definition are as follows:

1. *Aggression is evolutionarily adaptive.* The definition implies that aggression is a natural phenomenon which is a necessary component of the behavioral repertoire of animals. Resources are usually in short supply, and aggression is a highly efficient form of obtaining them. In evolutionary terms, non-aggressive individuals have lower chances to leave descendants, and their genes will gradually disappear from the gene pool. Unsurprisingly, aggression is present in every known

species that have the physiological means to perform it, e.g., adequate musculature and nervous system. Aggression is present even in worms [12], cephalopods [13], insects [14], and vertebrates.

Consequently, the definition implies that there is an evolutionary pressure on the perpetuation of aggression as a form of behavior.

2. *Aggression is governed by rules.* Although it does confer advantages, aggression is also costly in terms of both the risk of injuries and time and energy spent while performing it, for which cost–benefit relationships are important for fights and the strategy adopted [15].The risks associated with aggression are relevant not only from the point of view of the individual aggressor. Aggression can endanger the survival of the species if males, the aggressive gender in most species, inflict lethal wounds on each other when fighting for often trivial resources (e.g., small quantities of low-quality food), or if the competition by aggression was indiscriminately targeted towards reproductively valuable females and pups. Unsurprisingly, cost–benefit calculations play roles in aggression from lower animals, e.g., insects [16], up to communal range defense in primates [17]. Moreover, cost–benefit relationships have important roles in humans practicing martial arts or other sports [18]. In humans, such analyses can be done by the managers, trainers, and the competitors themselves in rational terms, and decisions can shape the career of the competitor.

In non-human animals, one cannot expect the capacity of evaluating costs and benefits cognitively. Yet, animals appear to follow certain rules which help minimizing risks while maximizing benefits. Such rules are as follows [19, 20]:

(i) Aggressive intent is signaled in advance to allow withdrawal by the opponent.
(ii) The intensity of aggression is kept below a certain limit to minimize injuries and excessive energy losses.
(iii) The most dangerous forms of aggression (e.g., bites) are targeted towards body parts that lack vital organs and are less exposed to infections (e. g., the back and flanks in rodents).
(iv) Aggression is rapidly deferred by submission or flight by the opponent.
(v) Reproductively valuable individuals (e.g., pups and females) are largely protected from attacks by males if the pups belong to those males.

As one cannot hypothesize that animals respect such rules by mental reasoning, one has to refer again to evolution, i.e., to evolutionary selected heritable action patterns.

Deviations from the typical rules of aggression do exist; these were observed either when the life of the subject was at risk or when natural aggressiveness was influenced experimentally to model harmful apparently abnormal aggression. For instance, small rat intruders preferentially target their bites at the head and throat of large colony males [21]. As such, their aggression is atypical, but only to save their lives, because small intruders are regularly killed in such conflicts. (For atypical aggression models, see the fourth section below.)

In conclusion, the costs and benefits of aggression are balanced by evolutionary pressure against dangerous forms of aggression. This pressure can be recognized and conceptualized as evolutionarily shaped "rules" that govern the behavior of non-human animals in conflict and help maintain the competitive advantages of the behavior without endangering the individual or the species. From the perspective of the rules that govern competitive forms of non-human animal aggression, it is worth mentioning that non-human animals – at least primates – show even rudimentary forms of social control of aggression, which control intragroup conflict to preserve social networks [22]. Thus, not only so called self-control but also social control was favored by the evolution of aggression.

3. *Biology applies to humans*. We know since Darwin [5] that man descends from apes, which descend from lower mammals. As such, people carry a series of genes and features that are common to mammals and vertebrates in general. Language and culture have a large role in defining human aggression; however, one can still ask the question: Does the biological/functional definition of aggression describe a behavior that is present in typical, non-criminal humans?

One reason to believe that the answer is affirmative is provided by studies in young children. Aggressive behaviors (e.g., pushing, kicking, hitting) occurs very early in toddlers at the age of 12 months [23]; 5 months later, 80% of children of both sexes show aggressive behaviors [24]. Aggression is elicited mostly by disputes over toys but may also take the form of dominance fights in the form of assertive interactions [25]. Toys are naturally major resources at early ages, whereas dominance is not only recognized by toddlers, but they also expect resources to be distributed along social dominance relationships [26]. As such, aggressive competition for resources (objects, rank) is present in children at ages when norms and laws have minimal influences on their behavior.

The second line of reasoning comes from studies on tolerated forms of aggression. Such behaviors will be summarized below as relational aggression and consist of rumor spreading, gossiping, or socially isolating others, which damage the social status of the victims. Tolerated forms of aggression are relevant here because its actors are not limited by legal consequences; the behavior is often normative within particular social groups and is widespread. Thus, this behavior is also in line with the definition presented above: relational aggression is used as a competitive strategy for the attainment of social goals from adolescence [27] into adulthood [28].

These examples show that aggression is often used by people as a form of resource competition, suggesting that the biological/functional definition also applies to humans. Importantly, this "biological" type of aggression is related to neither mental disorders nor criminal behavior and is present at various ages.

1.1.2 The Aims of Competition and Obtaining Resources

There are two types of competitive situations that elicit aggression. The first bridges the gap between limited resources on one side and the individual needs for survival on the other. Non-human animals may fight for food, water, and shelter (e.g., burrows or other places protected from predators), that is, for the daily necessities of life. Organism strives for biological fitness, the ability of the individual to maintain normal functioning, in this case by ensuring access to resources through aggression. The second type of competitive situation relates to the more general "evolutionary need" of leaving as many descendants as possible. Males fight for females and females fight for males in some species. Both genders – more often the female only – also fight to protect their offspring from attacks by conspecifics. Note that males have the predilection of killing other males' pups which maximizes the transmission of their own genes to the detriment of other males' genes [29]. The apparent goal is inclusive fitness, the ability of getting advantage in the contest for passing genes to the next generation directly through one's own offspring or through other relatives.

The two main aims – fitness and inclusive fitness – and the particular objects of competition can be reached by two major ways: territory ownership in solitary animals and high social rank in gregarious species. These two mechanisms ensure access to both the daily necessities of life and mating opportunities. As such, all types of aggression can be reduced to territorial and hierarchy fights. Note that the same species may be involved in both, being territorial during the breeding season and gregarious outside of it. In addition, some gregarious species (e.g., rats) may maintain a sub-territory or individual space within the territory of the colony. They defend their sub-territory within the group but also fight for rank and also cooperatively defend the colony's territory from members of other colonies.

These forms of competitive behavior are species-specific and range from bites through kicks to stabbing with horns. It is noteworthy that aggressive behavior also includes threatening postures and acts, as these may be just as effective as more harmful behaviors (e.g., bites) and at the same time minimize the risks of aggression (see above).

1.1.3 The Utilization of the Concept

The biological concept of aggression is amply employed by ecologically relevant research that studies free-ranging animals [22, 30–32]. These studies address issues that are highly relevant for the present book, e.g., the relationship between aggression on one side and social life, rules, and the enforcement of rules by group members on the other, all being conceptualized as behavior having competitive advantages. Neurobehavioral issues, however, are relatively rarely addressed in this line of research; for this reason, it will be only occasionally referred to in this book.

In the areas more fully reviewed here, laboratory animal research is closely related to the biological approach of aggression, albeit in most cases implicitly. Laboratory tests of aggression create competitive situations where animals fight for a resource, and aggression is understood to serve competition. These contests do have a touch of artificiality, but they may model everyday occurrences under natural conditions.

In the resident–intruder test, a standard laboratory test of aggression, for instance, animals compete for the ownership of the home cage, which is a territory, with obvious advantages for the owner in terms of access to food, shelter, and mating partners. True, intruders do not willingly interfere with the residents, because they are placed in the resident's cage by the experimenter and cannot leave the cage on their own accord as only when the experimenter removes them. Consequently, the resident–intruder test only *models* resource competition by making use of fixed action patterns (FAPs) that enable resource competition in real life.

Fights for social rank are sometimes modelled in rather realistic research enclosures, e.g., the visible burrow system of the Blanchard group [33]. The system hosts relatively large male–female colonies that live together for prolonged periods within large arenas, and they may even be allowed to raise pups. Although similar models are in use in other laboratories [34], the paradigm is labor-intensive for researchers, requires large laboratory space, and is costly. Some researchers substitute male only smaller colonies [35]. In this paradigm, however, aggression does not lead to practical advantages, because reproductive behavior is unavailable, food and water are available ad libitum and males still readily fight for social rank.

Finally, the maternal aggression paradigm is a laboratory equivalent of the violent defense of pups by females, who attack unfamiliar males placed into their home cage, as these males pose a real threat to the life of pups.

The third major area where the biological approach was utilized relatively frequently is psychology. As a rule, psychological definitions of aggression make no reference to competition; the focus is usually either on the behavior itself (e.g., its likelihood or intensity) or on its negative consequences, mostly for the victim or the social group. Nevertheless, the biological-like conceptualization of aggression gained attention in three areas as follows:

(1) The evolutionary origins of human aggression are often considered from the perspective of resource competition. The general belief is that the competitive advantages of intraspecific aggression are high in humans, which may serve as an explanation for human aggression and even crime. Furthermore, it has been repeatedly suggested that sexual selection – the evolutionarily relevant selection of traits based on sexual competition – is one of the major drivers of aggression that is also responsible for sex differences in aggression [4, 8, 36–38]. Moreover, efforts have been made to validate such claims experimentally [39]; however, these studies, which are at the interface of biology and psychology, aim to provide biological–evolutionary explanations of aggression and remain speculative. Usually, psychologists use their own definitions and measurements of aggression and study aggression regardless of its possible role in ensuring competitive advantages.
(2) Competitive situations are frequently used to study human aggression in the laboratory. In these studies, however, the competitive situation is used to trigger rather than to model aggression. The ensuing behavior is usually interpreted in terms of the general psychological trait of "aggressiveness" rather than by considering aggression as a form of competition. Explanations attributed to aggressiveness in these models stem from concepts like frustration, anger, hostility, etc. all being psychological notions that are not explicitly related to competitiveness although may derive from it.

(3) Psychologists often integrate findings obtained in animal research, especially when these refer to molecular, endocrine, and neural mechanisms. This implies that many biologists and psychologists consider animal aggression as a model of human aggression. Nevertheless, the ground of integration is the form of the behavior and not its function. It is assumed tacitly or explicitly that similar behaviors have similar mechanistic backgrounds irrespective to the importance attributed to the functionality of behavior. It is also worth mentioning that the overlap of the two fields is selective. Attitudes range from total indifference ("biological and psychological aggression show only superficial resemblances") to total unity ("animal findings are valid for humans").

The presence of the biological approach is even more restricted in psychiatry and law enforcement. One of the primary criteria of mental disorders is that they result in "impairments in social, occupational, or other important areas of functioning" (DSM-5 [40] p. 21). This notion is incompatible with any major gains resulting from aggression, because gains eliminated the criterion on impairment and the behavior could not be diagnosed as a mental disorder. Consequently, aggression is never dealt with as a natural form of competition in psychiatry. Finally, gain-oriented aggression, such as acquisitive offences, is considered aggravated forms of violent crime, and it is usually not acknowledged that violence can be a natural – even less so a legitimate – form of competition (see below). This is in line with the concept of "biological rules" that control competition and aggression. In humans, the rule is cooperation, which supports society. Consequently, the competition for resources by physical force is outlawed as such. Exceptions and their reasons will be discussed in Sect. 1.4.2.1 below. We only note here that one of the main exceptions cover the preservation of life, which is also exempt from biological rules, as shown by small intruders into large male colonies.

Recent studies try to use the biological concept to explain the gains from aggression [41–43]. It is noteworthy that many such studies address the issue from both psychiatric and law enforcement perspectives. These studies seek the motivations of aggression and suggest that the advantages of aggression explain its high frequency. This is to a certain extent similar to the evolutionary–psychological approach. The difference is that the latter tries to explain human aggression from a natural history point of view, while the former focuses on the immediate or short-term gains of behaving aggressively.

Taken together, the biological approach to aggression – it being a form of competition – is widely used in studies of free-ranging animals, is implicitly encompassed by the laboratory models of aggression, and serves as an aggression-triggering situation in experimental psychology. The latter uses models of competition rather than addressing aggression as a competitive phenomenon. In classical psychology, psychiatry, and law enforcement, the concept is used only when theoretical or mechanistic explanations are sought for the persistence and attractiveness of aggressive behavior.

1.2 Psychology: Aggression as a Form of Behavior

1.2.1 Definition and Implications

For psychologists and social psychologists, aggression is a behavior that aims to deliver harm: "Social psychologists define aggression as behavior that is intended to harm another individual who does not wish to be harmed" (see paragraph 2 of Chapter "Defining Aggression" in the e-book by Jhangiani and Tarry [44]). The first version of the definition likely belongs to Arnold Buss [45], who used the more objective phrase "the delivery of noxious stimuli" instead of the subjective "intention to harm." In later formulations of the same definition, harm and injury even occur as goals so that aggression is defined as any behavior directed towards the *goal* of harm and injury, which does not benefit the victim by any means ([46, 47]). More recently, authors have amended the definition with further details, e.g., "Like most psychologists, we define human aggression as behavior directed towards another individual carried out with the proximate (immediate) intent to cause harm. Furthermore, the perpetrator must believe that the behavior will harm the target, and that the target is motivated to avoid the behavior. Actual harm is not required" (p. 298 [48]). Note that the last sentence creates a certain degree of confusion, especially if considered together with the term "intent" that occurs in the first sentence. It may be implied that aggression is equaled with intention alone. Yet, this is excluded by the first part of the same definition ("We define human aggression as behavior"). The authors probably meant that unsuccessful behaviors – i.e., those that fail to cause harm – might also be aggression.

The examples cited above are excellent examples of the rewording of old definitions to make them more explicit and detailed. In essence, the definitions are built up from four components: (a) aggression is a behavior; (b) the essence of the behavior is harm; (c) the behavior is intentional, as such, accidental harm does not qualify as aggression; and (d) the harm does not serve the interests of the victim, for example, surgeons, dentists, etc. cause harm without being aggressive while delivering pain and injury. The victim may express their disinterest in harm by trying to avoid. As such, behavior in masochistic and other "games" where subjects seek harm does not qualify as aggression.

In these definitions, harm is understood broadly. It may include physical pain and injury but also psychological pain and sociopsychological injury. This stipulation may not directly derive from the above cited definitions but from the classification of aggression types that will be addressed below.

The lack of attributed function is an interesting feature of the psychological definition which may be due to the observed apparent meaningfulness of many forms of human aggression. Indeed, it is very difficult to find a function for uncontrolled outbursts of aggression, which are so frequent in humans. These are harmful for both the victim and perpetrator in terms of social and legal consequences, without apparently benefiting the aggressor in any way. Even when aggression confers the perpetrator a momentary competitive advantage, this will often be outweighed by negative outcomes in the long run. Due to the multitude of the situations when people are aggressive, it may seem better to restrict the definition to the behavior rather than assuming functions. One may hypothesize that aggression thus defined may be a human-specific behavior. Animals – driven by inherited FAPs – fight for definable goals, while people often employ behaviorally similar but apparently functionally senseless acts.

To sum this up in one sentence, the psychological definition broadly describes the category of behaviors that qualify as aggression without attaching any functional connotations to it.

1.2.2 The Classification of Behaviors

Harms delivered to another individual can be classified according to two criteria. The first relates to the motivation of performing the behavior, whereas the second concerns the behavioral tactic. Psychologists and others differentiate two types of aggression based on their motivations: reactive and proactive aggression. The former consists of uncontrolled aggressive outbursts that are elicited by real or perceived threat or provocation, whereas the latter is a goal-directed behavior involving the deliberate use of aggression for the purposes of the perpetrator. The two forms were differentiated in psychology about 50 years ago [49] although the distinction between "crimes of passion" and "cold blooded planned aggression" was differentiated by law much earlier. After its scientific formulation, the idea rapidly entered textbooks [50] and was taken up and developed further by a series of authors some of whom also renamed them. Reactive and proactive aggressions differ in a series of other attributes besides the motivation of being aggressive (see Table 1.1). These terms refer to essentially similar behaviors so that they can be considered synonyms.

Table 1.1 *Brief comparison of reactive and proactive aggressions*

	Aggression types (Synonyms)	
	Controlled	Impulsive [51]
	Instrumental	Hostile [52]
	Predatory	Emotional [53]
	Premeditated	Impulsive [54]
Features	Proactive	Reactive [55]
Motivation	Goal	Provocation
Aim	Reaching the goal	Revenge/defense
Behavior	Planned	Random
Emotionality	Weak	Intense
Stress-response	Weak	Strong
Primary brain area involved	Prefrontal cortex (hypofunction)	Amygdala (hyper-function)

(continued)

Table 1.1 (continued)

	Aggression types (Synonyms)	
	Controlled	Impulsive [51]
	Instrumental	Hostile [52]
	Predatory	Emotional [53]
	Premeditated	Impulsive [54]
Features	Proactive	Reactive [55]
Post hoc attitude (if successful)	Satisfaction	Repentance

Note: This is only a crude presentation. The issue will be developed in the following sections

Regarding the behavioral tactic, aggression can be verbal, physical, and relational. All three have the aim of inflicting harm but in different ways. Verbal aggression consists of threats that entail verbal warnings and threats, facial expressions, body language, etc. Due to the heterogeneity of these behaviors, we will call this type of aggression "intimidation" in the followings sections. This also includes aggression against inanimate objects if the goal was intimidation (e.g., beating the table, slamming the door, etc.) [56]. The harm inflicted on the subject is psychological in nature and may consist mainly of fear and feelings of helplessness. Physical aggression – harms delivered to the body – is the clearest from the point of view of the psychological definition as it inflicts pain, injury, or even death since the harm is self-evident in this case. Finally, relational aggression covers a series of behaviors that uses of the social influence of the perpetrator. This type of aggression covers three related but distinct behaviors [57]. Indirect aggression is "commissioned" in that the perpetrator instigates others to harm the victim on their behalf. Relational aggression consists in manipulating the social environment to disrupt the relationships and friendships of the victim. The third subtype, social aggression, aims at damaging the social status of the victim or at isolating them from the social group (ostracism). Although the harm inflicted by relational aggression is not very severe at the first sight – especially when compared to the consequences of physical aggression – this impression is false. Relational aggression may disrupt biological development [58] including the development of the neural system [59] and can lead to the emergence of aggression-unrelated psychopathologies (e.g., anxiety and depression [60, 61]) and to aggressiveness and antisocial attitudes [62, 63]. Moreover, it may endanger cardiovascular health [64]. Relational aggression is practiced and is harmful at all ages from childhood [65] through adolescence [66] to adulthood [64]. One is tempted to make a guess that relational is more damaging than many forms of physical aggression. It is used as an alternative strategy to inflict severe harm on victims, when the risks and costs of physical aggression are high in social and legal terms [57].

1.2.3 The Utilization of the Concept

The psychological definition captures the behavioral essence of aggression, and consequently, it is linked tightly to the biological approach. Although aggression is conceptualized as competition according to the latter, aggressiveness is measured by the frequency and intensity of aggressive behaviors in non-human animals, which is very similar to the psychological approach. This is especially clear when the forms of behavior are compared. Physical aggression may take species-typical forms but is similar in the delivery of harm in all species. Threats are frequently used by animals to intimidate competitors; they consist of vocalizations which are perhaps analogous to human verbal threats and body postures and movements reminiscent of human intimidation.

The approach to threats shows only minor differences. In biology, these are viewed as efficient but less risky forms of aggressive competition, whereas in psychology they are viewed as aggression that causes psychological harm. Yet, threats and intimidation are integral parts of aggressive behavior according to both approaches. Moreover, animals may even show relational aggression. The members of social groups form coalitions to prevent infanticide by males [29], guard mating partners [67], and support each other in social conflicts [68, 69]. Within groups, animals form alliances to increase their social rank and their mating opportunities, which are based on a rather complex gestural communication system, at least in monkeys and apes [70–72]. The place in a social hierarchy also affects social integration in macaques [74]. In addition, behaviors aimed at the disruption of social bonds and the prevention of the formation of new bonds were reported in ravens [73].

Taken together, these findings show that the biological and psychological concept of aggression are compatible; moreover, they cross-fertilize each other as animal behavior is often used as a model of human aggression, whereas psychological concepts are often used in biology, especially when aggression is studied in primates. In such studies, however, competitive advantages are still in focus.

Surprisingly, neither the *Diagnostic and Statistical Manual of Mental Disorders Fifth Edition* (DSM-5) [40] nor *International Classification of Mental and Behavioural Disorders Tenth Edition (ICD-10)* [75] define aggression explicitly while using the term frequently. The context suggests that its use is in line with the psychological approach. Specifically, DSM-5 employs terms suggestive of inspiration from psychological work including terms like verbal, relational, and physical aggression. In addition, although more sporadically, DSM-5 uses the terms reactive and proactive (in one place termed "predatory") aggression to characterize the nature of aggressiveness in particular disorders. No such word usages are apparent in ICD-10.

Law enforcement is as behavior-centered as psychology; yet, the major categories substantially differ from those used in psychology in terminology and conceptualization. The largest difference between the two approaches is that law enforcement covers only a subgroup of those behaviors that all are considered to be aggression by the psychological approach, because the embodiment of aggression is violent crime for the law enforcement approach.

These considerations suggest that the biological and psychological approach readily cross-fertilize each other; psychiatry seems to take inspiration from psychology tacitly, whereas law enforcement follows a largely different route.

1.3 Psychiatry: Aggression as a Symptom of Psychopathology

1.3.1 The Lack of Definitions and Their Implications

The reluctance to define aggression (see above) may indicate that this behavior is not viewed as being very important in the manuals of mental disorders. It is worth mentioning that DSM-5, unlike ICD-10, does provide definitions to its key terms in the section "Glossary of Technical Terms." This Glossary defines a series of terms associated with aggression, such as callousness, disinhibition, hostility, impulsivity, and temper tantrums, but not aggression. There is a term, "antagonism," that may have stood for aggression, defined as "Behaviors that put an individual at odds with other people." However, its examples cover inflated sense of self-importance, antipathy towards others, unawareness of others' needs and feelings, etc. These may all underlie aggression but are very different from the aggressive acts named in the descriptions of disorders in DSM-5. In many cases, the manual used the common psychological terms when referring to aggression (reactive–proactive; verbal–physical–relational); in other instances, it simply named the behavior (assault, fights, harm of others, use of weapon, yelling at people, etc.). In view of this, one might assume that the failure to define aggression was a simple technical mishap.

Another more important feature of the diagnostic psychological manuals is that they do not consider aggression itself as a mental disorder. In general, mental disorders are diagnosed when a perception, feeling, or behavior is inappropriate to the situation; it lasts too long or occurs too frequently over a prolonged period and causes distress or impairments in important areas of functioning. The fourth criterion is that the perception/feeling/behavior is not attributable to another, non-mental condition such as physical illnesses and drug-induced phenomena. For instance, fever may provoke hallucinations, but these are not indicative of a psychiatric problem. Aggression may fulfill all four criteria. It may occur in inappropriate situations; it may be a life-long characteristic; it does cause distress or impairments in functioning; and finally, most of the time, it is expressed independently of other, non-mental conditions.

Aggression seems to be the stepchild of psychiatry. Its exclusion in the glossary is difficult to comprehend, yet the reluctance to define it as a disorder may have explanations as follows. First, aggressiveness as a psychiatric problem never occurs alone, and psychiatric thinking has to consider the complexities of its subject matter. Second, aggression occurs as a symptom of many disorders, and, as such, it should always be viewed in context. Because contexts are variable, aggression can occur across a variety of disorders. Third, aggression has many faces, as shown in the previous section. In other words, one type of aggression may be typical in one disorder, and another type of aggression may be typical in another disorder. Consequently, aggression cannot be considered as a unitary phenomenon in psychiatry.

Whatever the reason was, aggression is not defined in DSM-5, and so it is not a distinct phenomenon of its own right in psychiatry as in biology or psychology. Rather, it is a component of several, unrelated or weakly related mental problems; however, one can establish correspondences between the aggression types recognized by psychology and the aggression-related mental disorders. Moreover, psychiatric notions may have their representations in animal models, which implicitly involve the biological approach to aggression.

1.3.2 Aggression-Related Disorders

Aggression-related disorders will be presented below mainly based on DSM-5. The primary reason is that DSM-5 is the basic reference point in much research [76].

DSM-5 describes disorders by their symptoms, which are organized into clusters identified by capital letters. The first or the first few clusters list the symptoms. For instance, cluster A of conduct disorder lists all the 15 symptoms of the disorder, whereas the 22 symptoms of posttraumatic stress disorder (PTSD) are organized into 4 different clusters (A–D). The manual also indicates how many symptoms need to be met for a formal diagnosis. For example, a patient may be diagnosed with conduct disorder if she/he shows at least 3 of the 15 symptoms. For PTSD, the diagnosis needs the presence of one symptom from each of the clusters A–C and two from cluster D. In addition, the condition must last a significant length of time and impairs functions, and it is not secondary to another condition. The symptom lists are followed by more lengthy description of the disorder, which covers issues like its prevalence, gender ratio, course, prognosis, etc. We will focus below on those clusters that are specific to the disorders, i.e., on the symptom lists.

There are a number of disorders characterized by symptoms related to aggression. We will group them according to the overall characteristics of patients and the nature of aggressiveness they show. Specifically, we will present three categories of disorders, those characterized by antisocial traits, impulse control deficits, and cognitive deficits. The ultimate aim is to find the order in the disorder and to investigate whether there are identifiable groups of aggressions within the manual or, indeed, whether aggression is just a symptom incorporated into innumerable different conditions.

1.3.2.1 Disorders Associated with Antisocial Behaviors

This class of disorders will be presented by taking conduct and antisocial personality disorders (ASPD) as examples. The former is typically diagnosed in children and adolescents, whereas the latter can be diagnosed only in adults. The two disorders are closely related, as ASPD can be diagnosed only if conduct disorder was present before the age of 15 years. This suggests that we are dealing with two age-related phases of the same psychopathology [77].

Both conduct and ASPDs include symptoms that describe behaviors identified as aggression by the psychological approach. In the case of conduct disorder, aggressive acts include bullying and intimidating others, initiating fights, using potentially dangerous weapons, and being physically cruel to people and robbery. Aggression-related features of ASPD are reduced to one single symptom described as follows: "Irritability and aggressiveness, as indicated by repeated physical fights or assaults" (page 659). Notably, neither descriptions nor functions are attached to these behaviors; the manual lists simply their common names.

In addition to aggressive acts, diagnosis may also be made based on moral attitudes and non-violent criminal activity. In the case of conduct disorder, such symptoms include lying for own benefit, staying out of or running away from home, truancy from school and steeling, sexual abuse, fire setting, and burglary. In the case of ASPD, such symptoms include failure to conform to social norms, failure to sustain consistent work behavior or honor financial obligations, deceitfulness, lack of remorse and empathy, and repeated acts that are grounds for arrest. (The manuals do not stipulate that these should be violent.)

The emphasis of symptom lists is obviously on non-aggressive symptoms, which represent 66% (10 out of 15) in the case of conduct disorder and 85% (6 out of 7) in the case of ASPD. Considering that the number of symptoms required for diagnosis is three for both disorders, this means that diagnosed patients are not necessarily aggressive.

To get closer to aggression within these disorders, one has to consider their subtypes, for instance, conduct disorder associated with callous–unemotional traits. Subjects belonging to this subgroup are more likely to be aggressive than those who lack these psychological traits, especially when the onset is in early childhood [78]. Concerning ASPD, the "primarily aggressive subtype" is called psychopathy. This is not recognized as a mental disorder in its own right by either DSM-5 or ICD-10. The latter uses the term as one of the many synonyms of ASPD, whereas the former vaguely mentions particular characteristics of ASPD subjects who qualify for this subgroup (e.g., boldness and lack of anxiety and proneness to criminal behavior and recidivism). Yet, psychopathy is intensely studied by psychiatrists, although the differentiation of its subtypes is not always similar [79, 80]. Similar to the aforementioned subtype of conduct disorder, psychopathy – as a subtype of ASPD – distinguishes by callous–unemotional traits and high aggressiveness [81]. It is noteworthy that conduct disorder with callous–unemotional traits is often portrayed as a childhood form of psychopathy [82], suggesting again that we deal with age phases of the same problem.

Thus, psychopathologies persistently associated with antisocial behavior cover people with deeply disturbed personalities, who are at odds with the society who may or may not be aggressive. However, some subtypes of ASPD are more strongly prone to aggressive and violent behavior. Importantly for the categorization of antisocially aggressive patients based on the psychological approach, even people belonging to the most aggressive subtypes (e.g., psychopaths) are prone to commit non-violent, for instance, economic crimes, which require careful planning [83].

1.3.2.2 Impulse–Control Disorders

Patients belonging to these disorders frequently lose control of their behavior and show outbursts of anger and aggression, which they apparently cannot restrain. We will discuss below two rather similar disorders: disruptive mood dysregulation and intermittent explosive disorders (IEDs).

Although DSM-5 symptoms are organized differently, and wording is different when the symptoms are described, the two disorders are highly similar. Both are characterized by frequent temper outbursts manifested as verbal and/or physical aggression towards people. Temper outbursts may also be directed towards property. It is required in both cases that the magnitude of aggressiveness be grossly out of proportion to the provocation or to precipitating psychosocial stressors. Two differences still exist. Subjects with disruptive mood dysregulation disorder should show persistently irritable mood between outbursts, which is not mentioned in the case of IED; however, the number of symptoms required for diagnosis makes it likely that many mood dysregulated patients lack this symptom. The other difference is that outbursts in IED should not be premeditated or motivated by tangible objectives (e.g., money, power, intimidation), which specification is missing from the description of disruptive mood dysregulation disorder; however, the clarifications that follow the symptom list specify that temper outbursts are associated with frustration in this disorder, which usually excludes premeditation and goal-directed behavior.

In theory, either disorder can be diagnosed from age 6 upwards. In practice, however, disruptive mood dysregulation disorder is diagnosed in children and adolescents [84], whereas IED is mainly diagnosed in adults. For instance, the DSM-5 states that IED is rare in children, despite the fact that the age limit for IED is 6 years. Both disorders show many similarities with bipolar disorder by shared features and comorbidity [84, 85]. One can hypothesize that, at least in practice, the two disorders represent age phases of the same dysfunction.

These two disorders are closest to be "aggression disorders"; they fail to do so only by a narrow margin, specifically by including symptoms that cannot be considered aggression. We refer here to the destruction of property, which may alone be sufficient for a diagnosis. Although wanton destructiveness may be called aggression in everyday language, it is not directed towards conspecifics (e.g., people), and, as such, it qualifies only for being a temper outburst (as the DSM-5 description states) rather than being an aggressive behavior. It may have been considered aggression if aimed at intimidation, but this is excluded by DSM-5 criteria, which require that temper outbursts have no tangible goal.

1.3.2.3 Disorders Associated with Cognitive Dysfunctions

Many disorders consist of or are associated with a split between the reality and its perception, which may lead to aggressiveness under certain conditions. For instance, patients suffering from sleep–wake disorders may injure themselves or others. This is mentioned among the symptoms of rapid eye movement sleep behavior disorder but is described as a feature of most sleep disorders in the more general sections that follow the listing of symptoms. Epileptic patients may also harm others in the post-ictal period [86]. Such instances of aggression are involuntary, for which they would not qualify as aggression according to the psychological approach. Yet, aggression is not defined in the diagnostic manuals of psychiatry; and so these behaviors may be considered aggressive because they are named as such by DSM-5. In other cases, aggression is a volitional act, albeit motivated by irrational thoughts or faulty representations of the environment. These include aggressive acts by neurocognitive disorders from Alzheimer disease to traumatic brain injury. This is mentioned but not listed among symptoms by DSM-5; however, aggressiveness in these disorders is clearly demonstrated by clinical research [87, 88]. Finally, aggression is present in neurodevelopmental disorders including intellectual disabilities (ID) and autism spectrum disorders [89]. In these disorders, aggression results from adherence to stereotypies and/or distorted theory of mind. The latter phrase refers to the ability of attributing intents, emotions, and cognitions to others; aggression may ensue from faults in such attributions.

Here we will analyze in some detail one single example of cognitive distortions, specifically that resulting from psychosis. The reason is that the phrase "psychotic aggression" has a long history [90] and a well-established status in aggression research. The concept in fact transforms the reactive–proactive dichotomy into the reactive–proactive–psychotic aggression triple distinction [91].

Psychosis is a state when the subject acts under internal imaginary impulses. The condition may occur in a variety of disorders from schizophrenia through bipolar disorder to PTSD. The two leading symptoms of psychoses are hallucinations and delusions. The former may take any form but usually are auditory; the subject may hear voices that may make demands. Rarely, the voice may demand aggression against certain people. Delusions may also be of many sorts but typically are paranoid in nature; in some instances, the subject may attribute evil intentions or actions to people or groups of people. Violent outburst are frequently prompted by either of these two symptoms [92]. Such outbursts may have a goal (e.g., the elimination of an evil force) but may also be prompted by a misunderstood or imagined external event, for instance, the perception of threat to self, others, or the society as a whole [93]. Accordingly, people may carefully plan the act or, conversely, may act impulsively. In either case, the intent or the reaction is not antisocial; on the contrary, the subject may perceive its actions as being beneficial to the society. Although public opinion assumes that the victims of such actions are mostly schizophrenic patients, some data indicate that psychotic aggression is more frequent in bipolar disorder than in schizophrenia [94].

1.3.2.4 Overview

In addition to the disorders presented above, there are many others where aggressive behaviors are listed among the symptoms or where research revealed a strong association with aggression. Each of these can be classified into one of the categories presented above. For instance, oppositional defiant disorder is rather similar to conduct disorder as it regards the norm-breaking nature of aggression, albeit the targets are authority figures rather than the society as a whole. Aggression in borderline personality disorder and attention-deficit/hyperactivity disorder is akin to that seen in IED in the meaning that aggression is due to deficient impulse control. Irrational aggression may be present in a variety of conditions from ID to Alzheimer disease and confused states related to sleep disorders or epilepsy.

The aim of this section was not the detailed overview of mental disorders associated with aggression but the identification of the main types of aggression associated with mental disorders. This overview of the main forms of psychopathology suggests aggression-related disorders can be organized into classes. In one class, we have people who are reluctant to observe social norms and are disposed to commit crime in their own benefit, without feeling remorse for the deed or empathy for the victim. Criminal behavior includes but is not limited to violent crime. In the second class, people cannot restrain their impulses. In legal terms, their actions may be criminal, but their behavior is not motivated by the prospect of gain. The lack of remorse and empathy is not among the DSM-5 symptoms; moreover, clinical research suggest that remorse and empathy are preserved or even higher than average in those diagnosed with impulse–control disorders [95, 96]. Finally, there are a series of disorders, where the subject loses contact with reality and endeavors aggression under irrational influences. These three classes appear distinct based on the symptoms of DSM-5.

Importantly, our classification does not respect the classification of disorders by DSM-5. For instance, intermittent explosive and ASPDs are grouped by DSM-5 into the same disorder group called "disruptive, impulse–control, and conduct disorders." Yet, aggressiveness in these two disorders is very different. By contrast, intermittent explosive and disruptive mood dysregulation disorders belong to different groups of disorders. The former is in the aforementioned mixed group, whereas the latter belongs to "depressive disorders." Yet, they are characterized by aggression so similar that their descriptions are interchangeable. It is noteworthy that aggressive outbursts are the leading if not the only symptom in both. We do not want to go too far with this argument, but it occurs that a more thorough consideration of aggressiveness as a phenomenon may help improving the classification of disorders by DSM-5, which is so frequently criticized.

1.3.3 The Utilization of the Concept

Aggression is not a subject matter of its own right in psychiatry; it is always addressed in the context of various other dysfunctions and is present in the description of widely different mental disorders. In addition, aggression is not defined or interpreted; aggressive acts are simply named when the symptom lists of disorders are compiled. This attitude is markedly different from the biological and psychological approach. At the same time, the psychiatric approach shows many similarities with the law enforcement approach, not least because psychiatric symptoms directly either refer to criminal acts (e.g., in "antisocial-like disorders") or are implicitly criminal (e.g., in impulse control and cognitive dysfunction-related disorders).

1.3.3.1 Biological Models of Aggression-Related Psychopathologies

The psychiatric approach does not seem to be inspired by the biological conceptualization of aggression. In their turn, however, laboratory studies on aggression did take inspiration from psychiatry, which ultimately lead to the modelling of aggression-related mental disorders by abnormal aggression models. This biological approach has a long history. In initial phases, researchers restricted themselves to study the impact of etiological factors. Twenty-seven years ago, it was shown that alcohol increases aggressiveness in one subgroup of rats, whereas it did not affect it or decreased it in other subgroups, which is very similar to the distribution of the effects of alcohol intoxication in humans [97]. This and similar studies had no psychiatric dimension and did not aim at modelling mental disorders. The idea that the application of human etiological factors to animals may be developed into psychopathology-oriented models of aggression is only 18 years old [98]. Initially, proactive forms of aggression were modelled with the assumption that the laboratory paradigm also models mental disorders belonging to the "antisocial type." [19, 99] Later, models for reactive aggression putatively associated with impulse–control disorders were also developed [20, 100, 101], and trials were made to integrate earlier findings into the concept [102]. Finally, it was proposed that the concept may not only model groups of aggression-related disorders (e.g., antisocial and impulse–control related disorders) but also particular disorders (e.g., conduct disorder and several others) [77]. The approach became reasonably popular over time, and a series of new models were developed, for instance, the peripubertal stress model of abnormal aggression [103].

The idea standing behind these models is that the etiological factors of aggression-related psychopathologies result in abnormal forms of aggression when applied to laboratory rodents. The abnormality of aggression was defined by criteria that also had a temporal evolution and were worked out by different groups [19, 104, 105]. In a recent article, we categorized such abnormal aggressive behaviors as in Table 1.2.

Table 1.2 Criteria rendering aggression abnormal in the laboratory [20]

Criterion	Symptom
Excessive aggression (considerably surpasses levels observed under similar conditions in normal individuals)	Persistent bursts of biting Intense, tissue damaging attacks (for instance, a shift from soft to hard bites and clinches. For a description of these attack types, see [100])
Qualitatively changed attack patterns that imply severe injuries for opponents	Deficient signaling of attack intentions by threats, which makes attacks unpredictable to opponent, and lowers their potential for defense Bites targeted towards vulnerable body parts of opponents (for instance, the head, throat, belly, paws, or testicles) Disregarded appeasement signals, which prevents the opponent from evading attacks by flight or submission
Aggressive behavior that involves excessive risks for the attacker on the short or the long term	Aggression initiated in inappropriate settings (for instance, in unfamiliar environments, which are not normally defended or on the territory of opponents) Attacks on larger, potentially dangerous opponents Harmful attacks on pups and females, which hinders reproduction and the transmission of genes to the next generation
Dysfunctional aggression is persistent and is associated with other behavioral disturbances This mimics comorbidities that are quite frequent in aggression-related psychopathologies	Attack pattern does not vanish on repeated exposure to opponents Altered sociability-, anxiety-, or depression-like behaviors, etc.

The nature of symptoms suggests that under the influence of factors that lead to aggression-related psychopathologies in humans, aggression becomes dysfunctional in non-human animals. Such aggression is said to be dysfunctional because it leads to unnecessary damage to opponents, involves risks for the perpetrator, damages valuable reproductive partners, and is associated with multiple deficits as with psychopathologies. Abnormal aggression is in fact dysfunctional aggression. Importantly for interpretation, the abnormality of aggressive behaviors per se is not indicative of their association with a particular mental disorder, because the symptoms of abnormal aggression are largely independent of the etiological factor. Correspondences between the mental disorder and the abnormal aggression model may be derived from the nature of the etiological factor (e.g., alcohol- or drug-induced abnormal aggression), alterations in aggression-induced stress responses, the age of subjects, additional changes in sociability and other behaviors, etc. Such models may be used to investigate the neural underpinnings of mental disorders by extrapolating findings from laboratory animals to disordered subjects, who are more difficult to study for ethical reasons. In addition, they may be used to study the relationship between environmental influences (e.g., stress) and abnormal aggression, critical periods for stress effects, etc. [106]

1.3.3.2 Psychology

It is obvious that those who compiled DSM-5 were heavily inspired by the psychological concept of aggression. This is evident from equating of aggression with a behavior and from the overtaking of psychological notions as shown above. These psychiatric manuals only omitted to incorporate the psychological definition. In addition, the distinction between reactive and proactive forms of aggression can be used to group mental disorders [20, 107]. Actually, the psychological notion of proactive aggression and mental disorders grouped above based on their antisocial features is rather similar. In both cases, aggression is motivated by a goal and is associated with low emotionality and low stress responses. In addition, ASPD subjects preferentially, albeit not exclusively, employ proactive forms of aggression. Likewise, impulse–control disorders describe a behavior that would be termed reactive by psychologists. Similar to the latter, aggression is elicited by a real or perceived challenge or provocation and is associated with high emotions and high stress responses. Unsurprisingly, patients showing impulse–control disorders preferentially show reactive forms of aggression [108]. On the other hand, the third type – psychotic aggression – originates from difficulties determining what is real and what is not. The concept started to penetrate psychological thinking, although most psychological textbooks and review articles still state that according to motivation, human aggression can be divided into two categories, namely, reactive and proactive aggression. A promising subgroup adds the third type, which might be proactive or reactive depending on the circumstances, but is in fact elicited by unrealistic motives, which detaches it from both other types.

1.3.3.3 Law Enforcement

Finally, there are so many correspondences between the psychopathological and law enforcement approaches that one tends to view the two in conjunction. In addition to mentioning criminality among symptoms by normative psychiatric manuals, clinicians often investigate the association of mental disorders with aggression in terms of crime [109, 110]. This is also explained by the preponderance of mental disorders among criminals as shown in the next section.

Here we present another example of the tight connections between psychopathologic and law enforcement approaches, specifically Megargee's [111–113] criminal classification system. This system classified criminals into ten groups and described their attributes and their expected behaviors under detention. The system was heavily based on the psychiatric features of detainees. Albeit not very frequently used in research, its validity was recurrently confirmed over time in several countries [51, 114]; moreover, the concept was extended to specific populations such as sex offenders [115] and adult probationers [116]. These endeavors demonstrate that the psychiatric concept can have meaningful uses in law enforcement.

1.4 Law Enforcement: The Selective Censuring of Aggression

1.4.1 Definitions as Behavior Lists

In law enforcement, aggression is dealt with as violent crime. In many cases, penal codes offer a general definition of violence, followed by an allegedly complete list of behaviors that are considered violent crime. The Hungarian Penal Code [117], for instance, defines violent conduct as "any act of aggression and undue influence exerted on a person by the application of physical force, also if it does not result in bodily injury" (section 459/4). Following this, it lists 31 behaviors that are punished by law as being violent crimes. The list includes items like assault, duress, extortion, genocide, homicide, illegal restraint, manslaughter, mistreatment, private justice, riot, robbery, sexual exploitation, terrorism, unlawful detention, violation of freedom, etc. (examples from Closing Provisions, Section 459). This is not unique. The Uniform Crime Reporting Survey of Canada [118] also provides a definition for "violent incidents" and exemplifies violence by naming crime types. It reads as follows: "Violent incidents involve offences that deal with the application, or threat of application, of force to a person. These include homicide, attempted murder, various forms of sexual and non-sexual assault, robbery and abduction" (section "Concepts and Incidents" item 1.21). Similarly, the FBI's Uniform Crime Reporting Program defines violence as "...those offenses which involve force or threat of force" (section Violent Crime subsection Definitions) and specifies that "violent crime is composed of four offenses: murder and nonnegligent manslaughter, forcible rape, robbery, and aggravated assault" (section Violent Crime subsection Definitions) [119]. In addition to these examples, violent crime was defined by a behavior list in Australia without a preliminary definition-like statement. The list includes murder, manslaughter, rape or other sexual assault, aggravated assault, and robbery [120]. In a UN report [121], violent crime as such was not defined, but each crime type included was defined. The list included intentional homicide, assault, rape, robbery, and kidnapping, whereas a Justice Policy Institute report [122] entitled "Defining violence" provided a comparative overview of violent crime types with behavior lists employed in various US states. The lists are state-dependent, which cannot be reproduced here but in principle are similar to that provided by the FBI.

The preliminary definitions of violent crime typically include the use of, or threatening with, force. Although present in almost all law enforcement definitions, it does not accurately demarcate violent crime. The police, for instance, uses threats of force on a daily basis. Yet, this is not violent crime, provided, naturally, that the police respect the laws and regulations specific to its activity. Although police activity may fulfill the definition of violent crime, policing activities are not included in the lists of crimes and as such are exempt from the definition. Civilians may also use force to defend themselves or others without committing violent crime. Such activities are not only free from punishment but can be considered prosocial acts. Athletes practicing various martial arts are also free to use aggression without becoming violent criminals. They may also threaten one another violently during prefight press conferences without committing any violent offense.

These definitions do not provide clear criteria but rather serve as a general interpretative framework for law enforcement. The essence of the definition lies in the lists that cover various forms of violent crime. Note that acts of relational aggression as defined in psychology – e.g., malicious rumor spreading, damaging someone's social status, or social exclusion (ostracism) – are missing from these lists. Relational aggression may break the law when extreme, but it is not considered a violent crime. Intimidation may qualify as violent crime only if it involved a real threat of violence. Raised voices, threatening looks, and empty threats – so frequent in everyday life – are not violent crimes.

These considerations imply that (1) the approach of law enforcement to aggression is restrictive. According to these definitions, all behaviors defined as aggression by the psychological approach should be considered violent crimes since the delivery of harm includes the use of force. A good deal of psychological aggression, however, is dismissed from the concept (2). The law enforcement approach is as behavior-centered as the psychological one, but instead of formulating an all-encompassing definition, it operates with lists, which putatively cover all the behaviors that are considered violent. These lists are often organized into a complex classification tree (see below).

1.4.2 Aggression from a Law Enforcement Perspective

1.4.2.1 Types of Aggression Covered and Subject Selection

According to the law enforcement approach, the use of force or threat of force outlines three major categories of behaviors characterized by their social impact and legal consequence:

1. *Prosocial aggression.* In this case, the threat or use of force aims at protecting the society as a whole from disturbances or at protecting one or more individuals from suffering harm. Overall, this is the obligation of the police, but the act is similarly prosocial if performed by anyone – provided that the behavior is performed within the boundaries of law. Such acts – for instance, the capture of criminals – are not considered violent crimes and, consequently, are outside the scope of the law enforcement approach.
2. *Neutral aggression.* In the case of martial arts, the perpetrator threatens or uses force against another person for personal gain (be that winning prize money or fame), but aggression closely follows preset legally approved rules. Failure to follow the rules may be illegal. Martial arts have a considerable entertaining value, may serve national pride, and are sources of legal incomes for many people besides the fighter. As such, fights by athletes may be viewed as being socially

useful. Yet, they cannot be considered prosocial in that they are not done for the direct benefit of others. Although not prosocial, martial arts are legal and consequently are outside the scope of the law enforcement approach to aggression.

3. *Antisocial aggression.* In this case, the aggression harms the members of the society physically, psychologically, and sometimes also economically and may destabilize the society if they are very frequent. This is the case with assault, robbery, etc. One can easily deduce from the lists of violent crimes that this is the subject matter of the law enforcement approach.

The principle that differentiates the three types of aggression is the law. Since the law is the main categorizing principle, authors often tend to study mixed groups where all subjects committed law infractions (being delinquents or criminals) but only part of the subjects would be considered aggressive according to the other approaches. That is, subjects who have violated the law by other, non-aggressive means are usually also included in the study populations. In one study, for instance [123], the participants were delinquents who deliberately damaged another's property, stole something worth more than $50, stole something worth less than $50, sold drugs, threatened or used a weapon to take something from someone, participated in a group fight, committed burglary in a home or other building, or got into physical fights. Obviously, violent acts were prominent in the list of criminal acts, which also included other types of non-aggressive criminal behaviors. In another study [124], the participants were delinquent children who showed wanton destructiveness, vandalism, simple theft, hooliganism, infractions of firework regulations, and minor forms of aggression, i.e., a similarly mixed set of violations of the law. In this study, however, the aggressiveness of subjects was measured independently of criminal records by the Buss–Durkee Hostility Inventory [125]. Based on this, subjects were classified as showing overt aggression (feeling angry and displaying verbal or physical aggression) or covert aggression (hostility and angry feelings without expressing aggression openly). Only the latter showed a significant correlation with cortisol, the endocrine endpoint of the study. Yet, the paper bore the word "aggression" in its title. Implicitly, covert aggression was defined here by feelings, which is contrary to the psychological definition of aggression. Although the instrument was a psychological one, it was originally devised to detect hostility, as its name shows, and items addressing aggression just clarified the various behaviors associated with hostility. It was definitely not devised to investigate violent crime.

These two examples illustrate that studies into violent crime or delinquency are not always easy to evaluate from the point of view of aggressive behaviors or violent crime. The two papers referred to were not singled out because they were erroneous in one or another way but because their approach was typical. In law enforcement studies, delinquent/criminal study groups are frequently of the mixed type, and their aggressiveness is often evaluated by using concepts different from the law enforcement approach.

Naturally, there are studies where the subjects were all violent criminals (e.g., committed murder [126] or assault [127]) and the main inclusion criterion was their violent criminal records, not just any criminal record. Although not rare, such studies constitute only a subgroup of those that address violent criminal behavior. Discarding studies where violent crime was one of the main but not the only type of crime would deprive the area from important findings. In addition, the situation is quite similar with the psychiatric approach as aggression-related psychopathologies cover both aggressive and non-aggressive subjects. Yet, such studies are integral parts of the aggression literature. It is noteworthy, however, that the methods section of each study should be carefully checked for the type of crimes subjects committed and for the actual measure of aggression employed (if any), as crimes that include violent crime should not be evaluated together with those which were restricted to it.

1.4.2.2 Crime Classification

To illustrate how violent crime such as aggression is addressed from the point of view of the law enforcement approach, we will refer first to a now classical book written by Douglas, Burgess, Burgess, and Ressler, four highly respected experts of the topic [128]. According to one of the enthusiastic reviewers (a well-known criminal psychologist himself), this book "emulates and reflects a functional equivalent of the *Diagnostic and Statistical Manual of Mental Disorders* (5th ed.; DSM-5; American Psychiatric Association, 2013) but is focused upon the erudite categorization and description of violent crimes" (p. 1 in [129]). A detailed presentation of the whole system is beyond the scope of this section, so we will restrict ourselves to outline its main features.

One important categorization principle in this system is the motive of crime. The main categories for homicides, for instance, are the following: criminal enterprise, personal cause, sexual, extremist and medical, and group cause homicides. These leading classes of motives are broken down into subclasses. For instance, within the broad category of criminal enterprises, homicide may be committed for financial gain. There might be a series of other subcategories; for instance, the financial gain may be insurance-related, and a supplementary motive might be having a sexual affair with a third person (e.g., when the victim was the spouse). In this case, the financial gain motive is supplemented by another personal interest, i.e., the desire to eliminate an unwanted relationship. Crimes may also be categorized according to the type of offense. In the case of homicide, for instance, there are two categories along this principle: spontaneous and planned homicides. The same two categories are present in many of the main categories (personal cause, sexual, extremist, homicides, etc.) and in violent crimes other than homicide.

Even more nuanced categorizations result from considering the aggravating factors of the crime. These were grouped by the authors of the system around intents, actions, attitudes, and the victim. As it regards the intents, an aggravator may be the intent of preventing arrest or escaping custody. Actions are aggravators, for instance, if they created grave risks to others or many persons. Utter disregard for human life may be an aggravator from the point of view of attitudes, whereas targeting vulnerable victims (e.g., people with disabilities such as ID) is an aggravator from the point of view of the victim. Some behaviors, for instance, "Heinous, atrocious, cruel, depraved, wanton, vile, outrageous" acts (e.g., some murders), carry all four types of aggravators, which together may be summed up as a depravity measure associated with a particular criminal act. Importantly, this classification system often makes reference to psychiatric categories such as personality disorders, paraphilias, etc.

Classification systems compiled for statistical purposes are similarly complex but seem to lack the moral component of the former system. For instance, one of the proposed statistical classification systems [130] first list the main categories of crime. The list includes acts leading to death or intending to cause death, acts causing harm or intending to cause harm to a person, acts of violence or threatened violence against a person that involve property, etc. Thereafter, it creates subcategories. For instance, the category "acts leading to death or intending to cause death" has a series of subcategories such as murder and intentional homicide, non-intentional homicide, unlawful killing associated with armed conflict, etc. Note that these subcategories implicitly refer to motives. Aggravators and depravity measures are mostly missing from this system. Aggravators were mentioned for assault only, and these are established mainly in merely technical terms (e.g., use of weapon). Expressions like "reckless indifference," "honor crime," "felony murder," etc., which are to a certain extent morally oriented, are only mentioned in the appendices.

A common conclusion deriving from these two classification systems is that within the law enforcement approach, the meticulous classification of behaviors conceptualized as violent crime is of great concern. This attitude is rather similar to that employed by psychiatry but is largely missing from the biological and psychological approaches. The biological and psychological approaches do classify aggressive behaviors, but only in more general terms. For psychology, for instance, specifying two or three types of aggression (proactive, reactive, and psychotic) seems sufficient, and there does not appear to be a need for creating subclasses and sub-subclasses. In psychiatry, by contrast, a large number of mental disorders are described which are unified into broader categories; for instance, disruptive mood dysregulation disorder is classified as a depressive disorder. In their turn, mental disorders are often divided into subclasses (e.g., conduct disorder with or without callous–unemotional traits).

1.4.3 The Use of the Concept

1.4.3.1 Biology and Psychology

The law enforcement approach neither takes inspiration from nor inspires work centered on the biological approach to aggression although certain correspondences still exist. The biological function of aggression – e.g., competition for resources – has its corresponding notions like "criminal enterprises" and "gain-oriented violent crimes." In fact, all the three types of aggression differentiated based on their social impact – prosocial, neutral, and antisocial aggressions – have a competitive dimension. In a sense, the police compete with criminals for territory and social stability and/or to ensure the competitive advantages of fellow citizens. On their turn, athletes compete for prize money and/or fame, whereas criminals may compete for resources. In addition, law enforcement-related papers sometimes do refer to competitiveness, specifically when theoretical explanations are sought for the persistence of violent crime [41–43]. However, the law enforcement approach as a whole does not consider violent crime from the perspective of competition.

Overall, the same applies to psychology. For instance, the differentiation of "spontaneous" from "planned" violent crimes is reminiscent of the psychological concepts of "reactive" and "proactive" aggressions. Yet, psychology does not judge behaviors according to social impacts; it defines aggression exclusively by the nature of the behaviors observed (i.e., the delivery of harm). As such, all three prosocial, neutral, and antisocial aggression types of aggression are integral parts of the psychological concepts of aggression, whereas the law enforcement approach is concerned with antisocial aggression. A subgroup of studies into criminals or violent criminals uses psychological inventories to investigate the level of aggressiveness in their subjects. This, however, seems to be a practical borrowing of tools rather than a sign of theoretical integration.

1.4.3.2 Psychiatry

In contrast to biology and psychology, the psychiatric and law enforcement approaches are interwoven in many ways. First, the symptoms of various mental disorders refer to crime and legal actions explicitly or implicitly. Symptoms A1 of ASPD, for instance, refers to "performing acts that are grounds for arrest," whereas 7 of the 15 symptoms of cluster A of conduct disorder are in fact criminal, but not necessarily violent criminal acts. Likewise, the presence of the main symptoms of impulse–control disorders would inevitably lead to arrests even if this is not mentioned in DSM-5 [40]. Second, both Megargee's [111] criminal classification system and the crime classification system of Douglas, Burgess, Burgess, and Ressler [128] are partly based on or at least make extensive reference to psychiatric concepts such as mental disorders. Note that the use of psychiatric concepts in crime classification systems has a long tradition as shown by a crime classification system created in 1910 [131]. For instance, the authors of this paper wrote "The slight degree of mental defect involved in instinctive criminality can be recognized, of course, only by experts, and hence the necessity of expert psychiatrists in connection with all our criminal courts and correctional institutions" (journal page 540). Third, the format of the crime classification system presented above was inspired by DSM-5's formats recognized by its reviewers (see above). Finally, and most importantly, the subjects of psychiatric and law enforcement studies overlap largely; subsequently, representatives of the two branches of aggression research frequently make reference to each other's work.

The overlap of subjects appears to be almost complete in the most dangerous criminals as exemplified by a death row sample studied in California [132]. This sample of 16 murderers (multiple murderers in most cases) was diagnosed with at least 2 mental disorders out of the 4 that were investigated (PTSD, depression, drug addiction, and psychosis). The average was three disorders per convict. In addition to mental disorders, developmental or acquired brain damages were also recorded, which increased the average number of psychiatric or neurologic problems to four. One-third of the sample showed all the investigated abnormalities. Other reports on death row samples are in line with the one presented in some detail above [133–136]. One can speculate that the precarious psychiatric state of inmates was due to the death sentence as a traumatic experience or to prison life [136], which may at least question the relevance of the findings for criminals prior to conviction. A few studies bypassed such confounds by studying the psychiatric histories of criminals such as murderers before sentencing [137] or established diagnoses in non-criminal populations and assessed convictions subsequently [138]. The conclusions of both types of studies confirm the high incidence of psychiatric disorders in criminals *before* the emergence of criminal behavior.

High incidence rates of psychiatric disorders were not typical merely to the most dangerous criminals. A study on adolescent delinquents [139] found that all of them had conduct disorder and around 90% also suffered from a comorbid disorder, including attention-deficit/hyperactivity disorder (62%), drug addiction (57%), and PTSD (31%). A Dutch study on over 20,000 criminal cases [140] showed that two-thirds of the criminals suffered from at least one clinical disorder and about half of them had a personality disorder. Thus, the share of comorbid psychiatric diagnoses was high. This study was referred to not only to illustrate the high incidence rates of psychiatric disorders found in criminal populations but also because subjects committed a variety of offences and those who committed serious violent crimes showed few differences in rates of psychiatric disorders from those whose crimes were less severe. Similar studies are countless, each demonstrating that the incidence of mental disorders in criminals is much higher than that of non-criminal populations.

In addition to differences in the prevalence of psychiatric disorders, the type of mental disorders is also different. For instance, ASPD is rare in the general population (prevalence ~3% [141]) but rather frequent in criminal populations (prevalence ~50% [142]). Importantly, about 70–90% of criminal populations had personality disorders including but not restricted to ASPDs [142, 143].

The overlap of study populations offers opportunities for further associations between the two fields. For instance, people having psychiatric diagnoses are often subdivided into classes by law enforcement criteria, and criminals are often subclassified based on the diagnoses they may or may not carry. In one study, psychopaths were divided into two groups based on their success to evade apprehension, and their neurobiology was compared [144]. Unsuccessful psychopaths – i.e., those caught by the police – had brain structural and functional impairments together with autonomic nervous system dysfunction, whereas successful psychopath who avoided apprehension were assumed to have intact or enhanced neurobiological functioning. Psychiatric instruments are also frequently used to evaluate the risk of violent crime perpetration [145].

Although the relationship between psychopathology and violent crime remains controversial and complex as will be discussed in the section on responsibility, it seems clear that the psychiatric and law enforcement approaches are deeply intertwined.

1.4.3.3 Violence in Groups

One distinctive characteristic of the law enforcement approach is the great emphasis it puts on cooperative aggression. These may take several forms, from riots through organized crime to terrorism. Although the latter is in fact organized crime, it has several particularities that separate it from mafia-like crimes and deserves a separate place in the group crime category because of the presence of ideology and the lack of the financial gain component.

Naturally, attention payed to cooperative aggression is not unique to the law enforcement approach. Group aggression is a topic in biology and a subject matter of the psychological approach, although it omits psychiatric symptoms. In biology, for instance, aggression between groups of various species from ants [146] to chimpanzees [147] is frequently studied, whereas in psychology, relational aggression is a group phenomenon. In biology and psychology, however, the main focus is on the individual and the factors that influence his/her choices. In law enforcement by contrast, rioting, organized crime, and terrorism are just as important as violent crimes perpetrated by isolated individuals. This separates the field from all the others.

1.5 Methodologies Employed

All the main four approaches study the risk factors and mechanisms that contribute to the expression and maintenance of aggressive behaviors, and in so doing, they use technologies borrowed from other scientific areas, such as genetics, endocrinology, and neuroscience. The four approaches are highly similar as regards such borrowed methodologies. In contrast, the area-specific methodologies, especially those that are used to measure aggression, are widely different, which affects the cross-validity of the findings obtained in different areas. Quite often, the differences in methodologies are explained by tradition, technical possibilities, and ethical considerations.

In biology, competition – the essence of aggression according to this approach – is measured in a competitive situation, i.e., while aggression unfolds. Sometimes only critical-dependent variables are investigated, for instance, the latency of attack (the time taken from the first contact to the first attack) or the number of attacks (for instance, the number of bites a rat delivers during a conflict). In most cases, however, researchers score the full spectrum of behaviors shown in a particular situation. These include aggression-related behaviors (threats, bites, dominance-related behaviors) and aggression non-related behaviors (exploration, grooming, social investigation, etc.). Analysis is based on ethogram, i.e., a complete catalog of behaviors that a species may show in a particular situation. Although it is tacitly assumed that the momentary behavior characterizes the individual, this is not necessarily so. For instance, animals submitted to a particular treatment show dramatically enhanced aggressiveness in a dyadic contest but behave fearfully when in larger social groups [101]. Likewise, certain mouse lines selected for aggressiveness are unusually aggressive in dyads but behave typically in groups [148, 149]. In general, the context has a great impact on how aggression is expressed and with what efficiency [150]. In summary, aggression is investigated in biology as it unfolds, and the results are valid for the moment of and the context in which aggression was investigated. These circumstances do allow for group comparisons but are only indirectly related to the general characteristic that may be labelled aggression.

Psychology has a dual approach: usually studies aggression as a habit but can also evaluate aggression while it is performed. The habit of delivering harms to another – the essence of aggression in psychology – is frequently measured by a variety of psychometric inventories. These are usually unselective to the context where the behavior occurred; for instance, the statement "I yell at people" refers to all the situations when one may yell at others, without further specifications. In addition, the scales are often imprecise as the frequencies are asked for in general terms only (e.g., often – rarely – never or daily – weekly – monthly, etc.), whereas the duration of behaviors are rarely if ever investigated. It is noteworthy that various inventories cover overlapping but not entirely similar sets of behaviors, although they are supposed to investigate aggression. In summary, the inventory-based psychological approach is somewhat imprecise, but, at the same time, it accounts for the aggression history of the individual, which is rarely studied in animal aggression. Experimental human paradigms on their turn measure human aggression in the laboratory under challenging conditions, which in a way is similar to the methodologies employed in biology. Nevertheless, aggression is usually measured by a single number, for instance, the frequency of punishment delivered to a provoking opponent, which fails to mirror the complexity of human aggression. At the same time, these methodologies allow the evaluation of emotional, endocrine, neural, and other phenomena that accompany aggression.

Psychiatric and law enforcement investigations follow the same route: researchers inquire about the past and characterize their subjects based on their behavioral history or employ the laboratory paradigms developed by experimental psychology to investigate aggressive responses in challenging situations. There still are some differences from the psychological approach. For instance, the psychiatric diagnosis of aggression-related psychopathologies includes, but is not restricted to, the evaluation of aggressiveness, whereas the law enforcement approach is limited by the availability of information, especially when official criminal records are used to assign participants to groups. Nevertheless, the general approach is similar: they can evaluate both the history of aggression and acute responses to social challenges.

In summary, methodologies can be divided into two groups. Experimental psychology – irrespective to the clinical or criminal history of their subjects – and the biological approach allow the investigation of the proximate mechanisms of aggression. The main reason is that the studies are made while participants are performing aggression. By contrast, psychological inventories, psychiatric diagnoses, and criminal records are indicative of the behavioral history of study participants, which may be appropriate for evaluating ultimate but not proximate mechanisms of aggression, because when the measurements are made, study participants are peaceful. The only difference between them and controls is their past.

1.6 Overview and the Chances for Integration

In the introduction of this chapter, as well as when comparing the four approaches, we asked a simple but important question: Is knowledge achieved in one area of aggression research usable by another?

The behavior of scientists – rarely articulated in explicit views – suggests that at one extreme, the area is considered as a unitary one and findings in one area, for instance, biology, may be usable for another, for instance, law enforcement. On the other hand, many scientists neglect areas other than their own to an extent that suggests that they consider the four main approaches as independent fields. Naturally, there are many shades of differences between these opposing approaches. For instance, some appear to consider findings in other areas inspiring without considering them usable as direct arguments. Below we will briefly summarize issues that bind the four areas together but will also outline the differences. This will be followed by an evaluation of the possibilities of integration.

Worth noting that here we do not compare professionals but compare approaches. Nothing stops a psychologist to study animals by adopting the biological approach or a law enforcement expert to use psychiatric inventories; however, there still are basic approaches that define how mainstream research is performed in a particular field.

1.6.1 Overview

1.6.1.1 The Form of Behavior

The form of behavior is formulated most clearly and comprehensively by the psychological approach. The essence of the definition is “harming others.” Although biological definitions include this specification only indirectly, for example, by giving examples, aggression is measured in biology by the harm one individual inflicts on another. Note that both psychology and biology include threats among aggressive behaviors. Neither approach differentiates different harms that are eligible from those that are not eligible for study. Consequently, the two approaches are rather similar as regards the basic form of behavior. Naturally, aggressive behaviors are species-specific: ants, cows, mice, and humans fight in different ways. Nevertheless, any harm delivered by ants, cows, etc. would be classified as aggression according to the psychological approach. Thus, the biological and psychological approaches appear to be similar, which is rather different from the other two.

According to the psychiatric approach, the "delivery of harm" is present among the symptoms of a variety of disorders, which links the approach to the previous ones. However, "harm to others" is always expected to take serious, in most cases physical, forms, and more importantly the behavior should be inappropriate and/or out of proportion in the context where it occurs. No rational, explicable uses of aggression are eligible for inclusion among the symptoms of mental disorders: rats fighting for rank will never be eligible for a diagnosis. Likewise, neither social games deemed aggression by the psychological approach, for instance, relational aggression, nor the so-called verbal aggression, renamed here "intimidation," can be considered symptoms of aggression-related psychopathologies unless they take extreme forms. Even in this case, such behaviors have the possibility to be classified among the symptoms of disorders other than those that are aggression-related.

The law enforcement approach is even more restrictive. One can harm others to any extent without being classified as a violent criminal – the embodiment of aggression in this field. A police officer is even allowed to kill an offender if the situation requires it, whereas a prizefighter is rewarded for his/her ability to harm others. The very same behaviors are deemed violent crime, however, if harm is delivered under conditions that are punishable by the law. In addition, minor forms of aggression are irrelevant from a law enforcement viewpoint. Similar to the psychiatric approach, the apprehended behaviors are deemed irrational, if not from the point of view of the individual, then from the point of view of the society. Similar to the psychiatric approach, explainable forms of aggression are not considered aggression, rather it is better to say violent crimes. An animal fighting for rank or people employing relational or mild forms of verbal aggression to the same end is outside the scope of the law enforcement approach.

The psychiatric and law enforcement approaches may also be considered similar based on two criteria:

1. Both focus on extraordinary manifestations of aggression. In one case, the behavior breaks accepted social norms, whereas it breaks the law in the case of the other.
2. Both address forms of aggression that seriously affect various areas of functioning, for instance, by psychological suffering (e.g., distress) or legal penalties.

In conclusion, "harming others" as a form of behavior binds the four areas together and separates them at the same time. It is present in all four approaches but is selected or not selected based on specific criteria. The very same behavior may be within or outside the scope of investigations depending on the characteristics of the approach.

1.6.1.2 Research Subjects

In contrast to the behavior studied, the subjects of research are quite different with the four main approaches. One can argue that the differences are the smallest in the case of the biological and psychological approaches, although the biological approach aims at investigating non-human animals, whereas the participants of psychological studies are usually humans.

This seems to be a major difference at the first sight, but actually, it is not. There are two reasons that support this view. First, aggression is dealt with as a natural phenomenon in both types of studies, as an inherent property of the population, be that animal or human. Participants may show aggressiveness at a higher or lower level and may undergo environmental influences or treatments that increase or decrease aggressiveness, but no hypothesis predicts the absence of aggression in any study population, because aggression is considered an integral part of the natural behavioral repertoire of the species. Second, subjects are not selected; they usually are the typical animal or the general population in biology and psychology, respectively. This does not mean that subjects may not undergo any selection process. They may be, for instance, laboratory animals of a certain type, or participants may have specific social characteristics. Nevertheless, they all are healthy in psychiatric terms and non-criminal from a law enforcement approach.

The links between the two approaches are further outlined by the fact that laboratory models of aggression are often viewed as models of human aggression. The phrase "comparative psychology" and its synonyms, which can be recognized in the name of many journals, refer to this connection. In such journals and studies, animals are often viewed as substitutes for humans or at least as study subjects, which are directly or indirectly illustrative for the psychology of human aggression. Animal studies are employed when experimental technologies cannot be applied in humans for ethical or practical reasons or when the origins or the basics of human aggression are investigated.

By contrast, the psychiatric and law enforcement approaches select their subjects. Neither mental disorders nor criminal behaviors are natural characteristics of the population as a whole. These approaches focus on those that demonstrably showed a mental disorder or committed a violent criminal act. These are small subgroups of the general population, which on their turn are the subjects of study for the psychological approach. Moreover, psychiatric and law enforcement studies need a comparison for their subjects. This comparison, often a control group, is the general population. It is better to say that the comparison group has no diagnosis or did not commit violent crime.

The same applies to the abovementioned animal models of abnormal aggression, which aim at modelling aggression-related psychopathologies. Control groups belong to the typical animal category, which in fact are the experimental subjects for the biological approach. Aggression is assumed to be functional in the typical animal as the biological approach stipulates but becomes dysfunctional in the models. Mechanisms underlying the change are supposed to model the mechanisms of psychopathology. The same applies to real psychiatric and law enforcement studies. Differences between the general population, such as participants of psychological investigations and the psychiatric patients or offenders, are supposed to be informative about the mechanisms involved in the generation of these dysfunctional states and behaviors.

To take the argument to the extreme, one might say that the psychiatric and law enforcement studies start where the biological and psychological approaches stop. Even if this is an exaggeration, one can confidently state that the subjects of research are different with the four approaches, and again the biological and psychological approaches, on one side, and the psychiatric and law enforcement approaches on the other form two distinct dyads.

1.6.1.3 Methods of Investigation

Different approaches need different tools of investigation, but the differences between the four approaches go beyond such technical differences. The biological approach and experimental psychology investigate aggression while it is actually performed; work adopting the classical psychological, psychiatric, and law enforcement approaches classifies subjects according to their aggression histories. The psychiatric approach investigates a state where aggression is just one, but not necessarily indispensable symptom. These are not merely technical but conceptual differences as shown above. The former type of studies allows the study of proximate whereas the latter the ultimate mechanisms of aggression. In addition, the four approaches differ largely as it regards their precision and reliability.

1.6.2 Is Integration Possible?

These four approaches study overlapping but different types of behavior and recruit widely different research subjects, which are investigated by conceptually different methodologies. At the first sight, such major differences preclude their integration into one single area of research and seem to do justice to those who are reluctant to overtake findings or concepts originating from another area of the field. It seems only natural that under such circumstances, one cannot take it for granted that findings obtained in one area are directly relevant for another.

Yet, should we isolate the four areas from one another altogether? This does not seem to be rational mainly because the essence of behavior – harm to another – still seems to link the four approaches. We will take the neurobiology of aggression as an example to formulate three hypotheses regarding the relationships between the main approaches.

1. The null hypothesis would be that the four fields are entirely different. One can hypothesize that attacking an intruder in the home range, manipulating the social environment to eliminate a competitor, showing uncontrolled aggressive outbursts frequently, and stabbing somebody for a purse are governed by entirely different neural mechanisms. That is, the differences between the neural controls of behaviors that are studied by the four approaches are qualitative in nature. If this was true, we were dealing with four independent areas of research.
2. We might, however, also assume that there is one basic neural mechanism of aggression, which is active in any of its manifestations, naturally with minor modifications depending on the aspect that is investigated. For instance, the neural mechanism underlying an attack by a resident rat on an intruder may be very similar to that operating during an uncontrollable outburst of human anger. The only difference might be quantitative only. For instance, the very similar neural circuit might be overactivated in the latter situation as compared to the former. Such quantitative but not qualitative differences involve that the field is unitary with area-specific variations. Consequently, one can confidently rely on findings obtained in other fields.
3. Another possibility is that there are several mechanisms of aggression, but these do not separate approaches but the types of aggression. For instance, emotional aggressions (reactive aggression, IED, spontaneous violent crimes) may have one, whereas "cold-blooded" aggression (proactive aggression, ASPD, premeditated violent crimes) may have another basic neural mechanism. This hypothesis would bind together rather than separate the four approaches, suggesting that findings are relevant across fields, but the type of aggression needs a careful analysis before overtaking concepts or findings.

The overall conclusion deriving from this section is that the possibility of integrating the four approaches should neither be taken for granted nor refuted, but investigated. This is one of the major aims of the subsequent chapters of this book. These will reveal that the three hypotheses mentioned above are not alternative but complementary. There are mechanisms that unify rather than separate the four approaches; others are specific to each, and there also are mechanisms that separate aggression types rather than approaches to aggression. A graphic summary of the main approaches to aggression is given in Fig. 1.1.

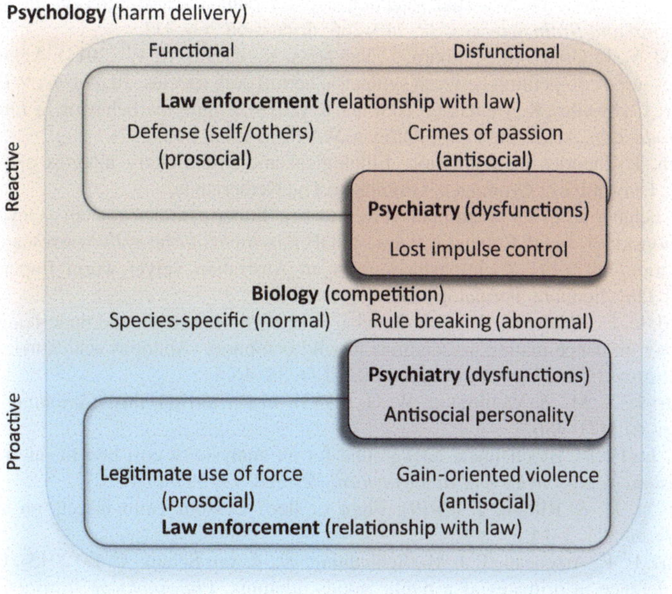

Fig. 1.1 Relationships between various approaches: a graphic summary. Due to its focus on behavior, the psychological approach encompasses all forms of aggression and violence but establishes the existence of two major forms: proactive and reactive. The functional–dysfunctional distinction comes from law enforcement, which classifies aggression according to its relationship with the law. According to the classical biological view, aggression is a form of competition which is functional; the so-called abnormal aggression, however, created dysfunctional aggression by submitting laboratory animals to the etiological factors of aggression-related disorders. Psychopathologic aggression is dysfunctional by definition but can be divided into two groups based on emotional and behavioral characteristics. Psychopathologies and crime overlap by virtue of their co-occurrence in a large share of people. They also overlap with abnormal aggression models as these were developed to model psychopathologies. For other differences and analogies between the approaches, see text

References

1. Siegel, A., & Victoroff, J. (2009). Understanding human aggression: New insights from neuroscience. *International Journal of Law and Psychiatry, 32*, 209–215.
2. Siegel, A., Bhatt, S., Bhatt, R., & Zalcman, S. S. (2007). The neurobiological bases for development of pharmacological treatments of aggressive disorders. *Current Neuropharmacology, 5*, 135–147.
3. Siegel, A., & Douard, J. (2011). Who's flying the plane: Serotonin levels, aggression and free will. *International Journal of Law and Psychiatry, 34*, 20–29.
4. Lindenfors, P., & Tullberg, B. S. (2011). Evolutionary aspects of aggression the importance of sexual selection. *Advances in Genetics, 75*, 7–22.
5. Darwin, C. (1859). *The origin of species by means of natural selection*. Penguin, London.
6. Darwin, C. (1871). *The descent of man and selection in relation to sex*. Murray, London.
7. Craig, W. *Appetites and aversions as constituents of instincts.*

8. Archer, J. (2009). Does sexual selection explain human sex differences in aggression? *Behavioral and Brain Sciences, 32*, 249–266; discussion 266–311.
9. Tran, M. V., O'Grady, M., Colborn, J., Van Ness, K., & Hill, R. W. (2014). Aggression and food resource competition between sympatric hermit crab species. *PLoS One, 9*, e91823.
10. Jalabert, C., Munley, K., Demas, G., & Soma, K. (2018). Aggressive behavior. In *Encyclopedia of reproduction*, Academic Press, Pullman, WA (Vol. 1, pp. 242–247).
11. Dennen, J. Theories of aggression: Ethological and evolutionary theories of aggression. (2005). University of Groningen, Groningen, The Netherlands.
12. Social behaviour in an Australian velvet worm, Euperipatoides rowelli (Onychophora : Peripatopsidae) | Judith Reinhard | Request PDF. *ResearchGate* https://www.researchgate.net/publication/43471391_Social_behaviour_in_an_Australian_velvet_worm_Euperipatoides_rowelli_Onychophora_Peripatopsidae.
13. Huffard, C. L., Caldwell, R. L., & Boneka, F. (2010). Male-male and male-female aggression may influence mating associations in wild octopuses (Abdopus aculeatus). *Journal of Comparative Psychology (Washington DC), 124*, 38–46.
14. Fitzpatrick, S. M., & Wellington, W. G. (1983). Insect territoriality. *Canadian Journal of Zoology, 61*, 471–486.
15. Haller, J. (1995). Biochemical background for an analysis of cost-benefit interrelations in aggression. *Neuroscience and Biobehavioral Reviews, 19*, 599–604.
16. Stevenson, P., & Rillich, J. (2019). Fight or flee? Lessons from insects on aggression. *Neuroforum, 25*, 3–14.
17. Willems, E. P., Arseneau, T. J. M., Schleuning, X., & van Schaik, C. P. (2015). Communal range defence in primates as a public goods dilemma. *Philosophical Transactions of the Royal Society of London. Series B, Biological Sciences, 370*, 20150003.
18. Hillman, K. L. (2013). Cost-benefit analysis: The first real rule of fight club? *Frontiers in Neuroscience, 7*, 248.
19. Haller, J., & Kruk, M. R. (2006). Normal and abnormal aggression: Human disorders and novel laboratory models. *Neuroscience and Biobehavioral Reviews, 30*, 292–303.
20. Haller, J. (2017). Studies into abnormal aggression in humans and rodents: Methodological and translational aspects. *Neuroscience and Biobehavioral Reviews, 76*, 77–86.
21. Blanchard, R. J., & Blanchard, D. C. (1981). The organization and modeling of animal aggression. In P. F. Brain & D. Benton (Eds.), *The biology of aggression*, Sijtoff and Noordhoff, Alphenaan den Rijn, The Netherlands. (pp. 155–174).
22. Flack, J. C., Girvan, M., de Waal, F. B. M., & Krakauer, D. C. (2006). Policing stabilizes construction of social niches in primates. *Nature, 439*, 426–429.
23. Hay, D. F., Castle, J., & Davies, L. (2000). Toddlers' use of force against familiar peers: A precursor of serious aggression? *Child Development, 71*, 457–467.
24. Tremblay, R. E., et al. (1999). The search for the age of 'onset' of physical aggression: Rousseau and bandura revisited. *Criminal Behaviour and Mental Health, 9*, 8–23.
25. Reebye, P. (2005). Aggression during early years - infancy and preschool. *The Canadian Child and Adolescent Psychiatry Review, 14*, 16–20.
26. Enright, E. A., Gweon, H., & Sommerville, J. A. (2017). 'To the victor go the spoils': Infants expect resources to align with dominance structures. *Cognition, 164*, 8–21.
27. Li, Y., & Wright, M. F. (2014). Adolescents' social status goals: Relationships to social status insecurity, aggression, and prosocial behavior. *Journal of Youth and Adolescence, 43*, 146–160.
28. Vaillancourt, T. (2013). Do human females use indirect aggression as an intrasexual competition strategy? *Philosophical Transactions of the Royal Society of London. Series B, Biological Sciences, 368*, 20130080.
29. Palombit, R. A. (2015). Infanticide as sexual conflict: Coevolution of male strategies and female counterstrategies. *Cold Spring Harbor Perspectives in Biology, 7*.

30. Bildstein, K. L., Golden, C. B., McCraith, B. J., Bohmke, B. W., & Seibels, R. E. (1993). Feeding behavior, aggression, and the conservation biology of flamingos: Integrating studies of captive and free-ranging birds. *American Zoologist, 33*, 117–125.
31. Baan, C., Bergmüller, R., Smith, D. W., & Molnar, B. (2014). Conflict management in free-ranging wolves, Canis lupus. *Animal Behaviour, 90*, 327–334.
32. de Waal, F. B. (2004). Evolutionary ethics, aggression, and violence: Lessons from primate research. *The Journal of Law, Medicine & Ethics, 32*, 18–23.
33. Blanchard, R. J., et al. (2001). Sexual and aggressive interactions in a visible burrow system with provisioned burrows. *Physiology & Behavior, 72*, 245–254.
34. Sachser, N., & Proöve, E. (1988). Plasma-testosterone development in colony and individually housed male Guinea pigs. *Ethology, 79*, 62–70.
35. Mikics, E., Barsy, B., & Haller, J. (2007). The effect glucocorticoids on aggressiveness in established colonies of rats. *Psychoneuroendocrinology, 32*, 160–170.
36. Georgiev, A. V., Klimczuk, A. C. E., Traficonte, D. M., & Maestripieri, D. (2013). When Violence pays: A cost-benefit analysis of aggressive behavior in animals and humans. *Evolutionary Psychology, 11*, 678–699.
37. Stockley, P., & Bro-Jørgensen, J. (2011). Female competition and its evolutionary consequences in mammals. *Biological Reviews of the Cambridge Philosophical Society, 86*, 341–366.
38. Buss, D. M., & Shackelford, T. K. (1997). Human aggression in evolutionary psychological perspective. *Clinical Psychology Review, 17*, 605–619.
39. Ainsworth, S. E., & Maner, J. K. (2012). Sex begets violence: Mating motives, social dominance, and physical aggression in men. *Journal of Personality and Social Psychology, 103*, 819–829.
40. American psychiatric association. (2013). *Diagnostic and statistical manual of mental disorders* (5th ed.). American Psychiatric Association, Washington.
41. Crombach, A., & Elbert, T. (2014). The benefits of aggressive traits: A study with current and former street children in Burundi. *Child Abuse & Neglect, 38*, 1041–1050.
42. Sommer, J., et al. (2017). The interplay between trauma, substance abuse and appetitive aggression and its relation to criminal activity among high-risk males in South Africa. *Addictive Behaviors, 64*, 29–34.
43. Nandi, C., Crombach, A., Bambonye, M., Elbert, T., & Weierstall, R. (2015). Predictors of posttraumatic stress and appetitive aggression in active soldiers and former combatants. *European Journal of Psychotraumatology, 6*, 26553.
44. Jhangiani, R., & Tarry, H. (2014). *Principles of social psychology – 1st international edition.* BCcampus, Victoria, British Columbia, Canada.
45. Arnold H. (1961). Buss. The psychology of aggression. https://www.worldcat.org/title/psychology-of-aggression/oclc/204291.
46. Baron, R. A. (1977). *Human aggression*. Plenum, New York.
47. Zillman, D. (1979). *Hostility and aggression*. Erlbaum, New York.
48. Anderson, C., & Husemann, R. (2003). Human aggression: a social-cognitive view. In M. A. Hogg & J. Cooper (Eds.), *The sage handbook of social psychology* (pp. 296–323). Sage Publications, London.
49. Berkowitz, L. (1967). Experiments on automatism and intent in human aggression. *UCLA Forum in Medical Sciences, 7*, 243–266.
50. Berkowitz, L. (1993). *Aggression: Its causes, consequences, and control*. Mcgraw-Hill Book Company, New York.
51. Sneyers, M., Sloore, H., Rossi, G., & Derksen, J. J. L. (2007). Using the Megargee system among Belgian prisoners: Cross-cultural prevalence of the MMPI-2 based types. *Psychological Reports, 100*, 746–754.
52. Atkins, M. S., & Stoff, D. M. (1993). Instrumental and hostile aggression in childhood disruptive behavior disorders. *Journal of Abnormal Child Psychology, 21*, 165–178.

53. Vitiello, B., Behar, D., Hunt, J., Stoff, D., & Ricciuti, A. (1990). Subtyping aggression in children and adolescents. *The Journal of Neuropsychiatry and Clinical Neurosciences, 2*, 189–192.
54. Barratt, E. S., Stanford, M. S., Dowdy, L., Liebman, M. J., & Kent, T. A. (1999). Impulsive and premeditated aggression: A factor analysis of self-reported acts. *Psychiatry Research, 86*, 163–173.
55. Dodge, K. A., & Coie, J. D. (1987). Social-information-processing factors in reactive and proactive aggression in children's peer groups. *Journal of Personality and Social Psychology, 53*, 1146–1158.
56. Bjorkqvist, K., Oesterman, K., & Kaukiainen, A. (1992). The development of direct and indirect aggressive strategies in males and females. In K. Bjoerkqvist & P. Niemelae (Eds.), *Of mice and women: Aspects of female aggression* (pp. 51–64). Academic Press.
57. Archer, J., & Coyne, S. M. (2005). An integrated review of indirect, relational, and social aggression. *Personality Social Psychology Review, 9*, 212–230.
58. Saylor, C. F., et al. (2013). Ostracism in pediatric populations: Review of theory and research. *Journal of Developmental & Behavioral Pediatrics, 34*, 279–287.
59. Sebastian, C., Viding, E., Williams, K. D., & Blakemore, S.-J. (2010). Social brain development and the affective consequences of ostracism in adolescence. *Brain and Cognition, 72*, 134–145.
60. Platt, B., Cohen Kadosh, K., & Lau, J. Y. F. (2013). The role of peer rejection in adolescent depression. *Depression and Anxiety, 30*, 809–821.
61. Epkins, C. C., & Heckler, D. R. (2011). Integrating etiological models of social anxiety and depression in youth: Evidence for a cumulative interpersonal risk model. *Clinical Child and Family Psychology Review, 14*, 329–376.
62. Ren, D., Wesselmann, E. D., & Williams, K. D. (2018). Hurt people hurt people: Ostracism and aggression. *Current Opinion in Psychology, 19*, 34–38.
63. Smart Richman, L., & Leary, M. R. (2009). Reactions to discrimination, stigmatization, ostracism, and other forms of interpersonal rejection: A multimotive model. *Psychological Review, 116*, 365–383.
64. Xu, T., et al. (2019). Workplace bullying and workplace violence as risk factors for cardiovascular disease: A multi-cohort study. *European Heart Journal, 40*, 1124–1134.
65. Galen, B. R., & Underwood, M. K. (1997). A developmental investigation of social aggression among children. *Developmental Psychology, 33*, 589–600.
66. Paquette, J. A., & Underwood, M. K. (1999). Gender differences in young adolescents' experiences of peer victimization: Social and physical aggression. *Merrill-Palmer Quarterly, 45*, 242–266.
67. King, S. L., Allen, S. J., Krützen, M., & Connor, R. C. (2019). Vocal behaviour of allied male dolphins during cooperative mate guarding. *Animal Cognition, 22*, 991. https://doi.org/10.1007/s10071-019-01290-1.
68. Loretto, M.-C., Fraser, O. N., & Bugnyar, T. (2012). Ontogeny of social relations and coalition formation in common ravens (Corvus corax). *International Journal of Comparative Psychology, 25*, 180–194.
69. Hemelrijk, C. K., & Puga-Gonzalez, I. (2012). An individual-oriented model on the emergence of support in fights, its reciprocation and exchange. *PLoS One, 7*, e37271.
70. Beisner, B. A., Jackson, M. E., Cameron, A., & McCowan, B. (2011). Effects of natal male alliances on aggression and power dynamics in rhesus macaques. *American Journal of Primatology, 73*, 790–801.
71. Scott, N. M. (2013). Gesture use by chimpanzees (Pan troglodytes): Differences between sexes in inter- and intra-sexual interactions. *American Journal of Primatology, 75*, 555–567.
72. Anderson, E. J., Weladji, R. B., & Paré, P. (2016). Changes in the dominance hierarchy of captive female Japanese macaques as a consequence of merging two previously established groups. *Zoo Biology, 35*, 505–512.

73. Massen, J. J. M., Szipl, G., Spreafico, M., & Bugnyar, T. (2014). Ravens intervene in others' bonding attempts. *Current Biology, 24*, 2733–2736.
74. Kawazoe, T., & Sosa, S. (2019). Social networks predict immigration success in wild Japanese macaques. *Primates, 60*, 213–222.
75. World Health Organization. (1992). *The ICD-10 classification of mental and behavioural disorders*. World Health Organization, Geneva.
76. Mezzich, J. E. (2002). International surveys on the use of ICD-10 and related diagnostic systems. *Psychopathology, 35*, 72–75.
77. Haller, J. (2018). Preclinical models of conduct disorder - principles and pharmacologic perspectives. *Neuroscience and Biobehavioral Reviews, 91*, 112–120.
78. Fairchild, G., et al. (2019). Conduct disorder. *Nature Reviews Disease Primers, 5*, 43.
79. Hicks, B. M., Markon, K. E., Patrick, C. J., Krueger, R. F., & Newman, J. P. (2004). Identifying psychopathy subtypes on the basis of personality structure. *Psychological Assessment, 16*, 276–288.
80. Murphy, C., & Vess, J. (2003). Subtypes of psychopathy: Proposed differences between narcissistic, borderline, sadistic, and antisocial psychopaths. *The Psychiatric Quarterly, 74*, 11–29.
81. Anderson, N. E., & Kiehl, K. A. (2014). Psychopathy and aggression: When paralimbic dysfunction leads to violence. *Current Topics in Behavioral Neurosciences, 17*, 369–393.
82. Frick, P. J., & Ellis, M. (1999). Callous-unemotional traits and subtypes of conduct disorder. *Clinical Child and Family Psychology Review, 2*, 149–168.
83. Hart, S. D., & Hare, R. D. (1997). Psychopathy: Assessment and association with criminal conduct. In D. M. Stoff, J. Brieling, & J. Maser (Eds.), *Handbook of antisocial behaviour* (pp. 22–35). Wiley, New York.
84. Krieger, F. V., & Stringaris, A. (2013). Bipolar disorder and disruptive mood dysregulation in children and adolescents: Assessment, diagnosis and treatment. *Evidence-Based Mental Health, 16*, 93–94.
85. McElroy, S. L., et al. (1996). Are impulse-control disorders related to bipolar disorder? *Comprehensive Psychiatry, 37*, 229–240.
86. Gerard, M. E., Spitz, M. C., Towbin, J. A., & Shantz, D. (1998). Subacute postictal aggression. *Neurology, 50*, 384–388.
87. Gallagher, D., & Herrmann, N. (2015). Agitation and aggression in Alzheimer's disease: An update on pharmacological and psychosocial approaches to care. *Neurodegenerative Disease Management, 5*, 75–83.
88. de Freitas Cardoso, M. G., et al. (2019). Cognitive impairment following acute mild traumatic brain injury. *Frontiers in Neurology, 10*, 198.
89. Visser, E. M., Berger, H. J. C., Prins, J. B., Van Schrojenstein Lantman-De Valk, H. M. J., & Teunisse, J. P. (2014). Shifting impairment and aggression in intellectual disability and autism spectrum disorder. *Research in Developmental Disabilities, 35*, 2137–2147.
90. Philipp, M. (1979). Psychotic aggression in the medical emergency service. *Medizinische Welt, 30*, 1436–1438.
91. McDermott, B. E., Quanbeck, C. D., Busse, D., Yastro, K., & Scott, C. L. (2008). The accuracy of risk assessment instruments in the prediction of impulsive versus predatory aggression. *Behavioral Sciences & the Law, 26*, 759–777.
92. van Beek, J., Vuijk, P. J., Harte, J. M., & Scherder, E. J. A. (2018). Symptom profile of psychiatric patients with psychosis or psychotic mood disorder in prison. *International Journal of Offender Therapy and Comparative Criminology, 62*, 4158–4173.
93. Hoptman, M. J. (2015). Impulsivity and aggression in schizophrenia: A neural circuitry perspective with implications for treatment. *CNS Spectrums, 20*, 280–286.
94. Volavka, J. (2013). Violence in schizophrenia and bipolar disorder. *Psychiatria Danubina, 25*, 24–33.

95. Kulper, D. A., Kleiman, E. M., McCloskey, M. S., Berman, M. E., & Coccaro, E. F. (2015). The experience of aggressive outbursts in intermittent explosive disorder. *Psychiatry Research, 225*, 710–715.
96. Fahlgren, M. K., Puhalla, A. A., Sorgi, K. M., & McCloskey, M. S. (2019). Emotion processing in intermittent explosive disorder. *Psychiatry Research, 273*, 544–550.
97. Miczek, K. A., Weerts, E. M., Tornatzký, W., DeBold, J. F., & Vatne, T. M. (1992). Alcohol and 'bursts' of aggressive behavior: Ethological analysis of individual differences in rats. *Psychopharmacology, 107*(551–563), 551.
98. Haller, J., van de Schraaf, J., & Kruk, M. R. (2001). Deviant forms of aggression in glucocorticoid hyporeactive rats: A model for 'pathological' aggression? *Journal of Neuroendocrinology, 13*, 102–107.
99. Haller, J., Mikics, E., Halász, J., & Tóth, M. (2005). Mechanisms differentiating normal from abnormal aggression: Glucocorticoids and serotonin. *European Journal of Pharmacology, 526*, 89–100.
100. Tóth, M., Halász, J., Mikics, E., Barsy, B., & Haller, J. (2008). Early social deprivation induces disturbed social communication and violent aggression in adulthood. *Behavioral Neuroscience, 122*, 849–854.
101. Toth, M., Mikics, E., Tulogdi, A., Aliczki, M., & Haller, J. (2011). Post-weaning social isolation induces abnormal forms of aggression in conjunction with increased glucocorticoid and autonomic stress responses. *Hormones and Behavior, 60*, 28–36.
102. Haller, J. (2013). The neurobiology of abnormal manifestations of aggression--a review of hypothalamic mechanisms in cats, rodents, and humans. *Brain Research Bulletin, 93*, 97–109.
103. Márquez, C., et al. (2013). Peripuberty stress leads to abnormal aggression, altered amygdala and orbitofrontal reactivity and increased prefrontal MAOA gene expression. *Translational Psychiatry, 3*, e216.
104. Miczek, K. A., de Boer, S. F., & Haller, J. (2013). Excessive aggression as model of violence: A critical evaluation of current preclinical methods. *Psychopharmacology, 226*(445–458), 445.
105. Haller, J., Halász, J., Mikics, E., & Kruk, M. R. (2004). Chronic glucocorticoid deficiency-induced abnormal aggression, autonomic hypoarousal, and social deficit in rats. *Journal of Neuroendocrinology, 16*, 550–557.
106. Sandi, C., & Haller, J. (2015). Stress and the social brain: Behavioural effects and neurobiological mechanisms. *Nature Reviews. Neuroscience, 16*, 290–304.
107. de Barros, D. M., & de Pádua Serafim, A. (2008). Association between personality disorder and violent behavior pattern. *Forensic Science International, 179*, 19–22.
108. Coccaro, E. F., Lee, R., & McCloskey, M. S. (2014). Relationship between psychopathy, aggression, anger, impulsivity, and intermittent explosive disorder. *Aggressive Behavior, 40*, 526–536.
109. Moran, P. (1999). The epidemiology of antisocial personality disorder. *Social Psychiatry and Psychiatric Epidemiology, 34*, 231–242.
110. Murray, J., et al. (2015). Childhood behaviour problems predict crime and violence in late adolescence: Brazilian and British birth cohort studies. *Social Psychiatry and Psychiatric Epidemiology, 50*, 579–589.
111. Megargee, E. I. (1977). A new classification system for criminal offenders. *Criminal Justice and Behavior, 4*, 107–216.
112. Megargee, E. I., & Carbonell, J. L. (1995). Use of the MMPI-2 in correctional settings. In Ben-Porath YS, Graham JR, Hall GCN, Hirschman R, Zaragoza MS (Eds.), *Forensic applications of the MMPI-2* (pp. 127–159). SAGE Publications, Inc.. https://doi.org/10.4135/9781452243771.
113. Megargee, E. I. (1984). A new classification system for criminal offenders, VI: Differences among the types on the adjective checklist. *Criminal Justice and Behavior, 11*, 349–376.
114. Nieberding, R. J., et al. (2003). MMPI-2 based classification of forensic psychiatric outpatients: An exploratory cluster analytic study. *Journal of Clinical Psychology, 59*, 907–920.

115. Davis, K. M., & Archer, R. P. (2010). A critical review of objective personality inventories with sex offenders. *Journal of Clinical Psychology, 66*, 1254–1280.
116. Shechory, M., Weiss, J. M., & Weinstain, R. (2013). Differentiating offenders by index offense and personality inventories: The characteristics of adult probationers in Israel. *International Journal of Offender Therapy and Comparative Criminology, 57*, 312–331.
117. Jogtár®. https://uj.jogtar.hu/#doc/db/62/id/A1200100.TV/ts/20190501/.
118. Government of Canada, S. C. Uniform Crime Reporting Survey (UCR). (2017). http://www23.statcan.gc.ca/imdb/p2SV.pl?Function=getSurvey&Id=380106.
119. Violent Crime. *FBI*. https://ucr.fbi.gov/crime-in-the-u.s/2010/crime-in-the-u.s.-2010/violent-crime/violent-crime.
120. Investigating Serious Violent Crime: What works, what doesn't and for what crime types? - UQ eSpace. https://espace.library.uq.edu.au/view/UQ:836d11a.
121. United Nations Office on Drugs and Crime & World Bank. (2007). Crime, violence, and development: Trends, costs, and policy options in the Caribbean.
122. [REPORTS 2016] Defining Violence: Reducing Incarceration by Rethinking America's Approach to Violence—Justice Policy Institute. http://www.justicepolicy.org/research/10708.
123. Roettger, M. E., Boardman, J. D., Harris, K. M., & Guo, G. (2016). The association between the MAOA 2R genotype and delinquency over time among men: The interactive role of parental closeness and parental incarceration. *Criminal Justice and Behavior, 43*, 1076–1094.
124. Popma, A., et al. (2007). Cortisol moderates the relationship between testosterone and aggression in delinquent male adolescents. *Biological Psychiatry, 61*, 405–411.
125. Buss, A. H., & Durkee, A. (1957). An inventory for assessing different kinds of hostility. *Journal of Consulting Psychology, 21*, 343–349.
126. Sajous-Turner, A., et al. (2019). Aberrant brain gray matter in murderers. *Brain Imaging and Behavior*. https://doi.org/10.1007/s11682-019-00155-y.
127. Shafi, R., Smith, P. M., & Colantonio, A. (2019). Assault predicts time away from work after claims for work-related mild traumatic brain injury. *Occupational and Environmental Medicine, 76*, 471–478.
128. Douglas, J. E., Burgess, A. W., Burgess, A. G., & Ressler, R. K. (2013). *Crime classification manual: a standard system for investigating and classifying violent crime*. Wiley, New York.
129. Kocsis, R. N. (2016). Book review: Crime classification manual: A standard system for investigating and classifying violent crime. *International Journal of Offender Therapy and Comparative Criminology, 60*, 1470–1473.
130. National Academies of Sciences, E. (2016). *Modernizing Crime Statistics: Report 1: Defining and Classifying Crime*. doi:https://doi.org/10.17226/23492.
131. Ellwood, C., & The, A. (1910). Classification of criminals. *Journal of the American Institute of Criminal Law and Criminology, 1*, 536–548.
132. Freedman, D., & Hemenway, D. (2000). Precursors of lethal violence: A death row sample. *Social Science & Medicine, 1982*(50), 1757–1770.
133. Lewis, D. O., et al. (1988). Neuropsychiatric, psychoeducational, and family characteristics of 14 juveniles condemned to death in the United States. *The American Journal of Psychiatry, 145*, 584–589.
134. Lewis, D. O., Pincus, J. H., Feldman, M., Jackson, L., & Bard, B. (1986). Psychiatric, neurological, and psychoeducational characteristics of 15 death row inmates in the United States. *The American Journal of Psychiatry, 143*, 838–845.
135. Evans, J., & Quantitative, R. (1997). EEG findings in a group of death row inmates. *Archives of Clinical Neuropsychology, 12*, 315–316.
136. Panton, J. H. (1976). Personality characteristics of death-row prison inmates. *Journal of Clinical Psychology, 32*, 306–309.
137. Frierson, R. L., Schwartz-Watts, D. M., Morgan, D. W., & Malone, T. D. (1998). Capital versus noncapital murderers. *The Journal of the American Academy of Psychiatry and the Law, 26*, 403–410.

138. Fazel, S., et al. (2015). Depression and violence: A Swedish population study. *Lancet Psychiatry, 2*, 224–232.
139. Gostisha, A. J., et al. (2014). Beyond physiological hypoarousal: The role of life stress and callous-unemotional traits in incarcerated adolescent males. *Hormones and Behavior, 65*, 469–479.
140. Vinkers, D. J., de Beurs, E., Barendregt, M., Rinne, T., & Hoek, H. W. (2011). The relationship between mental disorders and different types of crime. *Criminal Behaviour and Mental Health, 21*, 307–320.
141. Werner, K. B., Few, L. R., & Bucholz, K. K. (2015). Epidemiology, comorbidity, and behavioral genetics of antisocial personality disorder and psychopathy. *Psychiatric Annals, 45*, 195–199.
142. Fazel, S., & Danesh, J. (2002). Serious mental disorder in 23000 prisoners: A systematic review of 62 surveys. *Lancet, 359*, 545–550.
143. Fakhrzadegan, S., Gholami-Doon, H., Shamloo, B., & Shokouhi-Moqhaddam, S. (2017). The relationship between personality disorders and the type of crime committed and substance used among prisoners. *Addiction and Health, 9*, 64–71.
144. Gao, Y., & Raine, A. (2010). Successful and unsuccessful psychopaths: a neurobiological model. *Behavioral Sciences & the Law, 28*, 194–210.
145. Whittington, R., et al. (2013). A systematic review of risk assessment strategies for populations at high risk of engaging in violent behaviour: update 2002–8. *Health Technology Assessment, 17*, 1–128.
146. Sasaki, T., Pratt, S. C., & Kacelnik, A. (2018). Parallel vs. comparative evaluation of alternative options by colonies and individuals of the ant Temnothorax rugatulus. *Scientific Reports, 8*, 12730.
147. Feldblum, J. T., Manfredi, S., Gilby, I. C., & Pusey, A. E. (2018). The timing and causes of a unique chimpanzee community fission preceding Gombe's 'four-year war'. *American Journal of Physical Anthropology, 166*, 730–744.
148. Lagerspetz, K. M., & Lagerspetz, K. Y. (1971). Changes in the aggressiveness of mice resulting from selective breeding, learning and social isolation. *Scandinavian Journal of Psychology, 12*, 241–248.
149. Cairns, R. B., MacCombie, D. J., & Hood, K. E. (1983). A developmental-genetic analysis of aggressive behavior in mice: I. Behavioral outcomes. *Journal of Comparative Psychology, 1983*(97), 69–89.
150. Francis, R. C. (1988). On the relationship between aggression and social dominance. *Ethology, 78*, 223–237.

Chapter 2
The Heritability of Aggressiveness and Violence-Proneness

Introduction

Heredity is the passing on of traits from parents to their offspring. There is an age-old belief that just like other features aggressiveness can also be inherited.

The heritability of traits is mediated by genes, yet heritability of traits and genes can and should be studied separately. The reason is that all complex traits are influenced by many genes in parallel. Identifying all the genes involved and establishing their interactions are difficult as will be shown in the next chapter. Due to these difficulties, the separate study of heredity, which can be understood as the "summation" of the action of all genes, is especially important. Heredity studies do not clarify the nature or the number of the genes involved and provide no hints on how various genes interact or on the biological mechanisms they influence. Studies of heredity simply establish whether a trait is heritable and, if so, what the relative weight of inheritance is compared to other factors such as family and peer influences, environmental stressors, etc. Actually, no genetic analyses (e.g., gene-association studies) should be performed before researchers ascertain that the trait is heritable. This is why we discuss the issue of heredity first.

2.1 Background

2.1.1 Ethical and Theoretical Considerations

The heredity of aggression raises a host of ethical, legal, and social issues that need full attention. In legal terms, it questions culpability. In psychiatry and psychology, both heritability and genetic studies raise the perceived or the attributed stigma associ-

J. Haller, *Neurobiopsychosocial Perspectives on Aggression and Violence*, Advances in Preventing and Treating Violence and Aggression,
https://doi.org/10.1007/978-3-030-46331-1_2

ated with belonging to negatively affected populations. Indeed, a meta-analysis of 25 studies showed that laypeople holding biogenetic explanations for mental disorders tended to blame affected persons less for their problems but perceived them as more dangerous and desired a greater distance from them [1]. The relationship was weak but significant statistically. In other cases, by contrast, heredity explanations had positive impacts on perceptions. They reduced personal responsibility, e.g., in the case of eating disorders [2], and decreased the negative stereotyping of patients by medical students [3]. Taken together, these findings suggest that the stigma associated with behavioral heredity is of concern in psychology and psychiatry but the size of the problem is not very large and can be alleviated by seeking community consensus and by the education of fieldworkers, community members, and health workers [4].

Being aware of these ethical and legal problems, the aim of this and the following chapter is still the search for an answer to a question: "Is Crime in the Genes?" [5]. As such, the reason of addressing the issue is its importance. Associating heredity and aggression may improve the identification of social risks at the population level and personal risks at the individual level. It may also help the prediction of developmental trajectories, the design of more efficient prevention programs, and the development of novel effective treatments and/or improved resocialization strategies. In brief, genetics may help prevent the aggravation of psychological conditions into medical and/or legal problems. It might also help in the reduction of the medical and legal problems if they could not be prevented. However, studying genetics only makes sense if a trait is heritable. This chapter investigates whether aggression, aggression-related psychopathologies, and crime are heritable.

Unfortunately, it is not easy to establish what traits are inherited and what traits are not. Traits are influenced by a multitude of factors, and differentiating genetic from other factors is not easy. Difficulties are so numerous that some even labelled heritability studies as useless [6]. The starting point of this study was that heritability estimates for complex social behaviors, like aggression and crime, are so high as to be incredible. Consequently, the authors looked for and found various flaws in the methodologies by which heritability was currently estimated. Adherents of heritability studies naturally have refuted such criticisms and have claimed that heritability studies are scientifically sound [7], albeit the problems surrounding heritability estimates have never been denied. Thus, the quest for "perfect" heritability estimates continues. New approaches have been introduced; different approaches have been compared [8, 9], etc. Heritability estimates do indeed depend on the scientific approach used; yet, the heritability of aggression and related traits remains high in all approaches, and its share in shaping traits usually equals that of environmental factors.

2.1.2 *Technical Issues*

Heredity revolves around the transmission of genes. The familial aggregation of traits may be indicative of a heredity factor. It was found, for instance, that interpersonal violence aggregates among first-degree relatives [10]. In males, the odds ratio of being violent was 4.3 when the subject had a violent sibling but only 1.9 when his/her cousin was violent. The odds ratio was naturally one in unrelated subjects. In females, odds ratios were larger: 8.1 for siblings and 2.2 for cousins. Kidnapping and illegal confinement showed an even stronger family aggregation. If one sibling committed such an act, the odds ratio for doing the same was as high as 35.7 for the other sibling.

When such a study was done in very large populations, e.g., in 12.5 million people as in the study referred to, one tends to accept that heredity does indeed play a role. Yet, families not only share genes but also living conditions and life events and influence one another in various ways. Hence, the family aggregation of traits is important from an epidemiological or criminological but not from a hereditary point of view. The family aggregation of traits shows the combined effects of both heredity and environment that can be labelled together as the "family effect."

One way of differentiating hereditary from environmental factors is to investigate subjects who are similar genetically but live apart, i.e., are exposed to different environmental influences. This approach is employed in adoption studies, where offspring share genes with their biological parents but share living conditions with their adoptive parents. According to one author of this technology, adoptions "are natural experiments in which the effects of genetic and rearing influences may be separated to a relatively high degree" [11]. Typically, the aim of such studies is to establish the heritability component of a phenotype, this being an observable trait that is produced by both the genetic background (the genotype) and environmental influences. Aggressiveness, aggression-related psychopathologies, or the propensity to commit violent crime may all be phenotypes to be investigated. In such studies, both biological parents-adoptee and adoption parents-adoptee comparisons are relevant. Concordance with the biological parents indicates hereditary; concordance with the adoption parents indicates environmental influences. For instance, if the offspring was just as aggressive as his biological parents but much more aggressive than his adoption parents, then the trait would mostly be inherited and vice versa.

Finally, an even more subtle differentiation of the various factors that affect the heritability of a trait is shown by twin studies. This methodology exploits the fact that monozygotic (identical) twins share 100% of their genes, whereas dizygotic twins share just 50% like any other siblings. When the twins are raised together, they also share most environmental influences. The role of heredity is established by comparing the resemblance of monozygotic and dizygotic twins.

Classical twin studies provide a heredity estimate and an environmental influence estimate, which is usually broken down into a shared and a non-shared environmental effect. The logic of the analysis goes as follows. If monozygotic twins are more similar to each other regarding a particular phenotype (e.g., aggressiveness) than dizygotic twins, we infer that the phenotype was inherited to a certain degree. If, for example, heritability was complete (i.e., nothing else than genes affected the phenotype), then one would expect that monozygotic twins would be twice as similar to each other than dizygotic twins, because the former share twice as much genes than the latter (100% vs. 50%). Shared environmental influences are inferred from similarities between dizygotic twins. If their similarity was larger than that expected based on their genetic similarity (50%), then the additional similarity can be attributed to shared environmental influences. Non-shared environmental influences are inferred from dissimilarities between identical twins. As monozygotic twins are genetically identical, such differences are likely due to environmental influences they did not share.

There are a number of ways to calculate heritability estimates. In its simplest form, correlations are established between phenotypes in the two identical twins on one hand and in the two dizygotic twins on the other. The heritability estimate – usually called A, from additive genetic influences – is the difference between identical and nonidentical twin correlation coefficients multiplied by two. The non-shared environmental influence – usually called E, from unique environment – is one minus the correlation coefficient of identical (monozygotic) twins. Finally, shared environmental influences – usually called C from common environment – can be calculated by deducing the heredity estimate (A) from the correlation coefficient of monozygotic twins. In other cases, the gender concordance of dizygotic twins is also taken into account, and instead of correlations, subjects are classified into subgroups that show the trait at an unusually low or high level (e.g., are in the upper or lower 25%, respectively).

A special version of heredity investigations is the sibling studies, which take into account both the relatedness of siblings and their identified environmental influences. Naturally, the preceding paragraphs present just the basic premises and rudimentary ways of calculating estimates. Other research designs and mathematical models of such investigations are too complex to be presented here; those interested may wish to refer to detailed technical descriptions, e.g. [9, 12].

The complexity of twin studies has increased tremendously from early days, and the mathematics underlying them is now rather complex. New components of phenotypes were introduced, e.g., nonadditive genetic influences; twin and adoption studies are combined to assess similarities between twins who were reared together or apart, etc. In parallel, the establishment of zygosity (monozygotic or dizygotic) and measurement of phenotypes have also developed. We do not go into details here because such particulars are not necessarily important for understanding the findings although two factors are worth emphasizing. First, the estimates presented below are based on a complex methodology, which have evolved over time considerably. Developments were prompted by criticisms addressed either by improving the methodologies or by drawing conclusions based on several approaches. Second, studies use large samples. The smallest studies comprised several hundreds of subjects; the average study investigated several thousands, but studies performed in tens of thousands of subjects are not rare. In exceptional cases, scientists have studied 1–2 and even five million subjects. Large samples are used to make heredity studies as reliable as possible.

In the following sections, we will describe the main features and findings of human heredity studies. This will be followed by non-human studies into heredity, mainly rodent selection lines for aggressive traits. The last section will discuss heredity from a broader perspective.

2.2 Findings

2.2.1 Human Studies

The familial aggregation of aggression [13], aggression-related mental disorders [14], and crime [10] – and the liability to be exposed to particular life events [15] – are well established; however, aggregation studies do not clarify the mechanism of heredity. Therefore, we focus below on studies that tried to differentiate hereditary from environmental influences on aggression. As shown above, research paradigms can be divided into two classes: adoption and twin studies. Our primary focus will be on the latter. There are several reasons for this, most of them being technical. The number of adoption studies is lower than that of twin studies, and a good deal of twin studies incorporate approaches characteristic to adoption studies. Finally, adoption studies quite often provide estimates in the form of regression coefficients [16], which are more difficult to interpret than the figures derived from twin studies.

The weight of various factors in determining traits is expressed in twin studies by percentages of variance which is explained by a particular factor, in our case hereditary. A brief account of the "explanation of variance" is as follows. People are not similar; they show variation in all their characteristics. Some of the recorded variance is random or is due to measurement error, but some of it is due to – or explained by – a particular influence. If, for example, heredity explained 100% of the variance in aggression, then the aggressive phenotype would depend entirely on the genotype. If by contrast heredity explained 0% of the variance, then aggressiveness entirely would depend on other factors, e.g., environmental influences.

2.2.1.1 Everyday Aggression

First, we will briefly review findings on the heredity component of aggressiveness (see Table 2.1). In these studies, the phenotype was established based on various psychological instruments, e.g., by the *Child Behavior Checklist* [17], which contains items that are indicative of aggressiveness. Such items include "destroys things belonging to his/her family or other children," "gets in many fights," "physically attacks people," "hits others," and "hurts animals or people." The *Strength and Difficulties Questionnaire* [18] contains items like "often has temper tantrums or hot tempers," "often fights with other children or bullies them," "often lies or cheats," and "steals from home, school, or elsewhere." There are a variety of such instruments for all ages, and there are specific inventories that differentiate certain types of aggression, e.g., reactive and proactive aggression [19]. Each of the scales provides a score, based on which twin correlations can be calculated, and the percentage of variance explained can be estimated.

We took care to include in the table only studies where subjects had neither a mental diagnosis nor a criminal record. To make sure that findings were not influenced with subjects with psychiatric disorders, we excluded studies performed in clinical populations, even if no diagnoses were expressly mentioned. Thus, these findings refer to everyday manifestations of aggressiveness which may be disturbing, but do not reach the threshold for medical or law enforcement attention.

Table 2.1 reviews two types of findings. Where the phenotype was called "aggression," this was established either based on aggression-specific psychometric instruments or aggression-related items from more general questionnaires. Where the phenotype was called "conduct problems" or "externalizing behavior," the inventory covered a broader range of behaviors, but aggression had a major weight among the items. Table 2.1 and subsequent tables indicate heritability estimates only. Environmental influences will be addressed in later parts of the book.

Even a superficial glance at the table reveals that figures are very high. The mean is 56% (+/− one standard deviation between 44 and 68%). This suggests that most of the variance in aggressiveness is due to hereditary influences. Considering the methodological differences between studies and that they were done in different countries in very different populations, this variability is quite acceptable and rather small. Note that these calculations are not formal meta-analyses; they merely serve to indicate general trends.

Table 2.1 The percentage of variance explained by genetics in twin studies of everyday aggression, excluding psychiatric and criminal populations

Age (years)	Variance explained (%)	Gender differences	Phenotype
7 [20]	66	None	Aggression
7 [20]	62	None	Aggression[a]
10 [20]	68	Females: Smaller	Aggression
10 [20]	59	Females: Smaller	Aggression[a]
12 [20]	69	Females: Smaller	Aggression
12 [20]	57	Females: Smaller	Aggression[a]
10–19 [21]	55	n.d.	Aggression
19–60 [22]	72	n.d.	Aggression
7 [23]	53	Minimal	Aggression, direct
3 [24]	50	Minimal	Aggression, overt
7 [24]	57	Minimal	Aggression, overt
10 [24]	65	Minimal	Aggression, overt
12 [24]	67	Minimal	Aggression, overt
14 [24]	51	Minimal	Aggression, overt
16 [24]	58	Minimal	Aggression, overt
1–2 [25]	60	None	Aggression, physical
2–3 [25]	63	None	Aggression, physical
3–4 [25]	50	None	Aggression, physical
9–10 [26]	32	None	Aggression, proactive
11–14 [26]	48	None	Aggression, proactive
9–10 [26]	26	Minimal	Aggression, reactive

(continued)

Table 2.1 (continued)

Age (years)	Variance explained (%)	Gender differences	Phenotype
11–14 [26]	43	None	Aggression, reactive
26–85 [27]	17	None	Aggression, reactive
7 [23]	66	None	Aggression, relational
3 [28]	56	Minimal	Conduct problems
4 [29]	60	None	Conduct problems
7 [29]	64	None	Conduct problems
7 [30]	63	n.d.	Conduct problems
7 [28]	66	Minimal	Conduct problems
9 [30]	53	n.d.	Conduct problems
10 [28]	67	Smaller	Conduct problems
12 [29]	62	None	Conduct problems
12 [30]	48	n.d.	Conduct problems
12 [28]	67	Smaller	Conduct problems
16 [29]	73	None	Conduct problems
16 [30]	64	n.d.	Conduct problems
9–10 [31]	43	n.d.	Conduct problems
13–18 [31]	49	n.d.	Conduct problems
19–65 [31]	42	n.d.	Conduct problems
10–19 [21]	61	n.d.	Externalizing behavior

The term "aggression" stands here for a measure of aggressiveness as established by appropriate psychometric instruments. *Aggression direct* behavior overtly directed at victim, *aggression overt* outward or open confrontational acts *aggression physical* subject hits, bites, kicks, fights, and attacks another, *aggression proactive* self-initiated, purposeful aggressive acts, *aggression reactive* aggressive outbursts elicited by provocation, *aggression relational* damaging social relationships or status, *conduct problems* behavioral anomalies as evidenced, e.g., by *Achenbach System of Empirically Based Assessment*, where many but not all items are related to aggression, *externalizing behavior* in this study it is the sum of aggressiveness and rule breaking tendencies, [a] same study, different study population, *n.d.* not determined

There also are outliers. The lowest value (17% of variation explained) is likely due to an exclusive focus on reactive aggression. It is highly probable that the impact of heredity would have been larger if aggression was considered more broadly. The same might be true for studies where the heritability of reactive and proactive aggression was investigated separately. Values were somewhat higher if aggression types were considered together, as they have nonoverlapping heritability components [26]. As it regards high values, it is worth noting that the study by Pingault et al. [29] investigated heritability at four time points in the same subjects (at 4, 7, 12, and 16 years of age). At each time point other than the last one, heritability explained less than 65% of variability in aggression, which is in line with the rest of the findings in Table 2.1. At the age of 16, heritability increased to 73% (the highest among the studies) maybe because adolescence, unlike the earlier ages, is characterized by the stress of reaching independence from external influences, which may have increased the relative role of heredity. Without going into more details, one can state relatively confidently that the heritability component of aggression is in the range of the mean ± one standard deviation, and deviations from these values have logical explanations.

A careful inspection of Table 2.1 reveals three interesting features: The share of genetic influences depended neither on the presence of associated behavioral problems nor on gender or age. Similarities concerning conduct problems and aggression may be explained by the fact that aggression is a necessary component of conducts problems. The lack of gender influences is more surprising, as the level of aggressiveness did differentiate males and females in these studies. The heritability of aggression was independent of its intensity: both low and high aggressiveness can be inherited. The lack of age effects is more surprising, as one would expect that maturation would shift the weight of heredity to environmental influences; however, there was no obvious age trend in the data, despite the fact that the youngest and oldest subject were 7 and 85 years old, respectively, and that studies covered all age classes in-between.

To investigate the issue of age and heritability further, Table 2.2 summarizes those studies where the same subjects were investigated by the same authors more than once between the ages of 3–16 years. If anything, the findings show that the importance of heredity increases over time but differences are small and inconsistent across studies. The modest age-related trends in heredity are surprising because the age range covers two important windows of social influences: education within the family and socialization in the school. One would expect that with increasing educational environmental influences, the importance of heredity diminishes, which is not apparent in either Table 2.1 or Table 2.2. There are two explanations to this surprising finding: (i) family influences before the age of three are decisive, and no

Table 2.2 Age-related changes in the variance in aggression explained by heredity factors

	% Variance in aggression explained by heredity							
Age (years)	[20][a]	[20][a]	[26]	[26]	[30]	[29]	[28]	[24]
3							56	50
4						60		
7	66	62			63	64	66	57
9					53			
9–10			32	26				
10	68	59					67	65
11–14			48	43				
12	69	57			48	62	67	67
14								51
16					64	73		58
Phenotype	*AGG*	*AGG*	*PRO*	*REA*	*CON*	*CON*	*CON*	*OVE*

The second row contains references. The table should be read top-down; each column represents a study with assessments performed at various ages in the same subjects. *Age* the age of subjects in years, *AGG* aggressiveness, *CON* conduct problems, *OVE* overt aggression, *PRO* proactive aggression, *REA* reactive aggression, [a] same study, different populations

later influences can add to what occurred by that age; or (ii) family education and school socialization had mixed effects, which maintained the same level of heredity influences on average. Given sample sizes, it is very likely that subjects underwent both negative and positive educational influences, which averaged out each other at the population level.

Taken together, these studies show that the heritability of everyday aggressiveness is high and estimates are rather consistent. It is worth noting that the heritability of other psychological traits, e.g., altruism, empathy, nurturance, assertiveness, and irritability, is in the same range (56–70%) [22], suggesting that (i) psychological traits are heritable and (ii) aggressiveness is not different from other psychological traits in this respect.

2.2.1.2 Clinical Aggression

The next table summarizes findings obtained in subjects diagnosed with an aggression-related mental disorder. We excluded studies referring to "antisocial behavior" and similarly ambiguous labels to ensure that the study was psychiatrically relevant. An exception was psychopathy, which is not recognized as a mental disorder of its own right by either DSM-5 or by ICD-10. The former views psychopathy as a specific form of antisocial personality disorder; the latter uses the two terms synonymously. Thus, psychopathy is an aggravated form of antisocial personality disorder, which certainly deserves specific attention. As there are no valid diagnostic tools for psychopathy, we included here studies that used nondiagnostic psychometric instruments (Table 2.3).

The heritability of aggression-related disorders in psychiatric populations is also high, but it is not as high as with everyday aggression. While the average heritability estimate of the former was ~56% (SD = ~12%), the average heritability estimate of aggression-related mental disorders was ~41% (SD = ~11%). Again, approximately 80% of the findings were in the range of the mean ± the standard deviation. Thus, the inter-study variability was small, especially when one considers that the average was based on studies that investigated different mental disorders using different methodologies and with subjects of widely different ages.

There were some outliers. An exceptionally high heritability (75%) was obtained in one of the studies (the second highest value was 55%, which was close to the standard deviation range). This high heritability, however, was attributed to conduct disorder associated with callous-unemotional traits. (We will come back to this issue later.) The lowest heritability value (0%) was found in subjects showing weak attention deficit-hyperactivity disorder. (This will also be discussed below.) Three additional studies reported heritability estimates below the standard deviation range. Two were performed in subjects with psychopathic tendencies. We explain this by the difficulties and inconsistencies of establishing this quasi-diagnosis. Taken together, heritability estimates are close to 50% and are reasonably consistent.

The three most interesting features of the studies reviewed are the lack of differences related to gender, disorder, and age but a relatively large impact of the severity of the disorder. Many studies were reluctant to investigate gender differ-

Table 2.3 Mental disorders and heredity in twin studies. Diagnosis was established either by a psychiatrist or by diagnostic questionnaires. Criminal history was not reported in either case

Age (years)	Variance explained (%)	Gender differences	Diagnosis	Specification
12 [32]	41	n.d.	ADHD	
14–18 [33]	0	n.d.	ADHD	Weak symptoms
14–18 [33]	46	n.d.	ADHD	Strong symptoms
17 [32]	51	n.d.	ADHD	
18 [34]	40	n.d.	ADHD	
24 [34]	37	n.d.	ADHD	
25–75 [35]	36	n.d.	ADHD	
30 [34]	44	n.d.	ADHD	
19–36 [36]	39	None	ASPD	
19–36 [37]	51	n.d.	ASPD	
19–36 [37]	41	n.d.	ASPD	
30–42 [38]	40	n.d.	ASPD	
30–44 [36]	39	None	ASPD	
~32–37 [39]	41	n.d.	ASPD	
~44–45 [39]	37	n.d.	ASPD	
19–36 [36]	30	None	BPD	
19–36 [36]	34	n.d.	BPD	Self-damaging impulsive behaviors
30–42 [38]	38	n.d.	BPD	
30–44 [38]	30	None	BPD	
~32–37 [39]	36	n.d.	BPD	
~44–45 [39]	32	n.d.	BPD	
45–65 [40]	46	None	BPD	
7–9 [41]	75	n.d.	CD	CU traits
7–9 [41]	36	n.d.	CD	No CU traits
11–18 [42]	49	n.d.	CD	Aggressive domain
11–18 [42]	55	n.d.	CD	Non-aggressive domain
11–18 [42]	53	n.d.	CD	Full scale
12 [32]	46	n.d.	CD	
17 [32]	49	n.d.	CD	
30–42 [38]	41	n.d.	NPD	
~32–37 [39]	24	n.d.	NPD	
6–18 [43]	47	None	ODD	
11–17 [44]	46	Minimal	PP	Fearless dominance
11–17 [44]	52	Minimal	PP	Impulsive anti-sociality
19–20 [45]	26	None	PP	Complete

(continued)

Table 2.3 (continued)

Age (years)	Variance explained (%)	Gender differences	Diagnosis	Specification
29–35 [46]	46	Minimal	PP	Fearless dominance
29–35 [46]	51	Minimal	PP	Impulsive antisocial behavior
41–58 [47]	51	n.d.	PP	Fearless dominance
41–58 [47]	26	n.d.	PP	Impulsive antisocial behavior

References were indicated in column "Age (years)." *Disorders. ADHD* attention deficit-hyperactivity disorder, *ASPD* antisocial personality disorder, *BPD* borderline personality disorder, *CD* conduct disorder, *NPD* narcissistic personality disorder, *ODD* oppositional-defiant disorder, *PP* psychopathy. *Other explanations.* ~ the age of subjects not given in paper, age deduced from subjects' birth date and the date of publication, *n.d.* not determined: gender differences were either not mentioned or not addressed for the lack of statistical power, *none* gender differences were statistically non-significant, *minimal* significant differences that were around or smaller than 10%
Note: We found neither adoption nor twin studies for intermittent explosive disorder, likely because it is comorbid with other disorders (e.g., bipolar disorder, ADHD, PTSD, etc.); consequently, it is difficult to study the disorder separately [48]. Nevertheless, intermittent explosive disorder showed a strong familial aggregation when it was defined according to research criteria that excluded interactions with comorbid conditions [49]

ences due to lack of statistical power; yet, no large gender differences in heritability were reported when this was studied. This is interesting because the gender distribution of disorders is rather different. Antisocial personality disorder, for instance, is considerably more frequent in males, whereas borderline personality disorder is more frequent in females. Heritability is independent of the gender distribution of disorders. Something similar was observed with everyday forms of aggression, where heritability was independent of aggression intensity. Regarding disorders, the highest heritability estimates were observed in conduct disorder (~52%), whereas the lowest were in narcissistic personality disorder (~33%). These values appear different, but both are within the ± standard deviation range of disorders in general.

There were two studies where subjects were divided into subgroups. In Viding et al. [41], the heritability estimate for callous-unemotional conduct disorder was 75%, whereas the estimate for conduct disorder without callous-unemotional traits was just 36%. Greven et al. [33] studied extremes in attention deficit-hyperactivity disorder and found that heritability was considerable in subjects with strong symptoms (46%) but was zero in subjects with weak symptoms. These two studies suggest that the impact of heritability is larger in more severe mental disorders.

Taken together, these findings show that aggression-related mental disorders are heritable largely. In this respect, they are not much different from other mental disorders. For instance, heritability estimates were similar in autism spectrum, oppositional-defiant, and conduct disorder when these were studied by the same authors in the same twin sample [50]. Heritability estimates for these disorders were between 50 and 60%. The heritability of drug and alcohol abuse was found to be 54 and 61%, respectively, for males [8]; and heritability estimates for bipolar disorder were between 55 and 60% [51], etc. Thus, the heritability of aggression-related mental disorders is within the general range of the heritability of mental disorders, with the exception of schizophrenia, which has very high heritability estimates (~80%) [52]. If anything, aggression-related disorders are somewhat less heritable than other common disorders.

2.2.1.3 Criminal Populations

Finally, we review the heritability of crime and violent crime (see Table 2.4). In all the cited studies, criminality was established by convictions. Evidence for mental disorders was not provided although it is likely that a proportion of the subjects also showed mental disorders.

Table 2.4 Crime and heredity in twin and sibling studies. Group assignment was based on criminal records

Age (years)	Variance explained (%)	Gender differences	Type of offending
5 [53]	0	n.d.	Rule breaking
10–19 [21]	44	n.d.	Rule breaking
12–18 [54]	29	Large[a]	Crime, non-violent
6–10 [55]	25–70[c]	n.d.	Crime, non-violent
12–19 [56]	56	None	Crime, non-violent
Adult [57]	45	None	Crime, non-violent
Adult [57]	45	None	Crime, non-violent
Adult [58]	76	n.d.	Crime, non-violent
12–18 [54]	57	Large[a]	Crime, overall
15–19 [55]	59	n.d.	Crime, overall
20–24 [55]	42	n.d.	Crime, overall
25–29 [55]	41	n.d.	Crime, overall
25–55 [8]	50–71[d]	Moderate[b]	Crime, overall
25–55 [59]	39–56[d]	Minimal	Crime, overall
12–18 [54]	41	Large[a]	Crime, violent
25–55 [51]	58	n.d.	Crime, violent
Adult [57]	45 (sibling)	None	Crime, violent
Adult [9]	49 (twin)	None[e]	Crime, violent
Adult [9]	52 (sibling)	None[e]	Crime, violent
Adult [9]	41(adoptee-sibling)	None[e]	Crime, violent
Adult [9]	29 (adoptee-parent)	None[e]	Crime, violent
Adult [58]	50	n.d.	Crime, violent

Delinquency and crime were not separated for clarity; please see age as an indication of this difference. References were indicated in column "Age (years)." *Rule breaking* estimated by peers, parents, and/or teachers, rule breaking was not necessarily criminal behavior, *crime non-violent* property or white collar crimes included for comparison, *crime overall* criminal behavior including but not limited to violent crime, *crime, violent* various types of violence, from intimidation to homicide, *adult* precise age ranges could not be inferred from the study, [a]no heritability component in females, [b]the heritability component stronger in females, [c]depending on neighborhood, see below, [d]depending on the analysis type (relatedness, rearing etc.) which were taken into account in separate analyses, [e]variance explained by family environment was 15, 13, 2, and 0%, respectively

Table 2.4 is different from previous ones in several respects. It is shorter, because of the lower number of available studies. We note that the earliest studies used mathematical paradigms incompatible with those employed in later studies. Separate analyses of these studied will be presented below. In addition to violent crime, heredity estimates for non-violent crime were also presented for comparison. Rule breaking was also included as a prerequisite of crime. The heredity component of crime overall, including but not restricted to violent crime, was also shown. Finally, more attention was given to details such as methodological paradigms, social conditions, etc. The type of the study (twin, sibling, combination) was indicated in the column "Variance explained." If not indicated otherwise, the studies were twin studies.

One of the earliest adoption studies on the interaction between crime and heredity [60] established that adoptees are more similar to their biological than their adoptive fathers. A larger study [61] with about 15,000 subjects also established that siblings adopted separately into different homes were concordant for convictions, especially if the shared biological father also had a record of criminal behavior. A very early twin study [62] investigated the probability of crime for a twin whose co-twin was criminal. The authors called this a "twin coefficient." It was larger in monozygotic than dizygotic twins. There were a number of similar studies in the early years, which all pointed to the heritability of the propensity to commit crime.

A quick look at the table shows that figures, again, are high and are similar to those seen in aggression and higher than in those seen in mental disorder-related studies. Table 2.4 summarizes several interesting findings that need further comment. First, environmental factors have a large impact on the *heritability* of crime. When the subject lived in a law-abiding environment, the heritability of his/her criminal behavior was as high as 70%. This, however, decreased to 25% when his/her neighbors were also criminals. This outlines the delicate nature of heritability and environmental influences. These findings can be interpreted in two ways. First, crime can occur even in non-criminal environments if subjects inherit a strong propensity to commit crime. Second, criminal behavior may be shown even if the heritability component is low but environmental influences are strong. The alternative explanation is that the heritability component was masked if environmental influences were strong. One can hypothesize that the importance of heredity was independent of neighborhood but the strong presence of a potential environmental factor masked heredity influences.

The second interesting feature of the findings was revealed by a study that employed multiple approaches to investigate heredity [9]. According to the twin design, the heritability estimate was 49%. When siblings were compared by considering their degree of genetic similarity, the estimate was 52%, i.e., the difference was very small. When, however, the twin, sibling, and adoption approaches were combined, heritability estimates were lower. According to the adoptee-sibling model, the heritability estimate was 41% which was still not very different from the original 49%, but, according to the adoptee-parent contrasts, the estimate fell to 29%, which is a large difference; however, estimates of familial influences also decreased (see the legend in Table 2.4). Although the importance of the heredity component decreased, the importance of the family environment decreased even more. Such differences were observed in other studies which are not discussed here (see Rhee and Waldman [63]). The main conclusion deriving from comparisons of different paradigms is that differences in heredity estimates often represent an overall decrease in variability explained rather than a decrease in the role of heritability.

The third interesting feature of criminality estimates is that there are a few studies where moderate to large gender differences were reported. This is in contrast to findings in everyday aggression and aggression associated with mental disorders, where a minority of studies reported gender differences, and all those were minor; however, large differences were found in two studies related to criminality. In one of these studies, no heredity component was revealed in females committing either non-violent or violent crime, but the heredity component was relatively large in males (45%) [54]. In the other study, however, heritability was moderately higher in females than males [8]. Although these findings are contradictory, one cannot exclude the possibility that the heredity component of crime is gender-dependent as opposed to aggression and aggression-related mental disorders where differences in heritability between genders were minor.

Finally, it is worth noting that heredity estimates did not differentiate rule breaking, property, white collar, and violent crime. The only exception was a study done in five-year-old children, where the heredity estimate of rule breaking was zero. Possibly, children are not fully aware of rules at this age, which increased the role of environmental influences. That is, they acted impulsively or followed models. A meta-analysis showed that the heredity component of rule breaking is 48% in adults, who are more likely aware of rules [64]. The same study estimated that the heritability of broadly defined antisocial behavior was 65%, a figure somewhat but not exceedingly higher than that deriving from Table 2.4.

For a graphical representation of extremes in heritability and the overall heritability estimates of aggression (based on the studies reviewed), see Fig. 2.1.

2.2.2 *Selection for Aggression in Animals*

Studying heritability of aggression in non-humans has some advantages over human studies. Laboratory animals are kept under standard conditions, they eat the same food and are kept under the same temperature and day/night schedule, and their cages are regularly cleaned and are regularly inspected by veterinaries to prevent infections. Laboratory animals undergo similar environmental influences locally and worldwide. This is important because the evening of environmental influences reduces the environment factors that can affect behavior. Does this render the effects of heredity overwhelming? The answer to this question will be investigated by reviewing findings obtained in selection lines for aggression and anxiety.

The most aggressive mouse lines artificially selected for aggressive and non-aggressive traits were produced in the Netherlands in the 1980s [65]. Both the aggressive and the non-aggressive lines descended from the very same feral mouse

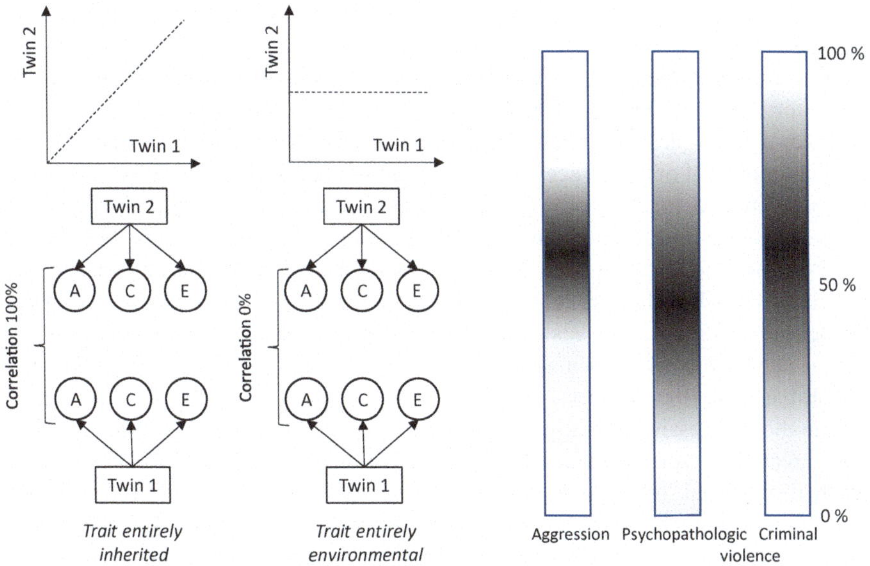

Fig. 2.1 Extreme examples and actual heritability estimates. The figure conveys principles (is very much simplified) and serves orientation. *Left hand panel.* If monozygotic twins are identical regarding a trait, e.g., their scores in an aggression test correlate perfectly irrespective of differences in living conditions, the trait is entirely inherited. The opposite, e.g., no correlation between the scores, denotes that the trait entirely depends on the environment. *A* additive genetic, *C* common environment, *E* unique environment components. *Right-hand panel.* The average heritability component (black) and its variability (decreasing shades of gray) based on the studies reviewed

population. Descendants of aggressive and docile parents showed differences even in the first generation, and their contrasting behavior reached maximal levels by the eighth generation [66]. Mice belonging to the aggressive line, called short attack latency mice, attacked unfamiliar opponents rapidly within seconds and sustained a high level of aggression while the intruder was present in their cage. Indeed, they may have killed opponents if the combatants were not separated for ethical reasons. On the other hand, the long attack latency mice were very docile. In some studies, they did not even attack opponents within the time frame allowed. During the same 10 min time period, the short attack latency mice bit their opponents 20–30 times [67]. The last study published on these mice was written about 35 years after the creation of the lines [68], which corresponds to approximately 100 generations. This strongly suggests that the lines can be maintained indefinitely if bred selectively, whereas crossbreeding reduced both aggression-related traits [69]. As a counterargument to the argument that environmental influences were attenuated by standardization of rearing practices, one may assume that maternal behavior may have still shaped the offsprings' phenotype. Cross-fostering experiments, however, reject this possibility as aggressiveness was independent of maternal phenotype [69]. These selection lines demonstrate that both extreme aggressiveness and extreme lack of aggressiveness can be created and maintained exclusively by heredity.

There are two other aggressive-non-aggressive selection line-pairs created in the laboratory. The one produced in the early seventies in Finland (Turku aggressive and Turku non-aggressive lines) [70] originated from laboratory mice and reached the maximal level of differences in aggression after just seven generations. The line has been studied for 45 years [68]. It differs from the Dutch line with respect to aggressiveness. Both Finnish lines can be maintained in groups where they do not show major differences in aggressiveness; yet their aggressiveness becomes markedly different when they are maintained in isolation for 1–2 weeks and tested in the resident-intruder test. The resident-intruder test is a standard laboratory test for rodent aggression where a male (the resident) is faced in its home cage with an unfamiliar male (the intruder).

Another aggressive-non-aggressive line-pair is the NC900 and NC100 selection lines created in North Carolina [71], where the aggressiveness of the two strains reached maximal differences just after four generations. As with the Turku aggressive-non-aggressive lines, phenotypic differences became evident only when mice were submitted to dyadic encounters after isolation (resident-intruder test); moreover, extended group living (socialization) eliminated the differences in aggression. Cross-fostering did not change aggressiveness, which excludes influences by maternal behavior. The phenotype is just as stable over time as the other selection lines [68].

Selection lines for aggression demonstrate that heredity can be responsible for aggressiveness alone – without any environmental influences. Thus, the aggressive phenotype is influenced exclusively by the genotype in these lines. This does not mean that the environment cannot affect aggressiveness in these strains. Life events do affect the phenotype, at least in some of the lines as shown below. However, the hyper-aggression phenotypes can be obtained exclusively by hereditary influences when the environment is controlled.

Two more issues need to be emphasized relative to the aggressive lines. First, their aggressive behavior is not the same, although all are aggressive [72]. Differences cover a series of properties from the level of aggressiveness to its response to environmental influences. For example, aggressiveness is an extremely stable, condition-independent, and life-long property of the Dutch lines; line differences are apparent only in dyadic encounters in the Finnish line, whereas socialization abolishes differences in aggressiveness in the North Carolina line. Obviously, the genotype of the founder stock had a great role. As the gene pools of the founder stocks were different, selection likely enriched different pro-aggression or pro-docility genes in the three line-pairs. This suggests that there are different "hereditary routes" to aggression; phenotypes characterized by increased aggressiveness may have a differential genetic background. This conclusion is relevant for and supported by human genetic findings as shown below.

The second important issue is that in parallel to increased aggression, the type of aggression also changed during the selection process and became highly similar to that seen in rat models of abnormal, psychopathology-like aggression. This was first observed in the short attack latency aggressive Dutch line. Abnormal aggression-like features ranged from behavioral characteristics to the particularities of brain function [67]. A detailed analysis of the traits of the three selection line-pairs and their corroboration with the general criteria for abnormal aggression in animals (detailed elsewhere in this book) demonstrated that only the short attack latency line fulfills the criteria for abnormal aggression [73]. The short latency line mice failed to signal attack intentions by threats, failed to stop attacks in response to submission signals by the opponent, attacked both familiar and unfamiliar females and pups, and aimed their attacks at vulnerable body parts of opponents. Their aggression was displayed during low basal heart rates and low adrenocortical stress responses suggesting a hypoarousal type during aggression [74]. The other two aggressive lines were considerably more aggressive than their non-aggressive counterparts, but their aggressiveness was normal, based on the above-mentioned criteria. This suggests that not only aggressive (Finnish and North Carolina lines) but also abnormal aggressive (psychopathology-like) phenotypes can be inherited (Dutch line).

The heritability of abnormal aggression is supported from an unexpected direction, particularly from studies into anxiety selection lines. A selection line-pair of rats showing low and high innate anxiety was created in Germany during the 1990s; the lines also differed in their anxiety responses to stress [75]. These properties of the selection lines can be observed about 20 years after their creation, which shows that the trait is stable [76]. The crossbreeding of the two genotypes produced intermediate phenotypes, whereas cross-fostering only partially affected the phenotypes, showing that maternal behavior had an impact but did not abolish inherited traits. In addition to altered anxiety, both lines showed signs of abnormal aggression in the resident-intruder test. One of the lines showed a hypoarousal whereas the other a hyperarousal type of abnormal aggression [77, 78]. This was still observed 5 years (about ten generations) after the initial observation by a different set of authors [79], which demonstrates that the phenotype was transmitted along the generations for a prolonged time, and thus it was determined by the genotype.

In conclusion, the phenotypes of both increased and abnormal aggression can be generated exclusively by the genotype as demonstrated by findings in four different selection line-pairs, three being mice selected for aggression, the fourth being rats selected for anxiety. This is a strong argument in favor of the heritability of aggression on one hand and of its psychopathology-like alterations on the other.

2.3 Overview and Interpretation

Heredity estimates of aggression are surprisingly high especially when judged from the perspective of criminological theories, which assume that crime including violent crime results from social conflicts of various kinds. For instance, the differential association theory of Sutherland [80] states that deviance is learned from association with the wrong people. According to the anomie theory of Merton [81], deviance results from the conflict between social goals and social means. Walter Reckless's control theory [82] assumes that deviance is due to inefficient self-control that ensues from the lack of proper socialization, whereas the labeling theory of Chambliss [83] proposes that people are deviant because the society labels them as deviant. How can genes code for norms, means, socialization, or labeling? Psychological theories also put a great emphasis on internal and inter-individual conflicts, whereas psychiatry attributes a great role to life events. How can one inherit conflicts and life events?

Heredity estimates of aggression are consistent. Studies are based on two natural experiments, e.g., adoption and twin studies. It might be better to say that these studies are based on environmental and genetic contrasts between parents and offspring in the case of the former and on the differential genetic relatedness in the case of monozygotic and dizygotic twins. The ensuing observational studies make use of reliable data on phenotypes and of the widely accepted rules of genetics; the system of thought standing behind these studies is highly consistent. The mathematics and the scientific approach may be and is continually improved; adoption and twin paradigms are combined to increase reliability, etc.; however, no methodological improvement has decreased heredity estimates. Animal studies consistently support the high heritability of aggression. Indeed, it is rather easy to obtain excessively aggressive and excessively docile animals by selective breeding. Differences were observable already at the first generation of offspring and maximized within a few generations. Inbreeding maintains the two phenotypes practically indefinitely under controlled environmental conditions, whereas mixed breeding reduces the differences. This confirms that aggression has a strong heritability component; moreover, abnormal – psychopathology-like – features of aggression are also highly heritable. It is notable that heritability of these features is 100% in selection lines, as their phenotype is independent of the environment, as documented above. The additional information from animal studies is that here we do not have to deal with phenomena like differential association, anomie, self-control, society labels, or environmental influences. Selection lines represent "biology" as purely as possible uncontaminated by other influences. These studies show that heritability can alone maintain aggression-related traits.

Thus, on one side, we have criminological theories that explain violence entirely in sociological terms and empirical evidence demonstrating that the heredity component of violence is at least 50%. It would be easy to argue for and against either side. One can point out that the four "nurture-oriented" criminological theories explain violence by completely different, sometime conflicting social and individual processes, whereas the "nature-oriented" heredity estimates belong to a unitary system of thinking. On the other hand, the nature-oriented heredity studies lack the explanatory power and social relevance of the other side. We do not think, however, that the nature-nurture debate should be revived here. The debate is hundreds of years old; some trace it back to Locke's 1690 "*An Essay Concerning Human Understanding,*" and this debate has led nowhere so far. Instead of arguing and counter arguing, we prefer an opinion that was formulated more than two decades ago [84]. The weight of nature and nurture is equal: both are 100% responsible for a trait. Neither genetics nor the society can influence aggression without the other. This idea will be developed further in later chapters. Before that, however, we will investigate how well we understand genetic alterations that must underlay heredity.

References

1. Kvaale, E. P., Gottdiener, W. H., & Haslam, N. (2013). Biogenetic explanations and stigma: A meta-analytic review of associations among laypeople. *Social Science & Medicine, 96*, 95–103.
2. Easter, M. M. (2012). "Not all my fault": Genetics, stigma, and personal responsibility for women with eating disorders. *Social Science & Medicine, 75*, 1408–1416.
3. Persky, S., & Eccleston, C. P. (2011). Impact of genetic causal information on medical students' clinical encounters with an obese virtual patient: Health promotion and social stigma. *Annals of Behavioral Medicine, 41*, 363–372.
4. Tekola, F., et al. (2009). Impact of social stigma on the process of obtaining informed consent for genetic research on podoconiosis: A qualitative study. *BMC Medical Ethics, 10*, 13.
5. Joseph, J. (2001). Is crime in the genes? A critical review of twin and adoption studies of criminality and antisocial behavior. *Journal of Mind & Behavior, 22*, 179–218.
6. (PDF) Pulling Back the Curtain on Heritability Studies: Biosocial Criminology in the Postgenomic Era. *ResearchGate.* Available at: https://www.researchgate.net/publication/260833911_Pulling_Back_the_Curtain_on_Heritability_Studies_Biosocial_Criminology_in_the_Postgenomic_Era. (Accessed 15 July 2019).
7. Barnes, J. C., et al. (2014). Demonstrating the validity of twin research in criminology. *Criminology, 52*, 588–626.
8. Kendler, K. S., et al. (2016). A novel sibling-based design to quantify genetic and shared environmental effects: Application to drug abuse, alcohol use disorder and criminal behavior. *Psychological Medicine, 46*, 1639–1650.
9. Frisell, T., Pawitan, Y., Långström, N., & Lichtenstein, P. (2012). Heritability, assortative mating and gender differences in violent crime: Results from a total population sample using twin, adoption, and sibling models. *Behavior Genetics, 42*, 3–18.
10. Frisell, T., Lichtenstein, P., & Långström, N. (2011). Violent crime runs in families: A total population study of 12.5 million individuals. *Psychological Medicine, 41*, 97–105.
11. Mednick, S. A., & Kandel, E. S. (1988). Congenital determinants of violence. *The Bulletin of the American Academy of Psychiatry and the Law, 16*, 101–109.
12. Neale, M. C. & Maes, H. H. M. Methodology for genetic studies of twins and families. 308.
13. Elmquist, J., et al. (2016). The relationship between family-of-origin violence, hostility, and intimate partner violence in men arrested for domestic violence: Testing a mediational model. *Violence Women, 22*, 1243–1258.
14. Faraone, S. V., Biederman, J., Jetton, J. G., & Tsuang, M. T. (1997). Attention deficit disorder and conduct disorder: Longitudinal evidence for a familial subtype. *Psychological Medicine, 27*, 291–300.
15. Middeldorp, C. M., Cath, D. C., Vink, J. M., & Boomsma, D. I. (2005). Twin and genetic effects on life events. *Twin Research and Human Genetics, 8*, 224–231.
16. Kendler, K. S., et al. (2014). A Swedish national adoption study of criminality. *Psychological Medicine, 44*, 1913–1925.
17. Achenbach, T. M. (2000). *ASEBA preschool forms & profiles: An integrated system of multi-informant assessment*. ASEBA, Burlington, VT.
18. Goodman, R. (1997). The strengths and difficulties questionnaire: A research note. *Journal of Child Psychology and Psychiatry, 38*, 581–586.

19. Raine, A., et al. (2006). The reactive-proactive aggression questionnaire: Differential correlates of reactive and proactive aggression in adolescent boys. *Aggressive Behavior, 32*, 159–171.
20. Porsch, R. M., et al. (2016). Longitudinal heritability of childhood aggression. *American Journal of Medical Genetics Part B Neuropsychiatric Genetics, 171*, 697–707.
21. Chen, J., Yu, J., Zhang, J., Li, X., & McGue, M. (2015). Investigating genetic and environmental contributions to adolescent externalizing behavior in a collectivistic culture: A multi-informant twin study. *Psychological Medicine, 45*, 1989–1997.
22. Rushton, J. P., Fulker, D. W., Neale, M. C., Nias, D. K., & Eysenck, H. J. (1986). Altruism and aggression: The heritability of individual differences. *Journal of Personality and Social Psychology, 50*, 1192–1198.
23. Ligthart, L., Bartels, M., Hoekstra, R. A., Hudziak, J. J., & Boomsma, D. I. (2005). Genetic contributions to subtypes of aggression. *Twin Research and Human Genetics, 8*, 483–491.
24. Lubke, G. H., McArtor, D. B., Boomsma, D. I., & Bartels, M. (2018). Genetic and environmental contributions to the development of childhood aggression. *Developmental Psychology, 54*, 39–50.
25. Lacourse, E., et al. (2014). A longitudinal twin study of physical aggression during early childhood: Evidence for a developmentally dynamic genome. *Psychological Medicine, 44*, 2617–2627.
26. Tuvblad, C., Raine, A., Zheng, M., & Baker, L. A. (2009). Genetic and environmental stability differs in reactive and proactive aggression. *Aggressive Behavior, 35*, 437–452.
27. Coccaro, E. F., Bergeman, C. S., & McClearn, G. E. (1993). Heritability of irritable impulsiveness: A study of twins reared together and apart. *Psychiatry Research, 48*, 229–242.
28. van Beijsterveldt, C. E. M., Bartels, M., Hudziak, J. J., & Boomsma, D. I. (2003). Causes of stability of aggression from early childhood to adolescence: A longitudinal genetic analysis in Dutch twins. *Behavior Genetics, 33*, 591–605.
29. Pingault, J.-B., Rijsdijk, F., Zheng, Y., Plomin, R., & Viding, E. (2015). Developmentally dynamic genome: Evidence of genetic influences on increases and decreases in conduct problems from early childhood to adolescence. *Scientific Reports, 5*, 10053.
30. Lewis, G. J., & Plomin, R. (2015). Heritable influences on behavioural problems from early childhood to mid-adolescence: Evidence for genetic stability and innovation. *Psychological Medicine, 45*, 2171–2179.
31. Wesseldijk, L. W., et al. (2018). Genetic and environmental influences on conduct and antisocial personality problems in childhood, adolescence, and adulthood. *European Child & Adolescent Psychiatry, 27*, 1123–1132.
32. Young, S. E., et al. (2009). Behavioral disinhibition: Liability for externalizing spectrum disorders and its genetic and environmental relation to response inhibition across adolescence. *Journal of Abnormal Psychology, 118*, 117–130.
33. Greven, C. U., et al. (2016). The opposite end of the attention deficit hyperactivity disorder continuum: Genetic and environmental aetiologies of extremely low ADHD traits. *Journal of Child Psychology and Psychiatry, 57*, 523–531.
34. van den Berg, S. M., Willemsen, G., de Geus, E. J. C., & Boomsma, D. I. (2006). Genetic etiology of stability of attention problems in young adulthood. *American Journal of Medical Genetics Part B Neuropsychiatric Genetics, 141B*, 55–60.
35. Polderman, T. J. C., et al. (2013). Attentional switching forms a genetic link between attention problems and autistic traits in adults. *Psychological Medicine, 43*, 1985–1996.
36. Reichborn-Kjennerud, T., et al. (2015). A longitudinal twin study of borderline and antisocial personality disorder traits in early to middle adulthood. *Psychological Medicine, 45*, 3121–3131.
37. Rosenström, T., et al. (2017). Genetic and environmental structure of DSM-IV criteria for antisocial personality disorder: A twin study. *Behavior Genetics, 47*, 265–277.
38. Torgersen, S., et al. (2012). The heritability of cluster B personality disorders assessed both by personal interview and questionnaire. *Journal of Personality Disorders, 26*, 848–866.

39. Czajkowski, N., et al. (2018). A twin study of normative personality and DSM-IV personality disorder criterion counts: Evidence for separate genetic influences. *The American Journal of Psychiatry, 175*, 649–656.
40. Skoglund, C., et al. (2019). Familial risk and heritability of diagnosed borderline personality disorder: A register study of the Swedish population. *Molecular Psychiatry*. https://doi.org/10.1038/s41380-019-0442-0.
41. Viding, E., et al. (2013). Genetics of callous-unemotional behavior in children. *PLoS One, 8*, e65789.
42. Gelhorn, H. L., et al. (2005). Genetic and environmental influences on conduct disorder: Symptom, domain and full-scale analyses. *Journal of Child Psychology and Psychiatry, 46*, 580–591.
43. Waldman, I. D., Rowe, R., Boylan, K., & Burke, J. D. (2018). External validation of a bifactor model of oppositional defiant disorder. *Molecular Psychiatry*. https://doi.org/10.1038/s41380-018-0294-z.
44. Hicks, B. M., et al. (2012). Psychopathic personality traits and environmental contexts: Differential correlates, gender differences, and genetic mediation. *Personality Disorders: Theory, Research, and Treatment, 3*, 209–227.
45. Tuvblad, C., et al. (2019). Genetic and environmental influences on disinhibition, boldness, and meanness as assessed by the triarchic psychopathy measure in 19-20-year-old twins. *Psychological Medicine, 49*, 1500–1509.
46. Brook, M., et al. (2010). Psychopathic personality traits in middle-aged male twins: A behavior genetic investigation. *Journal of Personality Disorders, 24*, 473–486.
47. Blonigen, D. M., Hicks, B. M., Krueger, R. F., Patrick, C. J., & Iacono, W. G. (2005). Psychopathic personality traits: Heritability and genetic overlap with internalizing and externalizing psychopathology. *Psychological Medicine, 35*, 637–648.
48. Coccaro, E. F., Kavoussi, R. J., Berman, M. E., & Lish, J. D. (1998). Intermittent explosive disorder-revised: Development, reliability, and validity of research criteria. *Comprehensive Psychiatry, 39*, 368–376.
49. Coccaro, E. (2010). A family history study of intermittent explosive disorder. *Journal of Psychiatric Research, 44*, 1101–1105.
50. Kerekes, N., et al. (2014). Oppositional defiant- and conduct disorder-like problems: Neurodevelopmental predictors and genetic background in boys and girls, in a nationwide twin study. *PeerJ, 2*, e359.
51. Sariaslan, A., Larsson, H., & Fazel, S. (2016). Genetic and environmental determinants of violence risk in psychotic disorders: A multivariate quantitative genetic study of 1.8 million Swedish twins and siblings. *Mol. Psychiatry, 21*, 1251–1256.
52. Hilker, R., et al. (2018). Heritability of schizophrenia and schizophrenia spectrum based on the nationwide danish twin register. *Biological Psychiatry, 83*, 492–498.
53. DiLalla, L. F., & DiLalla, D. L. (2018). Gene-environment correlations affecting children's early rule-breaking and aggressive play behaviors. *Twin Research and Human Genetics, 21*, 285–288.
54. Newsome, J., Vaske, J. C., Gehring, K. S., & Boisvert, D. L. (2016). Sex differences in sources of resilience and vulnerability to risk for delinquency. *Journal of Youth and Adolescence, 45*, 730–745.
55. Burt, S. A., Pearson, A. L., Rzotkiewicz, A., Klump, K. L., & Neiderhiser, J. M. (2019). It really does take a village: The role of neighbors in the etiology of nonaggressive rule-breaking behavior. *Development and Psychopathology, 31*, 713–725.
56. Stringaris, A., Zavos, H., Leibenluft, E., Maughan, B., & Eley, T. C. (2012). Adolescent irritability: Phenotypic associations and genetic links with depressed mood. *The American Journal of Psychiatry, 169*, 47–54.
57. Kendler, K. S., et al. (2015). A Swedish national twin study of criminal behavior and its violent, white-collar and property subtypes. *Psychological Medicine, 45*, 2253–2262.

58. Cloninger, C. R., & Gottesman, I. I. (1987). Genetic end environmental factors in antisocial behavior disorders. In *The causes of crime: New biological approaches* (pp. 92–109). Cambridge University Press, Cambridge, UK.
59. Kendler, K. S., Lönn, S. L., Maes, H. H., Sundquist, J., & Sundquist, K. (2015). The etiologic role of genetic and environmental factors in criminal behavior as determined from full- and half-sibling pairs: An evaluation of the validity of the twin method. *Psychological Medicine, 45*, 1873–1880.
60. Cadoret, R. J. (1982). Genotype-environment interaction in antisocial behaviour. *Psychological Medicine, 12*, 235–239.
61. Mednick, S. A., Gabrielli, W. F., & Hutchings, B. (1984). Genetic influences in criminal convictions: Evidence from an adoption cohort. *Science, 224*, 891–894.
62. Christiansen, K. O. (1977). A preliminary study of criminal-ity among twins. In *Biosocial bases of criminal behavior* (pp. 89–108). Gardner Press, Oxford, UK.
63. Rhee, S. H., & Waldman, I. D. (2002). Genetic and environmental influences on antisocial behavior: A meta-analysis of twin and adoption studies. *Psychological Bulletin, 128*, 490–529.
64. Burt, S. A. (2009). Are there meaningful etiological differences within antisocial behavior? Results of a meta-analysis. *Clinical Psychology Review, 29*, 163–178.
65. Benus, R. F., Bohus, B., Koolhaas, J. M., & van Oortmerssen, G. A. (1991). Behavioural differences between artificially selected aggressive and non-aggressive mice: Response to apomorphine. *Behavioural Brain Research, 43*, 203–208.
66. van Oortmerssen, G. A., & Bakker, T. C. (1981). Artificial selection for short and long attack latencies in wild Mus musculus domesticus. *Behavior Genetics, 11*, 115–126.
67. Haller, J., Tóth, M., Halasz, J., & De Boer, S. F. (2006). Patterns of violent aggression-induced brain c-fos expression in male mice selected for aggressiveness. *Physiology & Behavior, 88*, 173–182.
68. Malki, K., et al. (2016). Transcriptome analysis of genes and gene networks involved in aggressive behavior in mouse and zebrafish. *American Journal of Medical Genetics Part B Neuropsychiatric Genetics, 171*, 827–838.
69. Sluyter, F., van Oortmerssen, G. A., de Ruiter, A. J., & Koolhaas, J. M. (1996). Aggression in wild house mice: Current state of affairs. *Behavior Genetics, 26*, 489–496.
70. Lagerspetz, K. M., & Lagerspetz, K. Y. (1971). Changes in the aggressiveness of mice resulting from selective breeding, learning and social isolation. *Scandinavian Journal of Psychology, 12*, 241–248.
71. Cairns, R. B., MacCombie, D. J., & Hood, K. E. (1983). A developmental-genetic analysis of aggressive behavior in mice: I. Behavioral outcomes. *Journal of Comparative Psychology (Washington DC), 1983*(97), 69–89.
72. Natarajan, D., de Vries, H., de Boer, S. F., & Koolhaas, J. M. (2009). Violent phenotype in SAL mice is inflexible and fixed in adulthood. *Aggressive Behavior, 35*, 430–436.
73. Natarajan, D., & Caramaschi, D. (2010). Animal violence demystified. *Frontiers in Behavioral Neuroscience, 4*, 9.
74. Haller, J. (2017). Studies into abnormal aggression in humans and rodents: Methodological and translational aspects. *Neuroscience and Biobehavioral Reviews, 76*, 77–86.
75. Liebsch, G., Montkowski, A., Holsboer, F., & Landgraf, R. (1998). Behavioural profiles of two Wistar rat lines selectively bred for high or low anxiety-related behaviour. *Behavioural Brain Research, 94*, 301–310.
76. Chekmareva, N. Y., Umriukhin, A. E., Landgraf, R., & Sotnikov, S. V. (2019). Inborn vs. acquired anxiety in cross-breeding and cross-fostering HAB/LAB mice bred for extremes in anxiety-related behavior. *Behavioral Neuroscience, 133*, 68–76.
77. Neumann, I. D., Veenema, A. H., & Beiderbeck, D. I. (2010). Aggression and anxiety: Social context and neurobiological links. *Frontiers in Behavioral Neuroscience, 4*, 12.

78. Beiderbeck, D. I., et al. (2012). High and abnormal forms of aggression in rats with extremes in trait anxiety--involvement of the dopamine system in the nucleus accumbens. *Psychoneuroendocrinology, 37*, 1969–1980.
79. Lukas, M., & Wöhr, M. (2015). Endogenous vasopressin, innate anxiety, and the emission of pro-social 50-kHz ultrasonic vocalizations during social play behavior in juvenile rats. *Psychoneuroendocrinology, 56*, 35–44.
80. Sutherland, E. H. (1934). *Principles of criminology*. Lippincott, Oxford, UK.
81. Merton, R., & Social, K. (1938). Structure and anomie. *American Sociological Review, 3*, 672–682.
82. Reckless, W. C. (1961). A new theory of deliquency and crime. *Federal Probation*, 42–46.
83. Chambliss, W. J. (1973). The saints and the roughnecks. *Society, 11*, 24–31.
84. Ferris, C. F. (1996). Cultivating violence. *Annals of the New York Academy of Sciences, 794*, 318–328.

Chapter 3
Neurogenetics, Genome-Wide Association and Candidate Gene Studies

Introduction

Since the discovery of "warrior genes," the heritability of aggression is not an academic question anymore. Naturally, "warrior genes" do not exist as shown in this chapter. Nevertheless, the concept has entered public speech [1, 2], and the "genetic argument" is brought up quite frequently in court proceedings. The success of such arguments is mixed; some perceive that courts – in contrast to practitioners and scientists – refrain from considering warrior genes [3]. Others deem otherwise. A study, for instance, showed that the MAOA-low functionality genotype (*the* "warrior gene") lessened the criminal charge in one out of two cases, whereas it was considered by the court in four out of five other cases and lessened the sentence in one [4]. A review described 81 such cases [5]. When genetics was not brought up during the trial, defendants claimed retrial based on ineffective assistance of counsel. When genetics was considered, it provided proof of the defendant's mitigating condition. As time passes, the genetic argument becomes an issue in an increasing number of countries [6, 7] but cannot be addressed properly without sound information on the phenomenon [8]. With the advancement of behavioral genetics, the need for a genetic counterpart of the so called "neurolaw" movement (see later) is felt more and more.

J. Haller, *Neurobiopsychosocial Perspectives on Aggression and Violence*,
Advances in Preventing and Treating Violence and Aggression,
https://doi.org/10.1007/978-3-030-46331-1_3

3.1 A Brief Introduction to Neurogenetics

3.1.1 The Place of Genes in Information Transfer and Processing

To understand how genetic variation affects neural function, we first need to understand how information travels across and is processed within the nervous system. Subsequently, we will analyze the role of genetic variation in this process.

The first important notion to be understood is the synapse. Classical textbooks depict such contacts linearly; one neuron extends an axon towards another, which receives the signal via the synapse and transmits it further. The neural circuit is envisaged as a chain of such contacts. The synapse is the mechanism by which neurons communicate with each other.

The real situation is completely different. Each neuron establishes synaptic contacts with many thousands of neurons. It receives inputs from several thousands of neurons via synapses located on its surface and then sends information to several thousands of other neurons which subsequently influences their functions. Synapses are located on different segments of neurons, which deeply affect the consequences of the information received by them (input).

We will illustrate these by two simple examples although the issue is naturally much more complex. An inhibitory input on the dendrite can block excitatory inputs located upstream (i.e., above the point where the dendrite was inhibited), because information cannot go further. The neuron can still receive information from downstream synapses located on the same dendrite and via synapses located on other dendrites, the cell body, or the axon. The closer is the inhibitory input to the cell, the larger is the disabled dendritic segment. If, by contrast, an inhibitory input (synapse) targets the initial segment of the axon, the neuron is silenced: it will not send information out, because it is inhibited at its "base." If the inhibitory input targets only one of the branches of the axon, then the transmission of information is blocked for that branch, but not other branches.

In addition to synapses, the neuron receives information via signaling molecules that target extra-synaptic loci on the neuron. This so-called extra-synaptic or volumetric transmission originates from distant neurons, without synaptic contacts with the respective neuron. Some neurons, e.g., serotonergic neurons in the dorsal raphe, preferentially communicate extra-synaptically, whereas others – e.g., serotonergic neurons in the *median* raphe – preferentially communicate synaptically.

To sum up, the neuron is not a link in a chain as the classical textbooks suggest but a small processor that integrates thousands of pieces of information in a highly complex way and communicates with thousands of similar microprocessors.

The key elements of neurotransmission and information processing are neurotransmitters and neurotransmitter receptors. The former carries the message and the latter receives it. Neurotransmitters are synthesized in the neuron that sends the message (presynaptic neuron), by complex biochemical pathways operated by enzymes (proteins). On their turn, receptors are proteins synthesized by the postsynaptic (receiver) neurons. After binding the neurotransmitter, the postsynaptic neuron elicits various responses within the target cell. These range from initiating the transmission of information by changing the polarity of the neuronal membrane to a series of intracellular processes managed by proteins specialized for the specific task.

After the neurotransmitter is released into the synapse – i.e., the message is conveyed – it fulfilled its role; therefore, it should be eliminated. This is done by two types of proteins. Transporters remove neurotransmitters from the synapse by carrying them back into the cytoplasm. This process is called reuptake. Degrading enzymes on their turn inactivate neurotransmitters by metabolizing them.

Finally, it is noteworthy that each type of the proteins involved (synthesizing enzymes, receptors, transporters, metabolizing enzymes, and many more) are varied. The same neuron usually synthesizes one, two, or three neurotransmitters at maximum, but within the whole brain, there are around 200 neurotransmitters. The same neurotransmitter can bind to several receptor types (up to around 16 in in the case of serotonin), each having a specific effect on the functioning of the postsynaptic neuron. The coupling of neurotransmitters and receptors is specific. As a rule, no neurotransmitter binds to the receptor of another. Yet, the same neurotransmitter can bind to any of its own receptors; e.g., serotonin can bind to any of its 16 or so receptors. Although transporters and metabolizing enzymes are not as specific as the neurotransmitter-receptor coupling, there still are around 20 types of transporters in the brain and even more numerous metabolizing enzymes. Thus, the same protein may process several neurotransmitters that have related structures.

All the proteins enumerated above are synthesized based on information encoded in genes. Humans share these genes; yet, they have them in several variants that are called polymorphisms. A simple example: We all have genes for the proteins that determine eye color; yet, some have brown, whereas others blue eyes, because they carry genetic polymorphisms that result in proteins that induce the expression of one or another eye color. Some polymorphisms are carried by a larger share of people and others by a smaller share of people, but they are regularly present in the population. Importantly, polymorphisms are not equivalent. Certain polymorphisms are more difficult to be "read," i.e., protein synthesis can be initiated only with some difficulty. Consequently, the amount of proteins synthesized based on their information will be reduced. Other polymorphisms result in proteins that are less effective: they perform their task less well than proteins based on another polymorphism.

Returning to the neuron, a polymorphism may reduce the amount of neurotransmitters, receptors, transporters, degrading enzymes, etc. that play roles in neuronal communication. Others may encode a less effective synthesizing or degrading enzyme, transporter, or receptor. The result is that the receipt, processing, or transmission of information changes. If neurons were organized in chains, this had dramatic consequences for neuronal function. As, however, neurons are organized in very complex networks, the impact of "wrong" phenotypes is reduced. For instance, if one serotonin receptor works less well, there still are about 15 properly working serotonin receptors in the brain. The brain can even tolerate the total lack of some of its proteins. This may result from a polymorphism that completely inactivates the gene. Such polymorphisms are rare, but they do exist. In a chain-like neuronal organization, this would stop the flow of information, with fatal consequences for brain function. In a network-type of organization, this results in only a small deficiency. One input or output might be disrupted, but the neuron had many alternative mechanisms due to the inbuilt redundancy in the system.

Although polymorphisms do not cause severe disruptions in neuronal functioning, their consequences should not be minimalized. Changes in one department of functioning will alter the balance between the various processes that govern the receipt, processing, and transmission of information at neuronal level. As a result, the brain circuits that control emotion, cognition, and behavior will be altered, because these circuits are composed of neurons. Therefore, altered neuron functioning will alter emotional, cognitive, and behavioral responses to environmental challenges.

3.1.2 Genes, Circuits, and the Targets of Research

Very roughly, brain circuits can be divided into three main elements as follows. The basics of brain function are the neurons that "do the job," i.e., control the behavior directly. These are organized in hierarchical networks (pathways), within which each brain area receives information from other levels and transmits them to the subsequent levels after processing them. Ascending pathways originate from external and internal sensory organs and transmit information upwards via a series of relay and processing neural nodes. In the case of aggression, the ascending pathways may go as high as the frontal brain, where the ultimate decision on aggression is taken. Descending pathways follow the reverse route; they originate from decision-making brain centers and terminate at executory centers – ultimately in the spinal cord from where movements are controlled. Both these pathways use glutamate as their neurotransmitters, this being stimulatory in nature. Within pathways, information is transmitted very precisely, in a point-to-point manner. All ascending and descending pathways interact by lateral connections.

The next category is the local interneurons, which are present at each relay and processing node of the brain and control the functioning of the ascending and descending stimulatory pathways. They use gamma-aminobutyric acid (GABA) as neurotransmitter and inhibit the neurons of the above-mentioned pathways. They form extremely intricate networks and interact with each other and glutamatergic neurons in highly complex ways. Despite this, they still work in a point-to-point manner in most cases. GABAergic neurons are the inhibitory counterparts of stimulatory pathways; roughly, the functioning of pathways depends on the balance between stimulation and inhibition. Stimulatory (glutamatergic) and inhibitory (GABAergic) neurons constitute the overwhelming majority in the brain.

The third category is represented by neurons aggregated into small brainstem nuclei. The most important of these utilize either dopamine or norepinephrine or serotonin as neurotransmitters. Each of these neuron types is organized in different, small nuclei dispersed over the brainstem. They are not integral parts of the circuits, but influence the way the circuits behave. The number of dopaminergic, norepinephrinergic, and serotonergic neurons is almost negligible compared to the huge number of glutamatergic and GABAergic neurons. Nevertheless, their axons are extremely long and arborize richly at all levels of the brain. They also extensively communicate extra-synaptically. Accordingly, they do not work in a point-to-point fashion but rather influence a series of circuits in parallel. Their effects depend largely on the type of receptors that a particular neuron expresses. The innervation of various brain areas is not homogeneous, however, which means that the arborization of axons also guides their effects. The main role of these neurons is the fine-tuning of the above-mentioned pathways.

Finally, all the elements of brain circuits are under the control of hormones. Hormones are secreted in distant parts of the organism, and are carried to the brain by circulation. As blood reaches all organs and cells practically at the same time, their message is not targeted at all. Nevertheless, only those cells respond to hormonal influences, which express their receptors, i.e., can sense the signal.

Based on the above, one may assume that genetic analyses of aggression are preferentially focused on the neurons that "do the job" – which directly control emotions, cognition, and behavior. However, this assumption is false. For example, genome-wide association studies (GWAS) are not focused on the neurons that "do the job." In the case of more focused studies, the major targets are those systems that only fine-tune the function of circuits, particularly the dopaminergic, norepinephrinergic, and serotonergic, and the hormonal systems, especially the genes that control the stress response. The reasons for this are multiple and will not be presented here. We mention, however, that psychoactive medications also target these systems preferentially; therefore, information on their genetics is also relevant from a therapeutic point of view.

3.2 Genome-Wide Association Studies

GWAS are based on relatively new technologies, which in many ways revolutionized our view on how genes encode various traits from physical ones like eye color to disease vulnerability and aggression. Below we will summarize the essence and main features of the approach, after which we will briefly review the main findings, which appear rather disappointing at the first sight. However, we will show in the *Interpretation* section that, despite the problems, GWAS outline a specific and very important aspect of the genetic underpinnings of aggression. Particularly, GWAS offer a tool to understand the genetics of neural structure as opposed to candidate gene analyses, which so far has focused more on functional aspects of neuronal mechanisms.

3.2.1 Background

GWAS employ a "backward genetic strategy," the starting point of which is the phenotype, and the target is the genotype. Studies are typically performed in two groups of subjects, which differ in one particular trait. For an example, the phenotype might be conviction for violent crime. Members belonging to the control group are selected who have no convictions, whereas the members of the study group are selected to have been convicted for violent crime, possibly several violent crimes to increase the contrast between the groups. Expected inter-individual variance of gene polymorphism is high; therefore, sample sizes should also be high – around 1000 in the smallest studies but may be as high as several tens of thousands. The second step is genotyping the subjects. The number of DNA loci investigated depends on a series of factors (e.g., the technique employed) but usually is in the range of hundreds of thousands to millions. The third step is the genetic analysis, i.e., the determination of the frequencies of various polymorphisms present in the two groups. The result of the procedure is a number for each DNA locus, which shows the odds ratio of a particular polymorphism in the study group compared to the control group. For instance, an odds ratio of 2 means that the particular gene variant is twice as frequent in the study group as in the control group.

The polymorphisms studied differ typically in one single nucleotide. For example, the DNA may contain different nucleobases at a specific position: some individuals may have cytosine (C) at that position, whereas others may have thymine (T). This affects protein synthesis when the genetic code is translated into amino acid sequences such as polypeptides and proteins. The codon TCT, for instance, translates as the amino acid serine, whereas the codon TTT (C changed into T) translates as phenylalanine, an amino acid with a different polarity, i.e., a differential distribution of electric charge, which affects the folding of the amino acid chain into a functional protein. This may alter the conformation (or form) and functional characteristics of the resulting protein. The change is called *single-nucleotide polymorphism* if the variant was widespread, i.e., was present in more than 1% of the population. Less widespread variants that occur in less than 1% of the population are called *single-nucleotide variations*. Single-nucleotide polymorphisms are rather frequent. A study found more than 300 million such variations in the genome of only 1000 individuals who belonged to different populations [9]. Although other forms of genetic variation (e.g., short insertions/deletions) were also found in this study, slightly more than 96% of genetic variation were single-nucleotide polymorphisms. These are the major research targets of GWAS. Sometimes single-nucleotide polymorphisms are specifically studied in microsatellites, which are repetitive segments of the DNA in which several nucleobase motifs are repeated from a few to a few tens of times. These DNA segments are highly prone to mutation [10] and are a great source of variation, which is important when trait–gene associations are investigated.

The most attractive feature of GWAS is its unbiased nature. These studies are unbiased in two ways. First, they ignore all knowledge related to the control of the trait under investigation. For instance, the hormonal and neural mechanisms of aggression are reasonably well-known, and such information may be used to guide genetic investigations. We know from neuroscientific studies, for instance, that noradrenergic neurotransmission is one of the control mechanisms of aggression; therefore, one may be tempted to specifically study genes that encode proteins relevant to the noradrenergic system, e.g., norepinephrine receptors, transport proteins, and synthesizing enzymes. Although this so-called candidate gene analysis is a useful approach, and is widely employed (see next section), it hinders new discovery to a certain degree. Candidate gene association studies supplement known information by investigating the degree to which variation in noradrenergic neurotransmission depends on genes. GWAS reject this guidance to allow for the discovery of associations that cannot be predicted by available information. In fact, this approach intends to guide rather than being guided. Second, besides ignoring information on the phenomenon studied such as knowledge related to the brain mechanisms of aggression, GWAS are balanced also in the sense that they ignore a series of genetic information. The genome is huge and is composed of vast non-coding regions ("gene deserts"), coding regions with unknown roles (e.g., unknown products), and regions where the encoded protein is known, but its role is not. Of course, there also are DNA regions (genes), which encode something known such as a well-known protein. GWAS cover all these types of DNA regions without bias. The point in this approach is that we know very little about gene function. The tremendous progress in genetics we presently witness may be misleading in this respect. Naturally, there was a huge progress from Darwin's [11] hypothesized gemmules as the unit of inheritance through Mendel's laws of heredity [12] to the human genome project [13] and beyond. Yet, there still are many gaps in our knowledge. For instance, the role of non-coding regions is poorly understood. We do not know the product or role of a large number of coding regions, and, most importantly, we are just about to start understanding gene–gene, protein–gene, and protein–protein interactions. Gaps in our knowledge, however, do not diminish the importance of natural phenomena. Coding regions may be important, even if we are ignorant of the role of the protein that is encoded or if we do not know what the region encodes at this time. Even non-coding regions can affect gene function by the phenomenon called *epistasis*. The term means that a "modifier gene" or locus on the DNA influences the function of another gene (the target gene) or DNA locus [14]. Changes in either regions can affect gene function in an often nonlinear way. Epistasis was originally described for coding regions, but non-coding regions may alter chromatin structure and by this may regulate the expression of coding regions (genes) [15]. There are many examples where non-coding regions proved to be important risk factors for disease. The basic assumption of GWAS is that all DNA regions are important, irrespective to the amount of the knowledge we have on their role at the time of the investigation.

The only hypothesis standing behind GWAS is the assumption that the trait investigated *does have* a genetic foundation, which is easily supported or refuted by the findings. The functionally unbiased approach allows GWAS to discover unpredicted genetic associations, the role and significance of which may be the subjects of subsequent neuroscientific studies. The genetically unbiased approach of GWAS is a safeguard for the lack of knowledge, a precaution explained by our incomplete understanding of genetics. As such, GWAS may become a true, unbiased motor of progress.

The lack of bias is a great asset of GWAS; however, the approach also has three main drawbacks. First, *statistical significance is difficult to reach.* When two groups are compared with regard to one single variable (e.g., the gene of MAO_A, see below), differences can be considered significant when the p value is below 0.05, which means that the chance of having an accidental rather than a legitimate difference is below 5%. However, multiple comparisons are a source of statistical error, and the threshold p value should be corrected in accordance with the number of comparisons. The most frequently used correction of this type is the Bonferroni correction. According to this, the threshold for significance is 0.025 when two groups are compared with a third, control group. Genome-wide analysis works with a huge number of comparisons (polymorphisms); consequently, the threshold for significance becomes very low, generally as low as ~$1/10^8$ (i.e., $p < 0.00000001$). Note that the threshold depends on the number of DNA loci investigated, which differs from study to study. The above threshold, however, holds true for the majority of studies. The very low threshold means that crossing it becomes difficult, and the number of *significant* genome-wide associations will always be small. Quite often, one or very few associations reach significance; moreover, many studies find no significant gene–trait associations at all, despite the fact that p values are extremely low.

Second, *the polygenic nature of traits complicates interpretation.* Characteristics like everyday aggressiveness, antisocial personality disorder, and violent crime are certainly polygenic, that is, they are determined by many genes. This holds true for most traits. For instance, a bodily characteristic as simple as eye color is determined by at least six single-nucleotide polymorphisms at six different genes and by several other candidate genes [16]. Neither these genes alone determines eye color: the trait results from the interactive effects of the six or possibly more DNA loci. It is only natural that traits as complex as aggression have more complex genetics, with multiple interactions. Such interactions may occur on a wide scale from effects on chromatin morphology to protein–protein interactions in the cell, all which are poorly known at present. Moreover, it is unknown how many polymorphisms should be present for changes in aggression to be observable. If, for instance, the trait was influenced by 100 DNA loci, it is unknown whether 10, 50, or all the 100 loci should carry modifications for the expression of the phenotype. It is not even known whether there are polymorphisms of key importance, and, if yes, which are the ones that have a greater importance than the rest. Nevertheless, findings obtained so far suggest that an aggressive phenotype is expressed even if only a subgroup of the critical DNA loci carries the relevant polymorphisms. This is of major importance for the interpretation of GWAS findings. If only a subset of DNA loci needs to be affected to result in an aggression phenotype, this subset may show individual variations. If, for instance, only 5 out of the critical 100 polymorphisms are sufficient for an aggressive phenotype, an individual may have polymorphisms at DNA loci 10, 20, 30, 40, and 50, whereas another individual may carry polymorphisms at DNA loci 11, 21, 31, 91, and 100. If five polymorphisms were sufficient, the phenotype may be similar, despite the large differences in the underlying genetic determinants. Such individual variation may render a real association non-significant at population level. Put more simply, one specific set of polymorphisms may be important in a particular individual, but may be cancelled out by statistics at population level, because of these individual variations.

Third, *the road from genetic discovery to biological knowledge is difficult*. The studies performed so far show that a good deal of the polymorphisms associated with a trait occurs in non-coding DNA regions for which their biological significance remains a mystery. Some researchers tend to ignore these polymorphisms, but this means nothing less than abandoning the road opened up by the GWAS technology. Such authors introduce a bias where there should be no biases. Although the issue remains rather unsettled, there are new scientific approaches, which may gradually make the story told by the polymorphisms of gene deserts understandable [17]. Another but in certain cases lesser problem is posed by polymorphisms in genes that are associated with functions that are completely unrelated to the trait that is studied. Such examples will be abundant in the findings reviewed below. The phenomenon is not new. Pleiotropy, the ability of genes to influence apparently unrelated features, was discovered long before the GWA technology was developed [18]. Nevertheless, biological mechanisms linking together widely different traits remain poorly understood despite the "one hundred years of pleiotropy" [18]. The phenomenon complicates the interpretation of GWAS considerably.

These and other shortcomings are fully recognized by experts [19], and it is acknowledged that the road from GWAS to testable hypotheses and true biological knowledge is difficult. Nevertheless, a variety of novel research strategies were developed to overcome these difficulties [105], and the scientific community as a whole is enthusiastic about the prospect of discovering genetic associations which are entirely novel and are not influenced by knowledge existing in other areas of research.

3.2.2 Findings

3.2.2.1 Significant Associations

Table 3.1 summarizes *significant* genome-wide associations found in human studies that investigated traits associated with aggression. The table was based on a PubMed search with the search terms "genome-wide AND (aggression[Title/Abstract] OR violence[Title/Abstract])" and "genome-wide AND (crime[Title/Abstract] OR delinquency [Title/Abstract])" (searched 2019.05). The reference list of review publications and the "similar articles" window of PubMed abstract pages were also checked. Thus, efforts were made to cover the topic as exhaustively as possible. Studies pertaining to the psychological, psychiatric, and law enforcement approaches to aggression were presented together due to the small number of studies. Studies reporting "nominal" (i.e., non-significant) associations, studies in animals, and studies having a conceptual significance will be discussed separately.

Table 3.1 Significant genome-wide association studies for traits related to aggression

Chromosome number	Gene (rs number)	Role	Gender	Phenotype
1	ACBD6 [21]	Circulation [22]	Female	ASPD
1	LHX4 [21]	Development [23]	Female	ASPD
1	LHX4-AS1 [21]	Unknown	Female	ASPD
2	(rs11126630) [24]	Unknown	Both	Aggression
2	(rs11126630) [24]	Unknown	Both	Aggression
3	CCNL1 [25]	Unknown	Both	cSUD and CD
3	LEKR1 [25]	Unknown	Both	cSUD and CD
3	MECOM [26]	Proto-oncogene [27]	Both	Aggression
3 (3q24)	AGTR1 [25]	Circulation [28]	Both	cSUD and CD
3 (3q24)	PLSCR1 [25]	Apoptosis [29]	Both	cSUD and CD
4	C1QTNF7 [30]	Immunity [31]	Both	CD
4	LOC101929095 [30]	Unknown	Both	CD
6	(rs4714329) [32]	Unknown	Male	ASPD*
6	(rs9471290) [32]	Unknown	Male	ASPD*
6	(rs4714329) [33]	Unknown	Both	ASPD
9 (9q34)	LOC108281115 [25]	Unknown	Both	cSUD and CD
11	(rs7950811) [30]	Unknown	Both	CD
11	LOC105369506 [21]	Unknown	Female	ASPD
11	LOC105369506 [32]	Unknown	Female	ASPD†
12	AVPR1A [26]	**CNS** [34]	Both	Aggression
13	LINC00331 [35]	Unknown	Both	CD
16	RBFOX1 [35]	Development [36]	Both	Aggression
17	DEL17Q12 [25]	Unknown	Both	cSUD and CD
17	DUP17Q12 [25]	Unknown	Both	cSUD and CD
21	DYRK1A [37]	Development [38]	Both	Criminal offense
X	(rs41456347) [21]	Unknown	Male	ASPD
X	MAOA [32]	**CNS** [39]	Male	ASPD‡

Findings were ordered according to the number of the chromosome where the polymorphism was found. Numbers associated with additional information (e.g., 3q24) indicate the microsatellites studied

Gene identification. The gene was indicated only where the single-nucleotide polymorphism was within a known gene. For other DNA loci, we showed the "rs number," which stands for the reference single-nucleotide polymorphism cluster identity number. Indications of the type "nearby genes" (indicated by some authors) were disregarded, because non-coding regions may indeed influence a "nearby" gene, but such relationships are basically unknown. *Abbreviations*: *ACBD6* acyl-CoA-binding domain containing protein 6, *AGTR1* angiotensin II receptor type 1, *AVPR1A* vasopressin receptor 1A, *C1QTNF7* C1q and tumor necrosis factor-related protein 7, *CCNL1* cyclin L1, *D10Mit145* DNA segment, Chr 10, Massachusetts Institute of Technology (MIT) 145, *D15Mit46* DNA segment, Chr 15, MIT 46, *D5Mit254* DNA segment, Chr 5, MIT 254, *DYRK1A* dual specificity tyrosine phosphorylation-regulated kinase 1A, *LEKR1* leucine, glutamate and lysine-rich 1, *LHX4* LIM/homeobox protein Lhx4, *LHX4-AS1* LHX4 antisense RNA 1, *LINC00331* long intergenic non-protein coding RNA 331, *LOC105369506, LOC105369506, LOC108281115, LOC101929095* no other names, *MAOA* monoamine oxidase A, MECOM, MDS1, and EVI1 complex locus, *NTM* neurotrimin, *PLSCR1* phospholipid scramblase 1, *RBFOX1* fox-1 homolog A, *SPTLC3* serine palmitoyltransferase long-chain base subunit 3. *Aggression-related conditions*:

(continued)

Even a superficial look at the table suggests that the general features of GWAS (see section "*Background*") are also valid for associations with aggression for six reasons. First, the number of significant associations is very low. There were only 27 significant associations in all the studies we could find, each investigating hundreds of thousands of DNA loci. Indeed, statistical significance is a hurdle for discoveries. Second, there are practically no overlaps between studies. Each study discovered a unique association or set of associations. Third, a considerable share of associations is in non-coding regions (26%), or in coding regions with unknown roles (15%) (i.e., a combined share of 41%). Fourth, the rest of the associations refer to functions that cannot be directly linked to the brain mechanisms of aggression (52%). Fifth, only two studies (7%) found associations that can be interpreted in terms of underlying mechanisms (those referring to MAOA and AVPRT1). Finally, the effects on development and apoptosis may affect the neural circuits that underlie aggression, albeit indirectly. This aspect is especially important for the relevance of GWA findings (see below).

Animal studies do not necessarily improve the picture. A study in mice found that aggressiveness as measured by the intensity of inter-male aggression, a behavior closely linked to the biological approach to aggression, is associated with single-nucleotide polymorphisms in two genes suggestively called Aggr1 (aggression 1, chromosome 10) and Aggr2 (aggression 2, chromosome X) [40]. Findings were replicated by the same group in different mouse strains indicating that they are potentially reproducible [41]. The authors suggest that polymorphism at these loci affects five genes: Dagk1, Kif5a, and Olfr9 (Aggr1) and Gria3 and Hprt (Aggr2). According to the gene database of PubMed, however, Aggr1 and Aggr2 are DNA loci that do not associate with any known gene. The authors also suggested that these "aggression genes" are near a series of genes (e.g., MAOA), the products of which are implicated in the brain control of aggression. The possibility that a DNA locus affects a neighboring gene definitely exists; however, this interaction has not been proven for these two loci and the genes that are in their vicinity. As such, this study similar to the human studies presented in Table 3.1 describes two loci that are associated with aggression in an uncertain way. Even if we accepted the authors' conclusions regarding the affected genes, the role of the latter in aggression is not easy to understand. For instance, Dagk1 encodes diacylglycerol kinases, which are involved in the phosphatidylinositol signal transduction system that has a general

Table 3.1 (continued)

aggression publication-specific measure that differentiated aggressive from non-aggressive individuals, *ASPD* antisocial personality disorder, *CD* conduct disorder, *criminal offense* controls and study populations differentiated by criminal convictions, *cSUD* "criminal" substance use disorder, "criminal" being indicated by conduct disorder comorbidity. *Smoking by mother facilitated the association with ASPD; †maltreatment facilitated association with ASPD; ‡maltreatment weakened the association with ASPD. *Roles*. The role of the protein products of genes were only roughly indicated. *CNS* central nervous system. *References*. The column "Gene (rs number)" also contains references to studies that discovered the association. The column "Role" contains references to the roles of the protein product of the gene. The roles of genes were only summarily indicated; for more information, see the articles referred to

importance in neurotransmission [42], whereas Kif5a encodes the kinesin family member 5A, which is a molecular motor protein involved in the transport of membranous organelles along the axons of nerve cells, towards the synapse [43]. The Hprt gene encodes for hypoxanthine guanine phosphoribosyl transferase, associated with the Lesch-Nyhan syndrome which induces a series of behavioral abnormalities [44], whereas Gria 3 is associated with glutamateric neurotransmission. The link to aggression-related brain circuits is clear only in the latter case. Another study in mice found polymorphisms at DNA loci the function of which are poorly understood, particularly D5Mit254 (D5Mit254 DNA segment, Chr 5, and D10Mit145 (DNA segment, Chr 10) [45].

A study in fruit flies (*Drosophila melanogaster*) showed that aggression is associated with polymorphism in the gustatory receptor 63a (Gr63a), which encodes for a subunit of the receptor for CO_2 [46]. While one cannot exclude that chemoreception is important for aggression in flies, it is very unlikely that aggression depends mainly on gustatory receptors. A study in chickens revealed that aggressiveness is related to polymorphism in the gene SORCS2, which encodes the sortilin-related VPS10 domain containing receptor 2. The role of this receptor is unknown in birds. In mammals, however, it is involved in neural plasticity [47] and the development and regeneration of neuronal circuits [48]. Although these processes are only indirectly involved in the neural control of aggression, it is worth emphasizing that the protein still has effects on brain structure and consequently function. Finally, a study in dogs of diverse breeds found single-nucleotide polymorphisms in the genes for the high-mobility group AT-hook 2 (HMGA2, chromosome 10) and the insulin-like growth factor 1 (chromosome 15, IGF-1) [49]. Albeit neither protein is directly implicated in the brain mechanisms of aggression control, IGF-1 plays roles in in brain development, maturation, and neuroplasticity [50]. HMGA2 in its turn is involved in inflammation [51] but may also be involved in neural development, at least in lower animals [52]. This study [49] also identified polymorphisms in non-coding DNA regions on chromosomes 18 and X.

Taken together, human and animal GWAS *significantly* associated aggression with polymorphisms in (1) non-coding DNA regions, (2) coding regions with unknown roles, (3) coding regions related to processes that are unrelated to brain function and behavior, and (4) coding regions implicated in brain development and neural function. Although the latter may be promising, as argued below, the picture is rather disappointing because few studies identified genes controlling brain mechanisms of aggression. Candidate gene studies regularly find such associations as shown below, so why are they mostly missing from the results of GWAS studies?

3.2.2.2 Nominal Associations

One can hypothesize that the lack of associations with the putatively most important genes is explained by the difficulty of obtaining significant associations with GWAS technology. A solution to this problem would be to consider "nominal associations." This phrase indicates very low p values, which still do not cross the significance threshold after Bonferroni corrections. Although never stated explicitly, many studies have suggested in between lines that this approach is too strict and the researcher may violate the rules based on his/her judgment. Consequently, "nominal associations" are listed as findings in some studies and are perceived as information on the genetic underpinnings of aggression in certain reviews.

From a statistical point of view, this practice is entirely wrong. The many zeros in the expression $p < 0.00000001$ are misleading. Actually, this expression is equivalent with $p < 0.05$. Statistical significance is not *denied* by the Bonferroni correction. The correction was not invented to make the life of scientists difficult but was developed in the context of multiple comparisons. This means that the p value "0.00000001" is in fact just 0.05. Deceptively, p values in the 10^{-5}–10^{-7} range look very low but actually are several orders of magnitude *larger* than the p value that corresponds to 0.05. As such, they may indicate associations that are due to mere chance – at least the likelihood of this is high.

From a biological point of view, however, "nominal associations" may show something that is not revealed by studies that seek statistically significant associations. Aggression is a polygenic characteristic according to all four of the main approaches and is very likely that there is considerable individual variation regarding the genes affected (see above). Individual variations of this type may considerably lower the chance of finding statistically significant associations, which increases the discovery power of nominal associations. These may be associations that are valid for some individuals but not for many individuals. Those individuals, in which a particular polymorphism is not present, may show others that are also important.

To have a "feeling" on such "nominal" but potentially still important associations, we compared in Table 3.2 two studies, which reported nominal associations in two closely related psychiatric conditions (psychopathic and antisocial traits). One of the studies [53] found 30 such associations, with p value ranging from 0.005 to 0.00005, whereas the other [37] found 49 associations with p values ranging 0.00002–0.0000005.

This table looks as disappointing as the previous one for three reasons. First, there were virtually no overlaps between the two studies. Single-nucleotide polymorphisms were elsewhere according to rs numbers. In addition, polymorphism locations (rs identity, ID) coincident with a gene, were different in the two studies. Notably, the correspondence between the rs numbers and candidate genes was indicated by the authors, but we also checked this correspondence in the PubMed single-nucleotide database. Although small differences were observed, correspondences were reasonable overall. For example, correspondence was 70% in the first and 92% in the second study. Second, there were only two overlaps with the studies presented in the previous table where the trait–polymorphism association was significant (see Table 3.1). The genes in question were the dual specificity tyrosine phosphorylation-regulated kinase 1A (DYRK1A) and the RNA binding fox-1 homolog 1 (RBFOX1), both of which were shown to control development. This strengthens the notion that the association between aggression-related traits and polymorphisms is very poorly reproducible. Third, only one gene could be related to brain function, specifically the glutamate ionotropic receptor delta type subunit 2 (GRID2). In studies where the

Table 3.2 "Nominal associations" in two studies

Viding et al. [53]				Thielbeck et al. [37]			
	Gene name according to:				Gene name according to:		
rs ID	Author	Pubmed	Role	rs ID	Author	Pubmed	Role
10050093		GRID2	**CNS** [54]	11176629	–		
10103840		LOC105379351	Unknown	11860152	*COX4NB*	COX4NB	Unknown
10859716		LOC102724960	Unknown	11866179	*COX4NB*	COX4NB	Unknown
11088618				11901615			
11637779				11956931	*STK32A*	STK32A	Unknown
11682518	ARL6IP6		Nucleus [55]	12106331	*DYRK1A*	**DYRK1A**	Development [38]
12411132	KCND3	KCND3	Heart [56]	13202756	*AL590874.1*		Unknown
12647756				1385551	*VRK1*		*Nucleus* [57]
12761718				1657978			
13064369	ROBO2	ROBO2	Cell [57]	1676146			
1345959	BNIP3		Mitoch [58].	17008528			
1441990				17510310	*REEP1*	REEP1	Mitoch [60].
1490666	DCHS2	DCHS2	Cell [61]	17722374	*RP11*	–	*cell* [62]
17835633	CDKAL1	CDKAL1	Unknown	2277512	*TTC7B*	TTC7B	Unknown
1893815		LOC105369406	Unknown	2835702	*DYRK1A*	–	
2311846				2835771	*DYRK1A*	**DYRK1A**	Development [38]
2376016	LEPR	LEPR	Apetite [63]	2917849			
2514788	CDH17	CDH17	Cell [64]	346425			
293844				346431			
41516949	TBC1D14	TBC1D14	Cell [65]	349493			
4241597	SEPT11	SEPT11	Cell [66]	369747			
4383690		LINC02173	Unknown	373666			
4479686	FAM160A1	FAM160A1	Unknown	3751656	*SEMA4B*	SEMA4B	Unknown

6446569				3771684	*BAZ2B*	BAZ2B	Nucleus [67]
6560704				3829490	*CIB1*	CIB1	Cell [68]
6846114	PET112L	PET112L	Unknown	386661			
7531603				387996			
7640807	BTD	BTD	Cell [69]	392246			
8059231		**RBFOX1**	Development [36]	401859			
9343557		LOC101928570	Unknown	409363			
				418226			
				424672			
				427421			
				434640			
				443543			
				444037			
				455575			
				458362			
				460325			
				460949			
				462861			
				6119363	*C20orf114*	C20orf114	Immunity [70]
				6558776	*CSMD1*	CSMD1	n
				7561888	*IMMT*	IMMT	Mitoch [71].
				775313			
				896253	*COX4NB*	COX4NB	Unknown
				9287528			
				942746	*TTC7B*	TTC7B	Unknown
				9920862			

(continued)

Table 3.2 (continued)

Findings were ordered according to *rs ID* (the reference single-nucleotide polymorphism cluster identity number) the location of the polymorphism found. When the polymorphism is within a gene, the name of the gene was also indicated. ***Bold font***: genes identified earlier as significantly associating with a measure of aggression. Note that only two such genes can be found in the table

Gene identification. *ARL6IP6* ADP ribosylation factor like GTPase 6 interacting protein 6, *BAZ2B* bromodomain adjacent to zinc finger domain 2B, *BNIP3* BCL2 interacting protein 3, *BPI* fold containing family B member 1, *BTD* biotinidase, *CDH17* cadherin 17, *CDKAL1* CDK5 regulatory subunit associated protein 1 like 1, *CIB1* calcium and integrin binding 1, *COX4NB* ER membrane protein complex subunit 8, *COX4NB* ER membrane protein complex subunit 8, *CSMD1* CUB and Sushi multiple domains 1, *DCHS2* dachsous cadherin-related 2, *DYRK1A* dual specificity tyrosine phosphorylation-regulated kinase 1A, *FAM160A1* family with sequence similarity 160 member A1, *GRID2* glutamate ionotropic receptor delta type subunit 2, *IMMT* inner membrane mitochondrial protein, *KCND3* potassium voltage-gated channel subfamily D member 3, *LEPR* leptin receptor, *LINC02173* long intergenic non-protein coding RNA 2173, *LOC101928570*; *LOC102724960*; *LOC105369406*; *LOC105379351* no other name, *PET112L* glutamyl-tRNA amidotransferase subunit B, *RBFOX1* RNA binding fox-1 homolog 1, *REEP1* receptor accessory protein 1, *ROBO2* roundabout guidance receptor 2, *RP11* pre-mRNA processing factor 31, *SEMA4B* sema domain, immunoglobulin domain (Ig), transmembrane domain (TM), and short cytoplasmic domain, (semaphorin) 4B, *SEPT11* septin 11, *STK32A* serine/threonine kinase 32A, *TBC1D14* TBC1 domain family member 14, *TTC7B* tetratricopeptide repeat domain 7B, *VRK1* VRK serine/threonine kinase

Roles. The roles of the protein products of genes were only roughly indicated. *Cell* effects on the cytoskeleton, on functional proteins playing roles in cellular processes, etc., *CNS* central nervous system, *nucleus* proteins of the nuclear membrane, transcription factors, etc., *heart*, *immunity*, etc. protein products playing various roles, e.g., affecting cardiac transient outwards potassium current, *mitoch.* mitochondrial proteins regulating contacts with other organelles or mitochondrial processes

References. The reference to the two studies reviewed were shown in headings. References to roles are shown in the respective column

association was significant (i.e., in the previous section), two central nervous system-related genes were found, but both were different from GRID2. A gene for glutamatergic neurotransmission was found in mouse studies, albeit this was Gria3 not Grid2. (Note that these genes are present in both humans and mice and are differentiated by the capital letters in the abbreviation of human genes.) Thus, genes controlling brain function and those involved in the brain control of aggression are notably missing from GWAS. Importantly, nevertheless, genes involved in development and cell function in general are widely represented.

3.2.2.3 The Specificity of Associations

Aggression and violent crime are not the main targets of GWAS. On the contrary, there are very few GWAS studies of aggression compared to other areas of research. Most studies address the genetic underpinnings of diseases, particularly cancer. For instance, the search term "genome-wide [title/abstract] AND cancer [title/abstract]" returned almost 10,000 hits, which is well above the number of studies on aggression-related GWAS (search date 2019.05).

Interestingly, polymorphisms associated with aggression are often associated with completely different traits. One example is the development-related polymorphism of the gene LHX4, which associated significantly with antisocial traits (see Table 3.1) but also showed associations with lung cancer [72]. The RBFOX1 gene significantly associated with aggression was also associated with the responsiveness to the antipsychotic lurasidone [73], with susceptibility to rheumatoid arthritis in African Americans [74], and testicular cancer [75]. Even the most promising hit AVPR1A, which controls aggression via its effects on vasopressin neurotransmission [76], was also associated with blood pressure [77], and female infidelity [78]. Other genes from the Tables 3.1 and 3.2 are no better. Without unnecessarily going into details, one can state with confidence that all genes are "polymaths," and each is associated with many different traits.

Consequently, genome-wide associations for aggressiveness (aggression-related mental disorders, violent crime) are very far from being specific to aggression. On the contrary, these genes are associated with a series of very different traits. At the first sight, such findings question the utility of GWAS at least from the point of view of aggression and violent crime.

3.2.3 *Interpretation: Making Sense of Senseless Associations*

As shown above, aggression-related GWAS identify DNA loci, which encode for the following: (i) nothing according to present knowledge; (ii) something, but the role of this "something" is largely unknown; (iii) products that do not seem to be linked to neuronal communication; (iv) different genes in each study (findings are practically irreproducible); and (v) genes that are highly nonspecific to aggression as they are associated with a number of widely different conditions. Although those who run GWAS are very enthusiastic and highly optimistic regarding the future and utility of the technique, independent observers feel compelled to ask the following question: Did GWAS contribute to our understanding of aggression in any way?

Although one may feel the temptation to answer this question with a "No," one may be wrong, because a deeper analysis suggests that GWAS are important despite appearances. We advance below three hypotheses, which attempt to explain the problems outlined above, and tentatively integrate GWAS into the valid research which aims to understand the genetics of aggression. Before entering into details, however, we stress that non-coding regions and poorly understood gene products are in our opinion of little concern and will not be discussed below. One must acknowledge that genetics – despite its spectacular advancements in the past few decades – still has some secrets and mysteries. Future discoveries will likely explain currently unknown phenomena. The lack of directly relevant neural communication-related genes in GWAS lists is more disturbing in our view.

3.2.3.1 The "Incidence-Driven Chance" Hypothesis

This hypothesis attempts to explain why GWAS find so few associations with genes relevant from a neurobiological point of view. As mentioned above, the brain mechanisms of aggression are fairly well understood, and one would expect to see on GWAS lists those genes that generate proteins related to neuronal communication. Such genes may encode for enzymes, which produce neurotransmitters, or neurotransmitter receptors, transporters, etc. GWAS did find association with such genes but only rarely. Of the 114 associations revealed by the studies briefly reviewed above, only 4 (3.5%) encoded for proteins that may have a role in the neural control of aggression (significant and nominal association and animal and human studies combined). Most surprisingly, no significant associations were found for genes involved in dopaminergic, noradrenergic, and serotonergic neurotransmission, although these are deeply involved in the control of aggression. Genes related to the stress response are also lacking from the association lists of GWAS. One explanation to this curious phenomenon would be that the involvement of these in aggression is not controlled at the level of the genes; that is, it is not related to single-nucleotide gene polymorphisms. This is an attractive assumption but an illusion. If aggression was not controlled at the level of single-nucleotide genes, then why did more focused approaches such as candidate gene studies find a great number of polymorphisms on dopamine-, norepinephrine-, serotonin-, and stress-related genes in aggressive individuals?

The question may be asked more simply. Why do genes relevant for neural communication almost always show *significant* associations with aggression in candidate gene studies but almost never in GWAS? [79] Why are such genes mostly missing from the list of *nominal* associations? Although this contradiction cannot be explained at present, a hint may come from studies that classify genes according to the function of their protein products. These studies show that the number of genes underlying neuronal communication is very low compared to the number of those which have other functions [80, 81]. The overwhelming majority of genes encode proteins involved in translation and transcription (gene function), proteins that contribute to the making of the cytoskeleton, cell adhesion molecules, transport, and other protein types. Very few encode for signaling molecules. Moreover, there are still fewer "signaling molecules" which are directly involved in neural communication. Most signaling molecules are intracrine, autocrine, juxtacrine, paracrine, and endocrine factors, neuropeptides, growth factors, cytokines, and members of intracellular signaling pathways, like proteases, phosphorylases, messengers, etc. [82]. The number of genes encoding for such proteins grossly exceeds those that are directly involved in neural communication. One can hypothesize that they are prominent in GWAS studies simply due to their large number.

Looking at it from the other side, one can hypothesize that GWAS "lose sight" of the genes that are important from a neurobiological and neurobehavioral point of view. They fail to record polymorphisms in genes involved in neural communication because these are very few compared to other classes of genes. Consequently, one needs more targeted techniques such as candidate gene studies to find them. If true, this hypothesis ascribes GWAS findings to chance to a certain extent and suggests that GWAS are able to find single-nucleotide polymorphisms within the very large number of genes only accidentally, and the probability of finding an association is inversely proportional with the number of genes belonging to a certain type. As such, it is rather difficult to find single-nucleotide polymorphisms within a class of genes as rare as those that code for molecules involved in neural communication. In a way, this hypothesis may also explain why the findings of GWAS are so difficult to reproduce. Individual genes encoding subgroups of proteins are just as difficult to replicate as neural communication-related genes. As such, this hypothesis attributes GWAS a chance factor, which favors the finding of associations for frequent gene types on the expense of rarer ones.

3.2.3.2 "Pleiotropy by Neuronal Development" Hypothesis

This hypothesis aims to explain why aggression is so frequently associated with single-nucleotide polymorphisms that are also associated with other, often very different traits. We assumed above that such multiple associations are due to pleiotropy, the ability of genes to underlie several traits simultaneously.

In some instances, such pleiotropies are easily understandable, because the genes often encode for proteins that are used by the organism in different places and in different contexts. As an example, the vasopressin 1A receptor (VR_{1A}, encoded by AVPR1A) can be found on the membrane of smooth muscle cells in blood vessels, where they mediate the vasopressor (blood pressure-heightening) effects of vasopressin [83]. At the same time, however, the VR_{1A} can be found on various segments of the circuits that control aggression and affiliative behavior [34]. So, it is unsurprising that polymorphisms of the AVPR1 gene associate with aggression [76], blood pressure [77], and female infidelity [78], the latter being a social affiliation-related phenomenon. This pleiotropy is due on one hand to the fact that vasopressin is used as a communication tool by endocrine, paracrine, and neuronal cells concomitantly. On the other, its receptors are expressed by a variety of cells, e.g., muscle, endocrine, and neuronal cells. The number of such understandable pleiotropic traits is relatively large, and understanding these poses no problem.

In other cases, however, the common pleiotropic mechanisms cannot be easily envisaged. Is there, for instance, any explanation for the significant association between conduct disorder and the polymorphisms of the gene for "C1q and tumor necrosis factor-related protein 7" (encoded by C1QTNF7)? [36]. All we know is that the protein may play a role in inflammatory processes elicited by amyotrophic lateral sclerosis in humans [31] and in fat deposition in sheep [84]. This information is very difficult to reconcile with conduct disorder! To take a better-known gene and gene product, we refer to the ACBD6 gene, which encodes for "acyl-CoA-binding domain containing protein 6," which regulates processes as diverse as viral replication, stem cell self-renewal, organelle organization, and protein acylation [85]. At a molecular level, the protein stimulates the covalent attachment of a 14-carbon aliphatic tail on a glycine residue of nascent translated peptide chains [86]. It is very difficult if not practically impossible at present to imagine the long chain of causative relationships by which polymorphisms of this gene can associate with antisocial personality disorder. Yet, this association was found to be significant [21].

Clues on how such highly specialized proteins can affect behavior come from studies where genome-wide associations were looked for several traits in parallel. For instance, a single-nucleotide polymorphism in the RBFOX1, which encodes for "fox-1 homolog A," is associated with both aggression in conduct disorder and temporal lobe volume [35]. The gene product is in fact a splicing regulator, i.e., a protein that removes introns (non-coding regions) from messenger RNA, making the joining of exons possible [35]. We do not know how this process can affect aggression. We know, however, that the temporal lobe is deeply involved in aggression. For example, temporal lobe epilepsy is frequently associated with aggressiveness and more specifically with intermittent explosive disorder [87]. As such, the molecular role of the gene product cannot be related to aggression, but its neural "side effect" may explain the behavioral consequences of single-nucleotide polymorphisms in this gene.

A similar association was found for the gene MECOM, which is involved in the development of various cancer types [88, 89]. MECOM (also called EVI1) is in fact a transcription factor [90], which can hardly be linked to aggression according to present knowledge. Nevertheless, it was shown that its single-nucleotide polymorphisms are associated with both aggression and the volume of the nucleus accumbens [26], a brain area that is implicated in aggression via reinforcement [91]. Again, we do not know how the molecular roles of the gene affect aggression, but its neural "side effect" may give an explanation.

Another occurrence of "association explained by another association" may be exemplified by the AVPR1 gene. As shown above, the pleiotropic effects of this gene can fully explain its involvement in aggression and other traits. In addition to these mechanistic explanations, a single-nucleotide polymorphism in AVPR1 co-associates with aggression and amygdala volume [26]. As the role of the amygdala in aggression is well-known, one can hypothesize that AVPR1 influences aggression not only via the VR_{1A} receptors located on the aggression circuitry but also by affecting the development of the amygdala.

All these examples converge on one factor when the implications of single-nucleotide polymorphisms are being evaluated. In addition to the role played by a gene in adult animals, the very same gene may also affect neuronal development much earlier, even at embryonic stages.

Neuronal development is a highly complex process that will not be reviewed here. We will give, however, a few examples which demonstrate that proteins with well-described roles in adult organisms can affect development in a counterintuitive way. In adults, the bone morphogenetic protein 7, encoded by the gene BMP7 plays a role in the transformation of mesenchymal cells into bone and cartilage, thereby affecting bone homeostasis [92]. Surprisingly, however, the very same gene controls the development of the brain cortex during embryonic life [93]. The cyclin-dependent kinase p57Kip2 is a tumor suppressor gene in adults [94], but the very same gene significantly contributes to neural differentiation during embryonic life [95]. Finally, the monoamine oxidase A (MAO_A) gene, which encodes for an enzyme that degrades monoamines in the central nervous system (norepinephrine, serotonin, and dopamine) and consequently plays important roles in aggression [96], is also involved in the ontogenetic development of the prostate [97]. If the first discovery were that the MAOA is a factor in prostate development, today we would wonder how it could play a role in aggression. Some of the polymorphisms that associate with various indices of aggression are on genes that are known to play roles primarily in development (see Tables 3.1 and 3.2). In addition to DYRK1A, LHX4, and RBFOX1, primarily involved in development, there are others, which have other primary roles, but also affect neural development. In addition to MAOA, this was shown for AVP1R [98], GRID2 [99], HMGA2 [52], IGF-1 [50], LEPR [100], ROBO1 [101], and SORCS2 [47]. Thus, at least 11 of the genes that were associated with aggression affect brain development. This number is not very large but considering the large share of associations with unknown or poorly known DNA loci may allow generalization. Genes with dual roles suggest that genetic effects on the development of the neural system may explain unusual associations between single-nucleotide polymorphisms and aggression. The genes involved may not only be pleiotropic because the proteins they encode are involved in a large number of processes. They might be pleiotropic because they affect brain structure, including those circuits that underlie aggression. Such effects are likely structural rather than functional. They affect neural communication not by encoding for the synthesis, reception and elimination of neurotransmitters but by encoding for general particularities of neurons and circuits. Such general neuronal traits may include cortical thickness in regions relevant for aggression control, the volume of particular brain regions, brain area connectivity, synapse mobility, cytoskeletal properties, the efficacy of transcription and translation, proneness to epigenetic influences, etc.

As such, genome-wide associations that apparently have no link to aggression but still show significant associations with it may reflect effects on neural development and may contribute to the development of the circuits that control aggression. Such genes may influence the hardware of behavioral control.

3.2.4 "Quality by Quantity" Hypothesis

This hypothesis aims at explaining why findings are so difficult to reproduce and at drawing attention on a new approach that may resolve the problem.

As shown above, the number of DNA loci associated with aggression is likely very large, but only a subgroup of them may be necessary for the expression of the trait. This suggests that the genetic underpinnings of aggression are heterogeneous at individual level so that individuals with similar aggressive phenotypes may not be necessarily similar as it regards the placement and number of single-nucleotide polymorphisms they carry. This assumption is supported by a study on extreme impulsive aggression where almost half of the subjects showed copy number variations [102] (i.e., the number of repeats within repetitive gene segments showed individual variations), suggesting that these copy variations have roles in aggression. The mere presence of this copy number variation correlated significantly with aggression. This suggests that investigating the *frequency* of genetic variations at individual level may be more informative than evaluating the share of particular genetic variations within a population [103].

The authors adopting this strategy use GWAS only to generate polygenic scores, which are summations of genetic differences found in an individual compared to controls. In this case, researchers establish an association between a trait on one hand and a composite score of genetic differences on the other. Consequently, variation in a trait is explained by the number rather than by the nature of genetic differences. The approach appears viable in other areas of research and may also be applicable in aggression. For instance, polygenic scores predicted aggression in subjects comorbid for attention-deficit/hyperactivity and conduct disorders [104]. In another study, polygenic scores for academic attainment, i.e., which predicted education success, predicted at the time criminal record rather accurately [105]. Yet another study investigated the interaction between polygenic scores and social conditions and found significant associations between polygenic scores, aggression, and low family cohesion [106].

This approach, which so far has only been used sporadically, has the disadvantage of losing the connection between the finding and its biological significance. A mere number cannot be linked to biological functions. This drawback is somewhat diminished by the fact that GWAS are no better in general. Both approaches have provided little mechanistically relevant information so far. Despite being mechanistically irrelevant, such studies clearly illustrate that a certain number of genetic polymorphisms disrupt brain function, which probably together with other consequences increase the propensity to behave aggressively. As such, the quality looked for aggression is explained by a quantity, e.g., the total number of single-nucleotide polymorphisms.

It is notable that this approach offers a new type of analysis for GWAS, although this possibility has not been explored so far. Studies may look for genetic variance constellations that are specific to aggression, may identify "leading" polymorphisms, interactions between various polymorphisms, and ultimately may potentially make sense of seemingly senseless associations. In conclusion, in the future inferences from GWAS may focus on aggregate, gene-level analyses, rather than on trying to make causative inferences from single-nucleotide polymorphism-level analyses. Potentially, this new approach may reveal the role of polymorphism constellations rather than trying to establish the roles of particular polymorphisms. Several new approaches already exploit this route in the field of aggression research [107, 108] and may revolutionize our view on the genetics of aggression. We will come back to this issue in the last section of this chapter.

3.3 Candidate Gene Association Studies

In contrast to GWAS, which survey vast areas of the DNA indiscriminately, candidate gene association studies are focused: they look for associations where there should be associations. If the reasons for performing the study were reliable, the genes investigated become in fact candidates for a successful research project.

Sometimes, a gene becomes a candidate simply by chance. For instance, Brunner, who discovered the most famous "aggression gene," when he discovered the role of the gene for the MAO_A enzyme in aggression, in fact looked for X chromosome determinants of intellectual disability [109]. The authors had good reasons for investigating this gene for intellectual disability. By the time of their investigations, there already were many X chromosome-related genetic conditions associated with intellectual disability, and, based on urine samples performed in a family with congenital intellectual disability, it was reasonable to look into genes affecting norepinephrine, serotonin, and dopamine metabolism. Note that the MAOA gene is located on the X chromosome, and encodes the common degrading enzyme of these neurotransmitters. The role of MAOA in intellectual disabilities was indeed confirmed by subsequent studies; however, the extraordinary career of the gene started when a subsequent publication by an overlapping set of authors revealed that all those who were subject to the deleterious effects of a point mutation in the MAOA also had a dramatic record for violent crime [110].

With few exceptions, however, a gene becomes a candidate if we have a good reason to believe that its product affects a trait, and so we decide to target it specifically. This approach is evidence-driven, a word combination that is very appealing to scientists. Building new lines of research on existing knowledge is risky to a certain extent, as shown in the previous section, as it may bar the road to entirely new discoveries. At the same time, however, candidate gene analyses add a new dimension to earlier neuroscientific discoveries and avoid the statistical and the methodological traps of GWAS.

Typically, being extensions of neuroscientific studies, candidate gene studies have the potential of answering the question whether brain functional differences are inherited and if so, to what extent. Thus, they explain aggression in a biologically relevant way, which was seldom true for GWAS. The road from genetic discovery to biological knowledge is open – at least in theory.

3.3.1 Background

The general schematic of GWAS and candidate gene approaches is similar. Scientists study groups that differ in their phenotypes. For example, one research group showed higher scores in aggression inventories than the comparison group. One of the groups was incarcerated for violent crimes whereas the other was not, etc. Subsequently, researchers genotype subjects and look for polymorphism frequencies in the study groups. If these differed significantly, then researchers assume that the phenotype was associated with the genotype.

At the same time, the two approaches differ in several important respects. Candidate gene association studies focus on a few genes in contrast to GWAS that may survey millions of DNA loci. This simplifies the statistics and allows for the assessment of multiple genotype–phenotype associations and for the study of more than two groups. The low number of investigated genes also allows for lower sample sizes, which enables researchers to consider environmental influences more easily. Although this is possible with GWAS, such gene x environment interactions are investigated in the case of the candidate gene approach as a rule. Furthermore, one can investigate several such interactions in parallel. For instance, one can test whether a particular polymorphism associates with aggression in interaction with stressful life events or family functioning. By doing this, one differentiates critical from irrelevant environmental influences. Finally, the gene-focused approach allows for investigating genetic variations other than single-nucleotide polymorphisms (see below). Scanning the whole or a major part of the genome concomitantly for several types of polymorphisms is time-consuming and costly; thus, GWAS authors usually restrict their investigations to single-nucleotide polymorphisms that are relatively easy to study. The candidate gene approach enables researchers to choose the type of polymorphism that is most appropriate for a particular gene, and they can study several types of polymorphisms in parallel. Taken together candidate gene analyses are technically more flexible and provide more detailed results.

Another important difference between the two genetic approaches derives from the neurobiological foundations of the choice of candidate genes. Usually it is known how a particular polymorphism affects the function of the gene or its product, which enables pertinent assumptions about its biological consequences. In most cases, these assumptions are checked experimentally. This is important because genes do not code for behaviors but determine the structure and function of proteins that are essential to the neuronal processes that underlie behavior. Thus, candidate genes fill the gap between genetics and neural function, which is rarely the case with GWAS.

A full overview of candidate gene studies is beyond the scope of this book; therefore, we decided to employ a different approach. We will focus on the purportedly most important genes and will investigate on one hand their involvement in aggression, aggression-related psychopathologies, and violent crime, whereas on the other hand, we will investigate their involvement in non-aggressive psychological features, non-aggression-related mental disorders, and non-violent crime. This approach would allow the answering of two important questions, namely, (i) Do candidate gene polymorphisms differentiate the three main types to aggression? And (ii) Is the genetics of aggression specific to aggression? Those who work in this field rarely ask these questions, but we consider answering them more important than providing a complete list of genes and studies on the subject.

Before addressing these questions, however, we will investigate whether there are genes with "full" efficacy, which alone can dramatically affect aggressiveness.

3.3.2 *Findings*

3.3.2.1 The Quest for the "Warrior Gene"

The first and to date the most suspected candidate for an "omnipotent" aggression gene is the MAOA, sometimes also nicknamed the "warrior gene." (See next section for a detailed description of the gene and its functions.) It was shown by Brunner et al. [110] that all the members of a Dutch family who carried a dysfunctional form of the gene had a long history of violent crime. The main point was that there were no exceptions; those who had normal MAOA genes did not differ from the general population, whereas those who had a dysfunctional MAOA were aggressive. In the enthusiasm of the discovery, the authors went as far as to propose that "the frequency of MAOA deficiency in the population has to be determined," and "one could ask whether aggressive behavior is confined to complete MAOA deficiency" (*p.* 580). Later developments dampened enthusiasm a bit. A relatively recent review categorized the finding as "never replicated," [111] and we know of no replication since this review. A study focusing on X chromosome-linked intellectual disabilities found just one family out of 251 where a genetic mutation rendered both the MAOA and MAOB genes dysfunctional [112]. Note that the study by Brunner et al., the MAOB was not mentioned. The siblings of this MAOA-/MAOB-deficient family showed developmental delay, intermittent decreases in blood pressure, and stereotypical hand movements. No aggression was reported. Two further studies, reporting on two MAOA-/MAOB-deficient individuals each, recounted essentially the same deficits. Neither mentioned aggression [113, 114]. A recent study reporting on one single case of Xp11.3–11.4 mutations that affected among others the MAOA gene also revealed serious problems, which, however, did not include aggression [115].

The findings briefly reviewed above do not support the "warrior gene" status of MAOA, despite the fact that almost all studies on the genetics of aggression mention this gene as a still viable candidate. There are two reasons: (i) the gene deficit is as rare as nobody found a similar one ever since; the studies referred to above found deficits in both MAO genes. (ii) The co-occurrence of the gene deficit and aggression cannot be rendered causal as long as the original findings are not replicated, and the dual MAOA/MAOB deficits were not associated with aggression problems.

We emphasize that no study questioned the role MAOA in aggression so far. MAOA-knockout mice, i.e., mice lines where the gene was made dysfunctional experimentally, are more aggressive than their controls [116], and MAOA polymorphisms are regularly associated with aggression. (See below.) However, MAOA polymorphisms decrease the activity of the MAO_A enzyme rather than abolishing it, which is a large difference from the deleterious MAOA mutation. According to present knowledge, the MAOA is just one of the many cases of gene x environment interactions that affect aggression.

To our best knowledge, no gene was proposed to overtake the "warrior gene" status from the MAOA, and no gene dysfunction discovered to date would lead to aggression unconditionally. As such, we have to abandon the idea of "warrior genes" and focus on less spectacular genetic effects on aggression.

3.3.2.2 Gene Polymorphisms

As indicated above, the number of candidate gene association studies is huge, making it practically impossible to review the issue entirely. Here we will focus on three genes, specifically the MAOA that codes for the enzyme MAO_A and two genes that code for dopamine receptors. These are among the most studied candidate genes in gene association studies. What we lost in width (the number of genes investigated), we will try to regain in depth: the few genes selected will be discussed in detail. We will also present a few other important genes but more succinctly. In addition, we will briefly review the role of genes that code for cell adhesion molecules. Although data are scarce in this regard, the issue seems important because such molecules are among the very few where the target of candidate gene association studies was not neurotransmission.

The MAOA gene codes for MAO_A, a mitochondrial enzyme that catalyzes the deamination (deactivation) of the biogenic amines dopamine, norepinephrine, and serotonin in the brain. These are called monoamines. MAO_A also deaminates other compounds in the brain and elsewhere, but this is not important here. The enzyme is more effective with serotonin and norepinephrine than with dopamine. The latter is metabolized mainly by another enzyme, monoamine oxidase B (MAO_B). MAOA has a series of polymorphisms, which either affects the readability of the gene (affect the amount of the protein product) or confers a higher or a lower efficacy to the enzyme that it encodes. Due to the popularity of the enzyme, the number of studies investigating its role is very large. Therefore, we limited our focus to one particular type, particularly to variable number tandem repeat polymorphisms. These are in the promoter region of the enzyme, i.e., where the first step of protein secretion, e.g., transcription, is initiated. In this region, short nucleotide sequences are repeated, and the repetitions are directly adjacent to each other (tandem repeats). The number of repetitions show individual variation that affects the functionality of the gene, which gives rise to variants with a low or a high transcriptional activity, which leads to more or less enzymes in the cell [117].

When considering the evidence for $MAO_{A,}$ three facts should be considered. First, neither of the MAOA polymorphisms renders the gene dysfunctional as with the above-mentioned Dutch family. MAO_A activity may be lower or higher, but there always are functional MAO_A enzymes in the organism. Second, low MAO_A activity enhances monoamine neurotransmission because of a decreased degradation rate, and, conversely, high MAO_A activity diminishes it. Consequently, the MAOA-low activity genotype leads to enhanced norepinephrine and serotonin neurotransmission. Dopamine may also be affected, but with an intact MAO_B activity, this is of smaller magnitude. Finally, although some authors emphasize serotonin as the subject of MAOA deficiencies, norepinephrine and serotonin are equally affected, and there might be an effect on dopamine as well. For associations between MAOA polymorphisms and aggression, see Table 3.3.

The findings briefly reviewed in the table show that the MAOA gene does not differentiate the various types of aggression, which were conceptualized here as the psychological, psychiatric, and criminological approaches to aggression. All three of these are associated with the low-activity polymorphisms of the MAOA gene, when variable number tandem repeat polymorphisms were studied. It is notable that other variants of the MAOA gene that decrease the functionality of the enzyme, e.g., single-nucleotide polymorphisms, lead to similar conclusions [154]. While MAOA genotypes do not differentiate aggression types, they seem to differentiate aggression-related from other phenotypes. Table 3.3 presents a wide array of aggression-unrelated psychological traits, mental disorders, and crimes, in which either no associations were found with MAOA genotypes or the association was of the opposite type. Anxiety and depression, for instance, were associated with the genotype that conferred high functionality to the MAO_A. The main exceptions were feelings that are tightly linked to aggressiveness, e.g., anger, hostility, and impulsiveness. Some other exceptions also exist; we will come back to this when we interpret the findings in their totality.

In conclusion, low MAO_A activity is associated with aggression in general. As low MAO_A functioning enhances all three norepinephrine, serotonin, and dopamine neurotransmission, the latter only to a lesser degree, the interpretation of this finding is partly explainable and partly inexplicable. Norepinephrine enhances aggression and aggression-related bodily and neural functions [155] which explains why the downregulated MAOA genotype increases aggression. Serotonin by contrast is considered to be the sine qua non "anti-aggressive" neurotransmitter [156] which is at variance with the genotype–phenotype associations reviewed above. High serotonin availability that should result from low MAO_A activity in theory should decrease aggression, yet the low MAOA variant associates with increased aggression. Finally, dopamine is one of the neurotransmitters that contribute to the expression of aggression [157] which is again in line with the findings reviewed above. Thus, the scorecard shows two to one: MAOA gene association studies are consistent with two lines of neuroscientific evidence and are at variance with the third. Importantly, the

Table 3.3 The association of variable number tandem repeat polymorphisms in the promoter region of the MAOA gene with aggression-related and other traits

Aggression (Psychological, psychiatric, and criminological meaning)		Other traits	
Phenotype	Genotype	Phenotype	Genotype
Aggression, lifetime	↓ [118]	Anger	↓ [119]
Aggression, reactive	↓ [120]	Hostility	↓ [121]
Aggression, dating	↓ [122]	Impulsiveness	↓ [123]
Aggression in autism	↓ [124]	Non-violent suicidality	↓ [125]
		Lack of cooperation	↓ [126]
		Spatial memory	↑ [127]
		Agitation	Ø [128]
		Cooperativeness	Ø [129]
		Harm avoidance	Ø [129, 130]
		Novelty seeking	Ø [129, 130]
		Persistence	Ø [129]
		Reward dependence	Ø [129, 130]
		Sleepiness	Ø [131]
Attention-deficit/hyperactivity disorder	↓ [132]	Autism spectrum disorder	↓ [133]
Attention-deficit/hyperactivity disorder +Conduct disorder*	↓ [134]	Alcoholism	↓ [135]
Antisocial personality disorder*	↓ [136]	Pathological gambling	↓ [137]
Conduct disorder	↓ [138]	Autism spectrum disorder	↑ [138]
Oppositional defiant disorder	↓ [140]	Depression	↑ [141]
Psychopathic traits	↓ [142]	Panic disorder	↑ [143]
		Anxiety disorders	↑ [144]
		Substance use disorder	↑ [145]
		Schizophrenia	Ø [146]
Criminal behavior (including violence)	↓ [147]	Property offence*	↓ [148]
Violent crime (murder, battery, etc.)	↓ [149]	Property offense*	↓ [150]
Violent crime (shooting, stabbing)	↓ [151]	Drug selling, fire setting, etc.	Ø [152]
Violent crime (repeated, extreme)	↓ [153]	Property, drug driving, etc.*	Ø [154]
Violent crime (assault, fighting)*	↓ [148]		
Violent crime (physical attacks)*	↓ [152]		

Other MAOA polymorphisms were not reviewed here (see text for the reasons)

↓ the trait associates with the MAOA-low activity variant, ↑ the trait associates with the MAOA-high activity variant, Ø no association between the MAOA genotype and phenotype. *Significant only in gene–environment interaction. Where not indicated, the genotype association was investigated irrespective to environmental influences or was significant alone (main effect). References were indicated in the "Genotype" column. Note that violent and non-violent offending were investigated sometimes in the same study (recognizable by reference numbers), which increases the reliability of differences due to the similarity of the methodology employed

association of the MAOA-high genotype with depression and anxiety is in line with the noradrenaline–serotonin deficiency in these disorders, which are ameliorated among others by MAO_A inhibitors [158]. As such, the scorecard in fact shows 4 of 5.

We stress that the findings reviewed above do not restore the "warrior gene" status to MAOA. The associations presented above are significant but are not absolute. Many people have poorly functioning MAOAs without being aggressive, whereas other people are aggressive despite a normal MAOA functionality. We will come back to this issue later.

Dopamine receptors are almost as popular among aggression researchers as the MAOA, likely because of the important role of dopamine in aggression as will be shown in the neural system section. The most intensely studied polymorphisms, especially in aggression research are the following. The first is a single-nucleotide polymorphism in the Taq1 region of the gene encoding the dopamine 2 receptor (D2). The name of the gene is DRD2. There are two polymorphisms at this site, called the A1 *and* A2 allele*s*. The DRD2-A1 genotype is considered the "problem" variant as it is associated with fewer D2 receptors in the brain [159, 160] and also decreases the activity of the receptor (e.g., ligand binding) [161]. As such, D2 functions are downregulated in the DRD2-A1 as compared with the DRD2-A2 genotype. The second gene polymorphism reviewed here is the variable–number tandem repeat polymorphism in the DRD4 gene, which encodes the dopamine 4 receptor (D4). This polymorphism is of the same type that was studied with respect to MAOA, but it is on the DRD4 gene. The number of repeats varies between two and ten. Generally speaking, longer alleles are associated with diminished D4 receptor function [162], although the impact of the variants are not fully understood [163]. Some attribute specific features to particular alleles, e.g., the 7-repeat allele, which is present in approximately 15% of the population, but the issue remains unclear. Thus, the DRD2-A1 and the DRD4 long alleles downregulate dopamine neurotransmission mediated by the D2 and D4 receptors, respectively. Their relationship with aggression-related phenotypes was summarized in Table 3.4.

Both the DRD2-A1 and DRD4 long genotypes are associated with aggression-related phenotypes, but the relationship is not as clear as with the MAOA genotype. MAOA genotypes do not differentiate the aggression-related phenotypes from one another but differentiated aggressive from non-aggressive phenotypes rather clearly. Dopamine receptor polymorphisms differentiated neither. The only exceptions may be non-violent forms of criminal behavior, but for some reason these were less studied with respect to DRD2 and DRD4, and as such, findings remain inconclusive.

Another important feature of associations and of the studies is that they conflict to degrees. For example, some authors understood the DRD2-A1 genotype as the carrying the A1 allele on both chromosomes (A1/A1); for others both the A1/A1 and A1/A2 were indicative of a DRD-A1 genotype. Yet others pointed out that the "real problem genotype" was the A1/A2, the other two being "better" (i.e., did not associate with the trait under study). As it regards DRD4 long genotypes, many authors used this term to refer only to the 7-repeat allele, whereas for other authors it referred to any repeat above 2. The 9-repeat allele was in focus in another study. We know so little about these variants that either choice can be defended or refuted. In addition, the association went the wrong way in a few instances, i.e., the aggressive phenotype associated with the DRD2-A2/A2 or the DRD4 short variant; however, this was rare.

Table 3.4 Associations between dopamine receptor gene polymorphisms and aggression-related phenotypes

Aggression				Other traits			
Ref	Genotype	Phenotype	Assoc.	Genotype	Phenotype	Assoc.	Ref
[164]	DRD2-A1	Aggressiveness	S	DRD2-A1	Impulsiveness	S	* [165]
[166]	DRD2-A1	Aggressiveness	S	DRD2-A1	Disinhibition	S	[167]
[168]	DRD2-A1	Reactive AGG	S	DRD2-A1	Impulsiveness	S	# [169]
[170]	DRD2-A1	School fighting	S	DRD2-A1	Novelty seeking	S(M)	# [171]
[172]	DRD4-L	MMA fighters	S	DRD2	Harm avoidance	NS	# [171]
[166]	DRD4	Aggressiveness	NS	DRD2	Reward DEP	NS	# [171]
# [173]	DRD4	Aggressiveness	NS	DRD2	Persistence	NS	# [171]
				DRD2	Self-directedness	NS	# [171]
				DRD2-A1	Cooperativeness	S(F)	# [171]
				DRD4-L	Social problems	S	# [173]
				DRD4-L	Impulsiveness	S	* [170]
				DRD4-L	Short temper	S(M)	* [174]
				DRD4-L	Thrill seeking	S(M)	* [174]
				DRD4-L	Impulsiveness	S	# [169]
# [175]	DRD2-A1	ASPD	S	DRD2-A1	ALC severity	S	# [170]
*# [176]	DRD2-A1	ADHD	S	DRD2-A1	Drug abuse	S	# [170]
* [177]	DRD2-A1	ADHD	S	DRD2-A1	Schizoid	S	# [178]
*# [179]	DRD4-L	ADHD	S	DRD2-A1	Alcoholism	S	[180]
[181]	DRD4-L	PTSD	S	DRD2	Bipolar disorder	NS	[182]
[183]	DRD4-L	ADHD	S	DRD4	Autism	NS	[184]
[185]	DRD4	ADHD	NS	DRD4-S	Bulimia	S	# [186]
[187]	DRD2	Arrest	NS	DRD2	Paraphilic SexOff	NS	[188]
[189]	DRD2	Murder	NS	DRD2	Non-violent CRI	NS	# [190]

(continued)

Table 3.4 (continued)

Aggression				Other traits			
Ref	Genotype	Phenotype	Assoc.	Genotype	Phenotype	Assoc.	Ref
* [190]	DRD2-A1	Crime	S	DRD2	Non-violent CRI	NS	* [191]
* [192]	DRD2-A1	Crime	S	DRD4	Paraphilic SexOff	NS	[193]
[187]	DRD2-A1	Incarceration	S				
* [191]	DRD2-A1	Violent crime	S				
[170]	DRD2-A1	Violent crime	S				
* [193]	DRD2-A1	Violent crime	S				
[194]	DRD2-A1/ A2	Violent crime	S				
* [195]	DRD2-A2	Crime	S				
* [196]	DRD2-A2	IPV	S				
[187]	DRD4	Arrest	NS				
* [196]	DRD4	IPV	NS				
[197]	DRD4	Murder	NS				
* [174]	DRD4-L	Crime	S(M)				
# [173]	DRD4-L	Crime	S				
* [193]	DRD4-L	Violent crime	S				
[187]	DRD4-S	Incarceration	S				

Associations (Assoc.). NS association not significant, *S* significant association, *S(M)* significant association in males only, *S(F)* significant association in females only, * association significant only in interaction with environmental effects, # association significant only in interaction with other gene polymorphisms, *, # association significant only when both the environment and other gene polymorphisms were considered. *Genotypes. DRD2-A1* dopamine 2 receptor gene, A1 allele at the TAq1 locus, *DRD2-A2* dopamine 2 receptor gene, A2 allele at the TAq1 locus, *DRD2-A1/A2* dopamine 2 receptor gene, heterogenotype at the TAq1 locus, *DRD4-L* long variant at the of variable number tandem repeat promoter region, *DRD4-S* short variant at the of variable number tandem repeat promoter region. Note that the variant was not mentioned when the association was not significant. *Abbreviations in the column Phenotypes. ADHD* attention-deficit/hyperactivity disorder, *AGG* aggressiveness, *ALC* alcoholism, *ASPD* antisocial personality disorder, *CRI* crime, *DEP* dependence, *MMA* mixed martial arts, *PTSD* posttraumatic stress disorder, *SexOff* sexual offences. *Crime, arrest, incarceration* violent crime was included, but was not the only crime type

Finally, associations tended to be non-significant when the genes were considered alone. In the overwhelming majority of cases, the genotype–phenotype association became significant only when investigated in interaction either with environmental influences or with other genes. Note that environmental influences were not dealt with in general terms as with GWAS. Rather, various specific influences were studied, and many proved useful in making the effects of polymorphisms significant by interaction. However, polymorphisms did not point to a specific environmental influence. Psychosocial stress exposure [174] just as readily interacted with genotypes as parental support [195], school achievement [193], or religiousness [192]. Other genes that made genotype–phenotype associations significant by interaction were similarly variable and ranged from cell adhesion molecules [176], through genes regulating other neurotransmitters such as serotonin [173] to alcohol-processing enzymes in the case of antisocial personality disorder [175]. The association of DRD2 and DRD4 genes with aggression phenotypes is enhanced by any other problem the organism faces, be that genetic, such as another genetic deficit, or environmental.

The weak association of dopamine receptor polymorphisms alone with aggression phenotypes is supported by studies involving D2 and D4 knockout mice, where the genes in question were experimentally cancelled. Findings in these animals are illustrative from a human perspective in two ways. First, wild-type (genetically not engineered) and knockout mice differ in one gene only. Thus, we do not have to deal with concurrent genetic deficits. Second, the two genotypes are reared together, which rules out differential environmental influences. Both the DRD2-KO [198–200] and the DRD4-KO [198, 201] mice show a series of deficits that range from locomotor disturbances through impulsiveness in the case of the DRD2 and anxiety in the case of DRD4 to learning deficits (DRD2) and drug-related behavior (DRD4). Moreover, the two genotypes affect longevity in opposite directions (DRD2-KO mice live less [202]; DRD4-KOs live longer, a phenomenon also present in DRD4 long humans [203]). Despite the multitude of behavioral and other investigations, there are virtually no reports on the aggressiveness of these lines. This strongly suggests that their aggressiveness was normal or was not obviously different from the aggressiveness of wild types. The knockout lines were produced decades ago and were relatively well studied, but their altered aggressiveness was not noticed over the decades.

Taken together, the findings reviewed above point to the conclusion that neither the DRD2-A1 nor the DRD4 long polymorphisms play particularly important roles in aggression, when considered alone. Yet, the multitude of positive association studies show that they are important candidates for interactions. Regarding gene x gene interactions, it is worth emphasizing again that aggression is not monogenic; the findings clearly highlight the need to study genes in interaction. For example, the specifics of dopamine neurotransmission are not controlled by any dopamine-related gene alone. Therefore, studying subjects by a "cumulative dopaminergic gene index" [204] when the focus is on dopamine or in interaction with non-dopaminergic genes when one is interested in genetics overall appears a better approach than picking one or another gene to study. Dopamine receptor polymorphisms are object lessons to gene x environment interactions, which will be discussed later. Finally, the involvement of the same dopamine receptor polymorphisms in a wide variety of non-aggression phenotypes raises the question whether the "wrong" polymorphisms increase the risk of an aggression problem or increase the risk for a problem in general, the specific problem trait being determined by the course of events over the life of the subject.

3.3.2.3 Miscellaneous Other Genes Involved in Neurotransmission

We show in Table 3.5 the association of various genes with aggression. As with the previous tables, studies on a series of non-aggressive phenotypes were also included for comparison. The table is not an exhaustive account of the literature. We selected a few studies on the most investigated genes, particularly those that by their protein products affect dopaminergic, noradrenergic, and serotonergic neurotransmission as

Table 3.5 The association of various gene polymorphisms with aggression-related and aggression-unrelated phenotypes

Gene	Encoding for/clarification/(neurotransmission affected)	Phenotypes associated with the gene
ADRA2 [205, 206]	α2 adrenoreceptor/neurotransmitter receptor/(noradrenergic)	Reading abilities Prefrontal executive functions Memory Impulsiveness Irritability Hostility Verbal aggression Physical aggression Attention-deficit/hyperactivity disorder
COMT [197, 207–209]	Catechol-O-methyltransferase/catabolizing enzyme/(dopaminergic and noradrenergic)	Prefrontal executive functions Prefrontal cognitive functions Aggression Panic disorder Violence in antisocial personality disorder Violent crime in antisocial personality disorder Murder in schizophrenia
CRHR1 [200–202]	Corticotropin-releasing hormone receptor 1/controls the stress response but also has neural effects/(CRFergic)	Hostility Aggression Suicidality Anxiety Depression Violent crime
DAT1 [203–215]	Dopamine transporter 1/reuptakes dopamine into the cell/(dopaminergic)	Prefrontal executive functions Self-regulation Cocaine consumption Attention-deficit/hyperactivity disorder Violent crime
DRD1 [189, 216, 217]	Dopamine 1 receptor/neurotransmitter receptor/(dopaminergic)	Depression Drug addiction Psychotic aggression Prefrontal lesion-induced aggression Murder

(continued)

Table 3.5 (continued)

Gene	Encoding for/clarification/(neurotransmission affected)	Phenotypes associated with the gene
GABRA2 [220–224]	GABA receptor α2 receptor subunit/component of the multi-protein GABA receptor/(GABAergic)	Externalizing behavior Rule breaking Alcoholism Relapse after substance abuse abstinence Conduct disorder Crime
HTR1B [225–230]	Serotonin 1B receptor/neurotransmitter receptor/(serotonergic)	Aggression Alcoholism Attention-deficit/hyperactivity disorder Conduct disorder Psychopathic traits Alcoholic criminals
HTR2A [231–233]	Serotonin 2A receptor/neurotransmitter receptor/(serotonergic)	Impulsiveness Aggression Suicide Impulse control disorders Bipolar disorder
HTR2C [234–238]	Serotonin 2C receptor/neurotransmitter receptor/(serotonergic)	Stress responsiveness Social problems Aggressiveness Anxiety in irritable bowel syndrome Depression Theft Murder
NR3C1 [239–244]	Glucocorticoid receptor/mediates the effects of glucocorticoids/(stress response)	Attention Executive functions Emotion recognition Depression Attention-deficit/hyperactivity disorder Efficacy of intervention in alcohol abuse Violent crime
SLC6A4 [245–248]	Serotonin transporter/reuptakes serotonin into the cell/(serotonergic)	Neurosis Aggression Reactive aggression Drug addiction Alcoholism Stereotypy in autism Theft Drug crime Violent crime Murder

(continued)

Table 3.5 (continued)

Gene	Encoding for/clarification/(neurotransmission affected)	Phenotypes associated with the gene
TPH [248, 249]	Tryptophan hydroxylase/serotonin synthesizing enzyme/(serotonergic)	Aggression Violent suicide Depression Attention-deficit/hyperactivity disorder Violent crime

Phenotypes were listed in the following order: psychological attributes (e.g., aggression or neurosis); psychiatric disorders (e.g., depression and attention-deficit/hyperactivity disorder); and crime (e.g., theft or murder). Missing categories are due to the sparsity of data

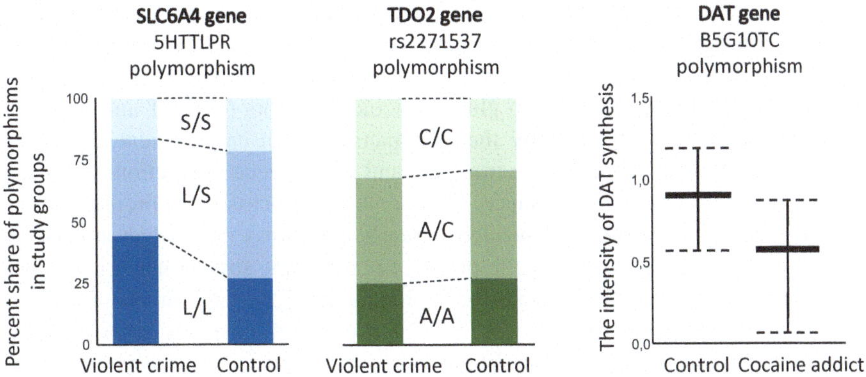

Fig. 3.1 The strength of associations in candidate gene studies. *Left-hand and middle panel*. A gene that did (left) and another that did not (middle) show association with violent crime (the genes for the serotonin transporter and tryptophan 2,3-dioxygenase, respectively, both involved in serotonin neurotransmission) [234]. S/S, L/S, and L/L variants of the 5HTTLPR polymorphism were expressed differently in violent criminals and controls, whereas the rs2271537 polymorphism were not. Yet, all polymorphisms were present in both groups i.e. differences were statistical only. *Right-hand panel*. The synthesis of the dopamine transporter did depend on the polymorphisms of its gene, and differences were significant, yet there were large overlaps between groups. This study was referred to show that even when the condition of participants was tightly related to the gene investigated, associations remained weak (dopamine neurotransmission is the major target of cocaine). As such, weak correlations are not specific to aggression

well as the stress response. As we have shown above, such genes rarely if ever associate with aggression in GWAS, despite that neuroscientific evidence clearly links aggressiveness to the neuroendocrine mechanism they influence. In the candidate gene approach, however, the expected associations are regularly found.

These and other studies show that genes relevant for dopaminergic, noradrenergic, and serotonergic neurotransmissions and for the stress response associate with aggressiveness as a rule. Very few studies failed to find significant associations, probably because candidate gene association studies are well funded theoretically. There always was a good reason to study one or another gene; consequently, the association was almost always found. Figure 3.1 was compiled to give a feeling of the strength of the association.

Associations, however, were rarely if ever valid for the polymorphism alone. Actually, all the genes (polymorphisms) that associated with aggression did so by an interaction with environmental influences or with polymorphisms in other genes. We illustrate such complex interactions by a few examples. In females, for instance, the CRHR1 GG genotype was associated with hostility in interaction with low familial warmth, whereas it associated with aggression in interaction with stressful life events [210]. Thus, the psychological and behavioral consequences of polymorphisms depended on particular environmental conditions, implying that the polymorphism alone did not matter, but the conditions under which its consequences developed were crucial. That is, the very same polymorphism may be associated with a feeling (hostility) under one condition and with aggressive behavior under another condition. Similar gene x environment interactions were the rule in all studies referred in Table 3.4. Regarding gene x gene interactions, individual associations are not significant as a rule but became significant, even without environmental influences, if gene x gene interactions were taken into account. An example to this is the genes encoding for the two glucocorticoid receptors (NR3C1 and NR3C2) associated with violent crime by their interactions with environment and other genes [240]. Moreover, gene x environment and gene x gene interactions are often present in combination. For instance, faulty emotion processing (a prerequisite of certain types of aggression) depended on early life stress only when studied in interaction with the additive genetic profile score of three stress-related genes; no polymorphism alone was sufficient for the interaction [242]. A similar interaction was valid for depression, which was associated with a multi-locus genetic profile score for stress-related genes in conjunction with acute or chronic stress exposure [244].

These findings show that no genetic polymorphism is a hallmark of aggressiveness; rather, polymorphisms only open a window to the environment and other genes to influence feelings or behaviors. To a certain extent, individuals with multiple genetic deficits are exceptions from this rule, although in many cases environmental influences are also required to make the association significant.

Regarding specificity, the very same polymorphisms that are usually associated with more than one type of aggression are also associated with non-aggressive features. For instance, the G–G polymorphism of the CRHR1 gene was associated in females with aggression, depression, and anxiety when assessed in combination with stressful life events [210]. Mostly similar associations were observed in males; however, the gene associated with aggression for men was the A-allele of the CRHR1 gene. In another study, the rs6318 polymorphism of the 5-HTR2C gene associated with both non-violent crime (theft) and murder [234]. The very same polymorphism (rs6318 – 5-HTR2C) also showed an association with liability to both stressful life events and depression [250].

Without developing this issue further, one can confidently state that gene polymorphisms are not associated with any specific type of aggression; moreover, the very same polymorphisms are usually associated with a variety of aggressive and non-aggressive phenotypes. The findings do not support the notion that candidate genes and their polymorphisms represent a risk factor for aggression. In fact, they may represent a risk factor for many problematic behaviors, but the nature of the risk depends on the environment. As noted above, multiple gene deficits may be the exception, but one cannot draw definite conclusions, as the number of relevant studies is low, and, even in these studies, interactions with environmental influences were studied frequently and found significant.

The last issue to be addressed in this section is the relationship between cause and effect. Candidate gene analyses are prompted by the roles of the gene products in neural function. Therefore, one is tempted to explain findings from this perspective. Yet, there is an alternative possibility. Out of the 12 genes listed in the table, at least 8 were shown to play roles in brain development, particularly CRHR1 [251], GABA [252], COMT [253–255], DAT1 [256], DRD1 [254], NR3C1 [257], SLC6A4 [255], and TPH [258]. The same may be true for other genes; their absence from this list is explained by either a general lack of evidence or the inability of the author to find them. Polymorphisms in these eight genes affected the development of the cortex, of prefrontal functions; the volumes of various brain areas, such as the hippocampus and amygdala; the developmental trajectory of hippocampal pyramidal neurons; or the functional connectivity of the amygdala. Alterations in these genes not only affect the ongoing processing of information before and during aggressive conflicts but also have effects on brain structure much earlier, even during fetal life. It is difficult to say whether the developmental or the brain functional consequences of polymorphisms are more important for defining the phenotype.

3.3.2.4 Cell Adhesion Proteins

Cell adhesion proteins – among them cadherins – are molecules that bind neighboring cells together. Although they do not play easily explained roles in aggression, there are a few candidate gene association studies which have investigated them in various populations. These studies have found that variants of the cadherin-13 gene are involved in extremely violent behavior (at least ten committed homicides, attempted homicides, or batteries) [153], whereas genetic variations in *neuronal* cell adhesion molecules are associated with aggressiveness in general [259]. Genetic variations in several other cadherins associate with attention-deficit/hyperactivity disorder, autism spectrum disorder, schizophrenia, bipolar disorder, and major depressive disorder [260]. This suggests that genetic variants of cell adhesion proteins do not specifically affect aggression; however, laboratory studies show that the genotype–phenotype association may be causal. For example, mice null-mutant for a specific neural cell adhesion molecule are highly aggressive, and this phenotype was reversed by the transgenic (re)expression of the very same cell adhesion molecule [261]. This finding does not make the genotype aggression-specific, because restoring the missing gene may have also corrected other behavioral deficits if these were studied. Yet, the study shows that a molecular event as difficult to relate to aggressiveness as the expression of cell adhesion proteins can be causally linked to the phenotype.

There might be other cell surface proteins important for aggressiveness. Animal studies suggest, for instance, that the proteins neuroligins and neurexins – molecules that by interaction bind not whole cells or neurons but synapses together [262] – may be similar to cell adhesion molecules. Thus, variations in their genetics may well associate with human aggression phenotypes. In animals at least, neuroligin expression is associated with both everyday aggression [263] and abnormal aggression elicited by peripubertal stressors [264, 265]. Moreover, mutations in neuroligin genes induce abnormal aggression [266]. These animal studies render neuroligin genes just as appropriate for human candidate gene studies as any of the genes discussed above.

One can argue that cell adhesion and "synapse adhesion" molecules are very far from the brain mechanisms of aggression and their role is very difficult to integrate into present knowledge. This is true, but GWAS lead to no better findings. More importantly, these molecules not only bind cells or synapses together but play roles in cell fate decisions during cell differentiation [267] and regulate the establishment of synaptic contacts between neurons [262]. Actually, they regulate brain network development [268], which is just as important for controlling aggression as the specifics of neurotransmission in the fully developed organism.

3.3.2.5 Knockout Mice

Gene knockouts are mouse lines in which one single gene was invalidated ("knocked out"). Comparisons with "wild-type" (genetically not engineered) mice may reveal the role of a particular gene in development, brain function, behavior, etc. Some gene knockouts are not viable, but, fortunately, most of the genes reviewed above can be knocked out, and the phenotypes of the resulting lines can be studied. We will use information in knockout mice to cross-check human findings, as these were highly dependent on environmental influences. Note that we selected here studies of knockouts for the genes that showed associations with human aggressiveness in previous tables.

In many cases, knockout mice show changes in aggression, which are expectable based on human findings and the known roles of the genes in brain function. For instance, decreased serotonin availability resulting from the knocking out of the TPH2 gene increases aggression, whereas increased serotonin availability in serotonin transporter knockouts decreases aggression. In 6 of the 12 gene knockouts presented in Table 3.6, however, there were no reports on aggressiveness perhaps due to a lack of interest by experimenters, but this is unlikely. The first research step after the creation of a knockout line is phenotyping, i.e., the search for the phenotypic changes induced by the novel genotype. One is reluctant to believe that aggressiveness was not investigated with genes that are associated with aggressiveness in humans and where neuroscientific evidence is suggestive for an effect on aggression. It is more likely that non-reporting is due to the well-known reluctance of scientists to report negative findings [287, 288]. Although we have no evidence for this assumption, we suggest that in most cases the phrase "no reports" can be

Table 3.6 Aggregession-related and aggression-unrelated phenotypes of gene knockouts

Gene	Aggression	Other phenotypes affected
ADRA2 [269]	Increased	Amphetamine-induced locomotion Startle reactivity Depression-like behavior Prepulse inhibition[a]
COMT [270, 271]	Increased in heterozygotes No change in homozygotes	Performance in various cognitive tasks
CRHR1 [272, 263]	No reports	Anxiety-like behavior Stress-related alcohol consumption
DAT1 [264]	Increase	Locomotion Learning Memory
DRD2 [198–200]	No reports	Locomotion Impulsiveness Learning Longevity
DRD4 [198, 201]	No reports	Locomotion Anxiety Drug-related behavior Longevity
GABRA2 [275–277]	No reports	Addiction Alcohol effects Anxiety-like behavior Anxiolytic action
HTR2A [278]	No reports	Antipsychotic action
HTR2C [279, 280]	No reports	Learned fear Sociability
MAOA [281]	Increased	Exploration Defense Fear
MAOA hypomorphic[b] [282]	Not changed	Locomotion Perseverance Anxiety-like behavior Sociability
SLC6A4 [283–285]	Reduced	Intestinal function Serotonergic drug response
TPH2 [286]	Increased	Metabolism Anxiety-like behavior Depression-like behavior Conditioned fear Impulsivity

[a]The inhibition of a response by a weaker pre-stimulus (prepulse). This response is typical to certain mental disorders, e.g., schizophrenia

[b]The MAOA gene is expressed but weekly. For other explanations, see previous tables

replaced with "no effect on aggression" in Table 3.6, especially when social behavior was studied, but no data on aggression were published. An exception is the MAOA hypomorphic mouse line. In these transgenic mice, the MAOA gene was not invalidated but was made less functional, which is similar to human genotypes depicted as the MAOA-low genotype (see above). Albeit this genotype was significantly associated with various types of aggressiveness in humans, MAOA hypomorphic mice showed no changes in aggressiveness despite significant changes in their social behavior. This negative finding was worth reporting likely because of the large interest of researchers in the MAOA gene.

Taken together, the findings reviewed in Table 3.6 strengthen the assumption that genetic variation requires an additional factor to result in an aggressive phenotype, particularly environmental influences. This assumption is strengthened by the fact that aggressiveness changed in the expected direction in many knockout mice. The reason is that in humans one has to deal with a polymorphism that confers a lower or a higher functionality to the gene or its product, but the respective protein is not lacking in the organism. Obviously, the total lack of a gene product has stronger effects than the presence of a non-deleterious polymorphism. The findings also reveal that the consequences of gene deletions are not restricted to aggression. A series of other traits were as strongly affected in knockouts as aggression. This strengthens the assumption that "warrior genes" do not exist and genetic variation induces a set of neural changes that manifest themselves in many domains of functioning, depending on the circumstances. In humans, these circumstances are called environmental influences, which are attenuated by their standardization under laboratory conditions.

The behavior of knockout mice is studied in various enclosures or test arenas which presents the animal with a different task. In the conditioned fear test, for instance, the animal receives an electric shock in an unfamiliar cage; the next day it is exposed to the same cage, where fear is expressed and measured by the amount of time spent in immobility. In the resident-intruder test, the animal is faced with an intruder in his home cage, and the ensuing aggressive behavior is recorded. A neural deficit manifests itself in both cases but differently, because the test situation is different. For example, the same knockout mouse may show increased conditioned fear in the first test and increased aggression in the second.

Knockout mice, in fact, exemplify one of the statements from the introduction of this section. Genes do not code for behaviors; they code for a protein that is relevant for brain function. On their turn, brain function controls responses to challenges and behavior. As such, the consequences of a gene deficit not only depend on conditions during development (called environmental influences in humans) but also on the specific challenges an animal or human is faced at a particular time.

3.3.3 Conclusions

We asked two questions in this chapter: (i) Do candidate gene polymorphisms differentiate the three main types to aggression? and (ii) Is the genetics of aggression specific to aggression? For graphical representation of the answer, see (Fig. 3.2).

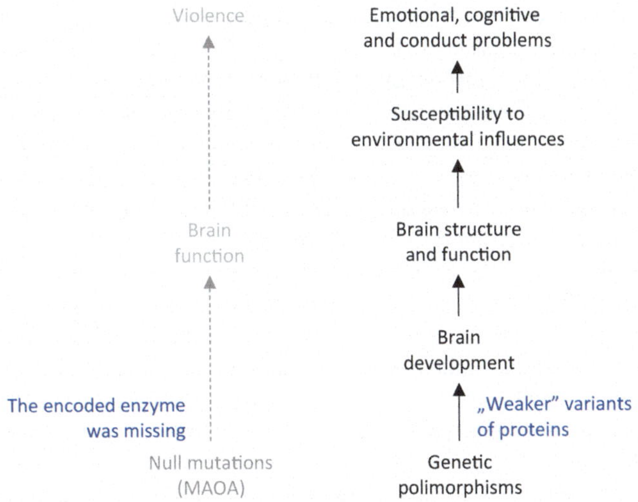

Fig. 3.2 Candidate genes – the general picture. Null mutations (left) may have large and possibly specific effects on aggression, yet only one such mutation was observed so far. This part of the figure was printed in gray to symbolize the rarity of the phenomenon. Gene polymorphisms are ubiquitous, yet none affects aggression very strongly. In addition, those that did associate with various forms of human aggression also showed associations with a series of other problems including non-aggressive psychopathologies and crime. It occurs that the impact of these gene variants on aggression is indirect and depends on gene x environment interactions

The answer to the first question is "no" for all the genes reviewed above. The very same polymorphisms are associated with, and consequently increase, the risk of all three: everyday manifestations of aggression that are at least tolerable, aggression-related psychopathologies that require professional attention and violent crime that is subject to legal proceedings. As such, no genes increase the risk of aggression-related psychopathologies or violent crime. There are, however, genes that increase the risk of responding a challenge aggressively.

The answer to the second question is also "no" for all the genes reviewed. The very same polymorphisms may increase the risk of anything from having disturbed social lives to novelty seeking, cooperativeness, drug abuse, psychopathology, and non-violent crime. Naturally, the risks for aggression, aggression-related mental disorders, and violent crime were also increased. MAOA is an exception to a certain degree, because the relevant polymorphism (the MAOA-low variant) associates preferentially with aggression. Nevertheless, it was also associated with impulsive, hostile, and angry feelings, which are related to aggression, but are not aggression themselves. In addition, these polymorphisms were also associated with autism spectrum disorder, property crime, refusal to cooperate with social partners, alcoholism, and pathological gambling. While the MAOA-low variant is closest to be an aggression-specific genotype, this specificity is by far not complete. Polymorphisms in other genes carry a greater risk of aggression in this respect and associate with a wide array of different phenotypes. Is there any explanation to this versatility?

One possibility resides in the widely accepted notion of gene x environment interactions. A genetic dysfunction, such as a poorly transcriptable gene or a poorly functioning gene product, just opens a window for environmental influences to exert their effects. It is common experience that people having very similar life histories have entirely different life trajectories. Some succumb and develop psychopathologies, whereas others prove to be resilient. Some become criminals when undergoing environmental influences predictive of criminality, whereas other do not. Gene polymorphisms may account for the difference.

Knockout animals – as a second explanation – reveal another important explanation for the variability of the consequences of genetic deficits. These suggest that the impact of genetic deficits may not only depend on the history of environmental influences but also on the challenge the individual faces at a particular moment. The very same deficit may be a risk factor for aggression when a situation calls for this behavior but may also be a risk factor for an exaggerated fear response when the situation is fearful.

The third explanation is related to the number and type of genetic changes and the relationships between them. A genetic deficit may be counteracted or amplified by another. Such interactions are poorly understood at present, but the first trials to address the issue have already been made as shown in the next section.

The overall conclusion from gene association studies is that a large number of gene polymorphisms significantly associate with aggression. These polymorphisms affect brain development in the long term, acute neural responses in critical situations, or both. However, all genetic variants studied to date seem to be "problem polymorphisms" rather than "aggression polymorphisms."

3.4 Overall Interpretation of Genetic Findings

Here we interpret the findings reviewed above from the perspective of a very general question. What did behavioral genetics teach us about the control of aggression? The answer is not simple.

On the positive side, we learned that all three forms of aggression are heritable and their heritability is rather high. We also identified a series of genes that are the carriers of heritability. These genes affect brain development, brain function, or both, revealing that it is not the behavior that is inherited but neural properties that affect the brain control of behaviors. We also learned that the environment has a large impact on the consequences of genetic polymorphisms and risks are due neither to genetics nor to the environment but rather to their interaction. Many well-conducted studies exemplify this general statement by evidencing interactions between particular genotypes and environmental conditions. These discoveries are important to biologists, psychologists, psychiatrists, and criminologists alike and in theory may help in identifying populations and individuals at risk, forecasting developmental trajectories, improving treatment strategies and reintegration programs, etc. Overall, these are important discoveries not only for science but also for the society as a whole; however, there is also a negative side of the discoveries.

One of the problems even has a name: It is called the "missing heritability," a general problem in all research on the relationship between heredity and genetics. The authors of an influential paper summarized the issue as follows. "Genome-wide association studies have identified hundreds of genetic variants associated with complex human diseases and traits, and have provided valuable insights into their genetic architecture. Most variants identified so far confer relatively small increments in risk, and explain only a small proportion of familial clustering, leading many to question how the remaining, 'missing' heritability can be explained" (see Abstract in [289]). We add that the very same problem is valid for candidate gene association studies. Associations are significant, but there is a considerable overlap in the genotypes of those who were aggressive and those who were not. This actually means that the genetics of heredity remains mostly unknown.

A second problem is the nonspecificity of associations. This was rarely if ever investigated or stated as a possibility, but our analyses clearly show that the very same polymorphisms are significantly associated with a wide array of psychological traits and with very different types of psychopathologies and criminal activity. The studies reviewed here did not identify genes related to aggression but genes that are associated with problem behaviors in general.

The essence of the findings can be summarized as follows. (1) Research into the genetics of aggression identified gene variants that make people vulnerable to long- or short-term environmental influences. (2) Vulnerability may result in problem behaviors under unfavorable environmental conditions. (3) Problem behaviors cover many domains of functioning, including but definitely not restricted to aggression-related traits. (4) Genetic vulnerabilities do not account for the large share of heritability observed in aggression-related and aggression-unrelated features. This is not exactly what one expects from studies into the genetics of aggression.

3.4.1 *Possible Solutions to the Failures*

The authors of the paper referred to above who primarily addressed the state of art in GWAS propose several ways to solve the problem of missing heritability. These include improvements in detection to evaluate the role of rare variants, increasing sample sizes, pooling variants of similar classes, finding proper control subjects, extending analyses to polymorphisms other than single-nucleotide ones, harnessing family studies, etc. These proposals are mostly methodological in nature and are addressed to researchers who perform such studies. Improved methodologies naturally lead to knowledge of higher quality. Ultimately, better studies may even account for a great deal of the missing heritability, but not necessarily.

The amount of data provided by genetic studies is overwhelming; it is much beyond human comprehension. This is especially clear in the genetics of complex phenotypes influenced by a very large number of genes and where interactions are probably more important than any information on individual genes. Assuming that improved methodologies would provide better data, one still has to solve the problem of their analysis.

People usually make use of artificial intelligence when human analytic capacities fail. Artificial intelligence may not understand things on our behalf but may organize findings to make them more comprehensible. This needs new mathematical approaches, some of which are available at present or may be developed in the future. One such approach is network science [290], which is widely used to understand the genetics of cancer [291] and already has its application in aggression research [26]. The available studies identified gene groups rather than individual genes as risk factors of aggression. Due to the functional relatedness of the genes, the groups are perceived as a "genetic pathways" that are centered on key genes, e.g., on NF-kB (nuclear factor kappa), which controls the transcription of the DNA, and MAPKs (mitogen-activated protein kinases), which control cellular responses to stimuli. Findings were essentially reproduced by the same [141] and a different set of authors [107], suggesting that the findings are reliable. Such gene network analyses can be extended to include other levels of organization, e.g., endocrine and brain functions and social interactions [292, 293]. This author considers that a detailed review of such findings is premature but expresses his opinion that gene network analyses are the future of aggression genetics, which may not only render immense datasets analyzable but may solve the problem of both missing and confusing heritability.

To summarize this in one sentence: Research methodologies should be improved and data analysis made as complex as the complexity of the phenomenon requires.

3.4.2 Expectations and Fulfillments: A Utilitarian Approach

The ultimate hope of the research endeavors reviewed above was that once the genetic underpinnings of aggression were recognized, we would know who would be at risk (e.g., in psychiatric or criminal terms), and we would be able to prevent the progress from risk to problem. In addition, genetic information may have helped to help those at risk for aggression. The hope was that genetic underpinnings were problem-specific. To exaggerate a bit, one could expect that the DNA of somebody be read, the specialist could tell whether he was prone to develop, let us say, attention-deficit/hyperactivity disorder or to become a violent criminal. This is reminiscent of a scene from the nineteenth-century play by Madách (*The Tragedy of Man*), where scientists of a remote future predicted the fate of people at birth.

At present, these hopes have not been not fulfilled. Studies did identify a series of genetic risks, but not sufficiently strong to determine "fate." In addition, genetic variants predict problems in general rather than aggression specifically. It is questionable whether gene association studies would meet expectations in the future and even whether it is wise to strive for this. However, new developments in the area suggest that the ultimate goals may be reached in an unpredictable future by employing improved research strategies and data-processing methods.

Although the ultimate goal was not reached, present knowledge may still lead to practical applications. One possibility was summarized in a study as follows. "… we suggest that the use of [the MAOA] genotype in trials should be limited to cases of impulsive (rather than premeditated) crimes, with clearly demonstrable risk factors (e.g., childhood severe adversity), and offering explicit and specific relationships between genetic makeup and the circumstances in which the offense occurred – such as provocation – that might have served as a trigger" (p. 196 [294]). In more general terms, the genetics of aggression should be viewed in the context of both life histories and acute triggering events. This is the subject of the next chapter.

References

1. Can your genes make you murder? *NPR.org*. Available at: https://www.npr.org/templates/story/story.php?storyId=128043329. Accessed 23 July 2019.
2. Pity the poor murderer, his genes made him do it. *Psychology Today*. Available at: http://www.psychologytoday.com/blog/the-human-beast/201007/pity-the-poor-murderer-his-genes-made-him-do-it. Accessed 23 July 2019.
3. Farahany, N. A., & Coleman, J. E. (2006). Genetics and responsibility: To know the criminal from the crime. *Law and Contemporary Problems, 69*, 115–164.
4. McSwiggan, S., Elger, B., & Appelbaum, P. S. (2017). The forensic use of behavioral genetics in criminal proceedings: Case of the MAOA-L genotype. *International Journal of Law and Psychiatry, 50*, 17–23.
5. Denno, D. W. (2011). Courts' increasing consideration of behavioral genetics evidence in criminal cases: Results of a longitudinal study. *Michigan State Law Review, 2011*, 967–1047.
6. Baum, M. L. (2013). The monoamine oxidase A (MAOA) genetic predisposition to impulsive violence: Is it relevant to criminal trials? *Neuroethics, 6*, 287–306.
7. Teodorovic, S., & Uzelac, B. (2015). Genetic basis of aggression: Overview and implications for legal proceedings. *Romanian Journal of Legal Medicine, 23*, 193–202.
8. Sabatello, M., & Appelbaum, P. S. (2017). Behavioral genetics in criminal and civil courts. *Harvard Review of Psychiatry, 25*, 289–301.
9. 1000 Genomes Project Consortium, et al. (2015). A global reference for human genetic variation. *Nature, 526*, 68–74.
10. Brinkmann, B., Klintschar, M., Neuhuber, F., Hühne, J., & Rolf, B. (1998). Mutation rate in human microsatellites: Influence of the structure and length of the tandem repeat. *American Journal of Human Genetics, 62*, 1408–1415.
11. Holterhoff, K. (2014). The history and reception of Charles Darwin's hypothesis of pangenesis. *Journal of the History of Biology, 47*, 661–695.
12. Henig, R. M. (2000). *The monk in the garden: The lost and found genius of Gregor Mendel, the father of genetics*. New York: Houghton Mifflin.
13. Green, E. D., Watson, J. D., & Collins, F. S. (2015). Human genome project: Twenty-five years of big biology. *Nature, 526*, 29–31.
14. Gros, P.-A., Le Nagard, H., & Tenaillon, O. (2009). The evolution of epistasis and its links with genetic robustness, complexity and drift in a phenotypic model of adaptation. *Genetics, 182*, 277–293.
15. Li, G., Pan, T., Guo, D., & Li, L.-C. (2014). Regulatory variants and disease: The E-Cadherin -160C/A SNP as an example. *Molecular Biology International, 2014*, 967565.
16. Liu, F., et al. (2009). Eye color and the prediction of complex phenotypes from genotypes. *Current Biology: CB, 19*, R192–R193.

17. Schierding, W., Cutfield, W., & O'Sullivan, J. (2014). The missing story behind Genome Wide Association Studies: Single nucleotide polymorphisms in gene deserts have a story to tell. *Frontiers in Genetics, 5*, 39.
18. Stearns, F. W. (2010). One hundred years of pleiotropy: A retrospective. *Genetics, 186*, 767–773.
19. Gallagher, M. D., & Chen-Plotkin, A. S. (2018). The post-GWAS era: From association to function. *American Journal of Human Genetics, 102*, 717–730.
20. Edwards, S. L., Beesley, J., French, J. D., & Dunning, A. M. (2013). Beyond GWASs: Illuminating the dark road from association to function. *American Journal of Human Genetics, 93*, 779–797.
21. Tielbeek, J. J., et al. (2017). Genome-Wide Association Studies of a Broad Spectrum of Antisocial Behavior. *JAMA Psychiatry, 74*, 1242–1250.
22. Soupene, E., Serikov, V., & Kuypers, F. A. (2008). Characterization of an acyl-coenzyme A binding protein predominantly expressed in human primitive progenitor cells. *Journal of Lipid Research, 49*, 1103–1112.
23. Xatzipsalti, M., Voutetakis, A., Stamoyannou, L., Chrousos, G. P., & Kanaka-Gantenbein, C. (2019). Congenital hypopituitarism: Various genes, various phenotypes. *Hormone and Metabolic Research = Hormon- und Stoffwechselforschung = Hormones et métabolisme, 51*, 81–90.
24. Pappa, I., et al. (2016). A genome-wide approach to children's aggressive behavior: The EAGLE consortium. *American Journal of Medical Genetics. Part B, Neuropsychiatric Genetics, 171*, 562–572.
25. Stallings, M. C., et al. (2005). A genome-wide search for quantitative trait Loci that influence antisocial drug dependence in adolescence. *Archives of General Psychiatry, 62*, 1042–1051.
26. van Donkelaar, M. M. J., et al. (2018). Pleiotropic contribution of MECOM and AVPR1A to aggression and subcortical brain volumes. *Frontiers in Behavioral Neuroscience, 12*, 61.
27. Connelly, J. A., et al. (2018). Identification of novel MECOM gene fusion and personalized therapeutic targets through integrative clinical sequencing in secondary acute myeloid leukemia in a patient with severe congenital neutropenia: A case report and literature review. *Cold Spring Harbor Molecular Case Studies, 4*, a002204.
28. Singh, K. D., & Karnik, S. S. (2016). Angiotensin receptors: Structure, function, signaling and clinical applications. *Journal of Cell Signaling, 1*(2), 1–4. https://doi.org/10.4172/2576-1471.1000111.
29. Luévano-Martínez, L. A., & Kowaltowski, A. J. (2017). Topological characterization of the mitochondrial phospholipid scramblase 3. *FEBS Letters, 591*, 4056–4066.
30. Dick, D. M., et al. (2011). Genome-wide association study of conduct disorder symptomatology. *Molecular Psychiatry, 16*, 800–808.
31. Berjaoui, S., et al. (2015). Complex inflammation mRNA-related response in ALS is region dependent. *Neural Plasticity, 2015*, 573784.
32. Ruisch, I. H., Dietrich, A., Glennon, J. C., Buitelaar, J. K., & Hoekstra, P. J. (2018). Interplay between genome-wide implicated genetic variants and environmental factors related to childhood antisocial behavior in the UK ALSPAC cohort. *European Archives of Psychiatry and Clinical Neuroscience, 269*, 741. https://doi.org/10.1007/s00406-018-0964-5.
33. Rautiainen, M.-R., et al. (2016). Genome-wide association study of antisocial personality disorder. *Translational Psychiatry, 6*, e883.
34. Cataldo, I., Azhari, A., & Esposito, G. (2018). A review of oxytocin and arginine-vasopressin receptors and their modulation of autism spectrum disorder. *Frontiers in Molecular Neuroscience, 11*, 27.
35. Fernàndez-Castillo, N., et al. (2017). RBFOX1, encoding a splicing regulator, is a candidate gene for aggressive behavior. *European Neuropsychopharmacology, 30*, 44. https://doi.org/10.1016/j.euroneuro.2017.11.012.
36. Bill, B. R., Lowe, J. K., Dybuncio, C. T., & Fogel, B. L. (2013). Orchestration of neurodevelopmental programs by RBFOX1: Implications for autism spectrum disorder. *International Review of Neurobiology, 113*, 251–267.

37. Tielbeek, J. J., et al. (2012). Unraveling the genetic etiology of adult antisocial behavior: A genome-wide association study. *PLoS One, 7*, e45086.
38. Tejedor, F. J., & Hämmerle, B. (2011). MNB/DYRK1A as a multiple regulator of neuronal development. *The FEBS Journal, 278*, 223–235.
39. Xu, M. K., et al. (2017). Monoamine Oxidase A (MAOA) gene and personality traits from late adolescence through early adulthood: A latent variable investigation. *Frontiers in Psychology, 8*, 1736.
40. Brodkin, E. S., Goforth, S. A., Keene, A. H., Fossella, J. A., & Silver, L. M. (2002). Identification of quantitative trait Loci that affect aggressive behavior in mice. *Journal of Neuroscience: The Official Journal of the Society for Neuroscience, 22*, 1165–1170.
41. Brodkin, E. S. (2005). Quantitative trait locus analysis of aggressive behaviours in mice. *Novartis Foundation Symposium, 268*, 57–69; discussion 69–77, 96–99.
42. Topham, M. K., & Prescott, S. M. (1999). Mammalian diacylglycerol kinases, a family of lipid kinases with signaling functions. *The Journal of Biological Chemistry, 274*, 11447–11450.
43. Hirokawa, N. (1997). The mechanisms of fast and slow transport in neurons: Identification and characterization of the new kinesin superfamily motors. *Current Opinion in Neurobiology, 7*, 605–614.
44. Ernst, M., et al. (1996). Presynaptic dopaminergic deficits in Lesch-Nyhan disease. *The New England Journal of Medicine, 334*, 1568–1572.
45. Dow, H. C., et al. (2011). Genetic dissection of intermale aggressive behavior in BALB/cJ and A/J mice. *Genes, Brain, and Behavior, 10*, 57–68.
46. Shorter, J., et al. (2015). Genetic architecture of natural variation in Drosophila melanogaster aggressive behavior. *Proceedings of the National Academy of Sciences of the United States of America, 112*, E3555–E3563.
47. Glerup, S., et al. (2016). SorCS2 is required for BDNF-dependent plasticity in the hippocampus. *Molecular Psychiatry, 21*, 1740–1751.
48. Glerup, S., et al. (2014). SorCS2 regulates dopaminergic wiring and is processed into an apoptotic two-chain receptor in peripheral glia. *Neuron, 82*, 1074–1087.
49. Zapata, I., Serpell, J. A., & Alvarez, C. E. (2016). Genetic mapping of canine fear and aggression. *BMC Genomics, 17*, 572.
50. Dyer, A. H., Vahdatpour, C., Sanfeliu, A., & Tropea, D. (2016). The role of Insulin-Like Growth Factor 1 (IGF-1) in brain development, maturation and neuroplasticity. *Neuroscience, 325*, 89–99.
51. Huang, H., et al. (2017). HMGA2, a driver of inflammation, is associated with hypermethylation in acute liver injury. *Toxicology and Applied Pharmacology, 328*, 34–45.
52. Macrì, S., et al. (2016). Hmga2 is required for neural crest cell specification in Xenopus laevis. *Developmental Biology, 411*, 25–37.
53. Viding, E., et al. (2010). In search of genes associated with risk for psychopathic tendencies in children: A two-stage genome-wide association study of pooled DNA. *Journal of Child Psychology and Psychiatry, 51*, 780–788.
54. Cendelin, J., Tuma, J., Korelusova, I., & Vozeh, F. (2014). The effect of genetic background on behavioral manifestation of Grid2(Lc) mutation. *Behavioural Brain Research, 271*, 218–227.
55. Cheng, L.-C., et al. (2019). Identification of new transmembrane proteins concentrated at the nuclear envelope using organellar proteomics of mesenchymal cells. *Nucleus (Austin, Tex.), 10*, 126–143.
56. Oudit, G. Y., et al. (2001). The molecular physiology of the cardiac transient outward potassium current (I(to)) in normal and diseased myocardium. *Journal of Molecular and Cellular Cardiology, 33*, 851–872.
57. Sevilla, A., Santos, C. R., Barcia, R., Vega, F. M., & Lazo, P. A. (2004). c-Jun phosphorylation by the human vaccinia-related kinase 1 (VRK1) and its cooperation with the N-terminal kinase of c-Jun (JNK). *Oncogene, 23*, 8950–8958.

58. Anbalagan, S., et al. (2019). Robo2 regulates synaptic oxytocin content by affecting actin dynamics. *eLife, 8*, e45650, 1–28. https://doi.org/10.7554/eLife.45650.
59. Ney, P. A. (2015). Mitochondrial autophagy: Origins, significance, and role of BNIP3 and NIX. *Biochimica et Biophysica Acta, 1853*, 2775–2783.
60. Lim, Y., Cho, I.-T., Schoel, L. J., Cho, G., & Golden, J. A. (2015). Hereditary spastic paraplegia-linked REEP1 modulates endoplasmic reticulum/mitochondria contacts. *Annals of Neurology, 78*, 679–696.
61. Li-Villarreal, N., et al. (2016). Dachsous1b cadherin regulates actin and microtubule cytoskeleton during early zebrafish embryogenesis. *Development (Cambridge, England), 143*, 1832.
62. Guo, K., et al. (2019). Long noncoding RNA RP11-547D24.1 regulates proliferation and migration in papillary thyroid carcinoma: Identification and validation of a novel long noncoding RNA through integrated analysis of TCGA database. *Cancer Medicine, 8*, 3105–3119.
63. Leibel, R. L. (2008). Molecular physiology of weight regulation in mice and humans. *International Journal of Obesity, 2005*(32 Suppl 7), S98–S108.
64. Long, Z.-W., Zhou, M.-L., Fu, J.-W., Chu, X.-Q., & Wang, Y.-N. (2015). Association between cadherin-17 expression and pathological characteristics of gastric cancer: A meta-analysis. *World Journal of Gastroenterology, 21*, 3694–3705.
65. Lamb, C. A., et al. (2016). TBC1D14 regulates autophagy via the TRAPP complex and ATG9 traffic. *The EMBO Journal, 35*, 281–301.
66. Moreno-Castellanos, N., et al. (2017). The cytoskeletal protein septin 11 is associated with human obesity and is involved in adipocyte lipid storage and metabolism. *Diabetologia, 60*, 324–335.
67. Kostrhon, S., et al. (2017). A histone-mimicking interdomain linker in a multidomain protein modulates multivalent histone binding. *The Journal of Biological Chemistry, 292*, 17643–17657.
68. Leisner, T. M., Freeman, T. C., Black, J. L., & Parise, L. V. (2016). CIB1: A small protein with big ambitions. *FASEB Journal : Official Publication of the Federation of American Societies for Experimental Biology, 30*, 2640–2650.
69. Canda, E., et al. (2018). Single center experience of biotinidase deficiency: 259 patients and six novel mutations. *Journal of Pediatric Endocrinology and Metabolism, 31*, 917–926.
70. De Smet, E. G., et al. (2018). Association of innate defense proteins BPIFA1 and BPIFB1 with disease severity in COPD. *International Journal of Chronic Obstructive Pulmonary Disease, 13*, 11–27.
71. Gieffers, C., Korioth, F., Heimann, P., Ungermann, C., & Frey, J. (1997). Mitofilin is a transmembrane protein of the inner mitochondrial membrane expressed as two isoforms. *Experimental Cell Research, 232*, 395–399.
72. Rauch, T., Li, H., Wu, X., & Pfeifer, G. P. (2006). MIRA-assisted microarray analysis, a new technology for the determination of DNA methylation patterns, identifies frequent methylation of homeodomain-containing genes in lung cancer cells. *Cancer Research, 66*, 7939–7947.
73. Li, J., Yoshikawa, A., Brennan, M. D., Ramsey, T. L., & Meltzer, H. Y. (2018). Genetic predictors of antipsychotic response to lurasidone identified in a genome wide association study and by schizophrenia risk genes. *Schizophrenia Research, 192*, 194–204.
74. Laufer, V. A., et al. (2019). Genetic influences on susceptibility to rheumatoid arthritis in African-Americans. *Human Molecular Genetics, 28*, 858–874.
75. Wang, Y., et al. (2018). Subphenotype meta-analysis of testicular cancer genome-wide association study data suggests a role for RBFOX family genes in cryptorchidism susceptibility. *Human Reproduction (Oxford, England), 33*, 967–977.
76. Malik, A. I., et al. (2014). The role of genetic variants in genes regulating the oxytocin-vasopressin neurohumoral system in childhood-onset aggression. *Psychiatric Genetics, 24*, 201–210.

77. Sung, Y. J., et al. (2019). A multi-ancestry genome-wide study incorporating gene-smoking interactions identifies multiple new loci for pulse pressure and mean arterial pressure. *Human Molecular Genetics, 28*, 2615. https://doi.org/10.1093/hmg/ddz070.
78. Cherkas, L. F., Oelsner, E. C., Mak, Y. T., Valdes, A., & Spector, T. D. (2004). Genetic influences on female infidelity and number of sexual partners in humans: A linkage and association study of the role of the vasopressin receptor gene (AVPR1A). *Twin Research: The Official Journal of the International Society for Twin Studies, 7*, 649–658.
79. Fernàndez-Castillo, N., & Cormand, B. (2016). Aggressive behavior in humans: Genes and pathways identified through association studies. *American Journal of Medical Genetics. Part B, Neuropsychiatric Genetics: The Official Publication of the International Society of Psychiatric Genetics, 171*, 676–696.
80. *PANTHER – Whole genome pie chart*. Available at: http://www.pantherdb.org/chart/summary/pantherChart.jsp?filterLevel=1&chartType=1&listType=1&type=1&species=Homo%20sapiens. Accessed 21 June 2019.
81. Beck, M., et al. (2011). The quantitative proteome of a human cell line. *Molecular Systems Biology, 7*, 549.
82. Cooper, G. M. (2000). Signaling molecules and their receptors. In *The cell: A molecular approach* (2nd ed.). Oxford: Sinauer Associates.
83. Holmes, C. L., Landry, D. W., & Granton, J. T. (2004). Science Review: Vasopressin and the cardiovascular system part 2 – clinical physiology. *Critical Care, 8*, 15–23.
84. Li, B., et al. (2018). Transcriptome analysis of adipose tissues from two fat-tailed sheep breeds reveals key genes involved in fat deposition. *BMC Genomics, 19*, 338.
85. Soupene, E., & Kuypers, F. A. (2019). ACBD6 protein controls acyl chain availability and specificity of the N-myristoylation modification of proteins. *Journal of Lipid Research, 60*, 624–635.
86. Soupene, E., et al. (2016). Association of NMT2 with the acyl-CoA carrier ACBD6 protects the N-myristoyltransferase reaction from palmitoyl-CoA. *Journal of Lipid Research, 57*, 288–298.
87. van Elst, L. T., Woermann, F. G., Lemieux, L., Thompson, P. J., & Trimble, M. R. (2000). Affective aggression in patients with temporal lobe epilepsy: A quantitative MRI study of the amygdala. *Brain: A Journal of Neurology, 123*(Pt 2), 234–243.
88. Tang, Z., et al. (2019). Data on MECOM rearrangement-driven chromosomal aberrations in myeloid malignancies. *Data in Brief, 24*, 104025.
89. Sorrentino, A., et al. (2018). PR/SET domain family and cancer: Novel insights from the Cancer Genome Atlas. *International Journal of Molecular Sciences, 19*, 3250.
90. Yatsula, B., et al. (2005). Identification of binding sites of EVI1 in mammalian cells. *The Journal of Biological Chemistry, 280*, 30712–30722.
91. Chester, D. S., & DeWall, C. N. (2016). The pleasure of revenge: Retaliatory aggression arises from a neural imbalance toward reward. *Social Cognitive and Affective Neuroscience, 11*, 1173–1182.
92. Chen, D., Zhao, M., & Mundy, G. R. (2004). Bone morphogenetic proteins. *Growth Factors, 22*, 233–241.
93. Segklia, A., et al. (2012). Bmp7 regulates the survival, proliferation, and neurogenic properties of neural progenitor cells during corticogenesis in the mouse. *PLoS One, 7*, e34088.
94. Matsuoka, S., et al. (1995). p57KIP2, a structurally distinct member of the p21CIP1 Cdk inhibitor family, is a candidate tumor suppressor gene. *Genes & Development, 9*, 650–662.
95. Tury, A., Mairet-Coello, G., & DiCicco-Bloom, E. (2011). The cyclin-dependent kinase inhibitor p57Kip2 regulates cell cycle exit, differentiation, and migration of embryonic cerebral cortical precursors. *Cerebral Cortex (New York, N.Y.: 1991), 21*, 1840–1856.
96. Holz, N., et al. (2016). Evidence for a sex-dependent MAOA× childhood stress interaction in the neural circuitry of aggression. *Cerebral Cortex (New York, N.Y.: 1991), 26*, 904–914.
97. Yin, L., Li, J., Liao, C.-P., & Jason Wu, B. (2018). Monoamine oxidase deficiency causes prostate atrophy and reduces prostate progenitor cell activity. *Stem Cells (Dayton, Ohio), 36*, 1249–1258.

98. Wang, J., et al. (2016). Sex-specific mediation effect of the right fusiform face area volume on the association between variants in repeat length of AVPR1A RS3 and altruistic behavior in healthy adults. *Human Brain Mapping, 37*, 2700–2709.
99. Smith, D. I., Zhu, Y., McAvoy, S., & Kuhn, R. (2006). Common fragile sites, extremely large genes, neural development and cancer. *Cancer Letters, 232*, 48–57.
100. Carter, T. C., et al. (2011). Evaluation of 64 candidate single nucleotide polymorphisms as risk factors for neural tube defects in a large Irish study population. *American Journal of Medical Genetics. Part A, 155A*, 14–21.
101. Guerrero-Cazares, H., et al. (2017). Brief report: Robo1 regulates the migration of human subventricular zone neural progenitor cells during development. *Stem Cells (Dayton, Ohio), 35*, 1860–1865.
102. Vevera, J., et al. (2018). Rare copy number variation in extremely impulsively violent males. *Genes, Brain and Behavior, 18*, e12536. https://doi.org/10.1111/gbb.12536.
103. Dudbridge, F. (2013). Power and predictive accuracy of polygenic risk scores. *PLoS Genetics, 9*, e1003348.
104. Hamshere, M. L., et al. (2013). High loading of polygenic risk for ADHD in children with comorbid aggression. *The American Journal of Psychiatry, 170*, 909–916.
105. Wertz, J., et al. (2018). Genetics and crime: Integrating new genomic discoveries into psychological research about antisocial behavior. *Psychological Science, 29*, 791–803.
106. Elam, K. K., Chassin, L., & Pandika, D. (2018). Polygenic risk, family cohesion, and adolescent aggression in Mexican American and European American families: Developmental pathways to alcohol use. *Development and Psychopathology, 30*, 1715–1728.
107. Feldker, D. E. M., et al. (2003). Serial analysis of gene expression predicts structural differences in hippocampus of long attack latency and short attack latency mice. *The European Journal of Neuroscience, 17*, 379–387.
108. Malki, K., et al. (2014). Genes and gene networks implicated in aggression related behaviour. *Neurogenetics, 15*, 255–266.
109. Brunner, H. G., et al. (1993). X-linked borderline mental retardation with prominent behavioral disturbance: Phenotype, genetic localization, and evidence for disturbed monoamine metabolism. *American Journal of Human Genetics, 52*, 1032–1039.
110. Brunner, H. G., Nelen, M., Breakefield, X. O., Ropers, H. H., & van Oost, B. A. (1993). Abnormal behavior associated with a point mutation in the structural gene for monoamine oxidase A. *Science, 262*, 578–580.
111. Piton, A., Redin, C., & Mandel, J.-L. (2013). XLID-causing mutations and associated genes challenged in light of data from large-scale human exome sequencing. *American Journal of Human Genetics, 93*, 368–383.
112. Whibley, A. C., et al. (2010). Fine-scale survey of X chromosome copy number variants and indels underlying intellectual disability. *American Journal of Human Genetics, 87*, 173–188.
113. Saito, M., et al. (2014). MAOA/B deletion syndrome in male siblings with severe developmental delay and sudden loss of muscle tonus. *Brain & Development, 36*, 64–69.
114. O'Leary, R. E., et al. (2012). De novo microdeletion of Xp11.3 exclusively encompassing the monoamine oxidase A and B genes in a male infant with episodic hypotonia: A genomics approach to personalized medicine. *European Journal of Medical Genetics, 55*, 349–353.
115. Hinds, A.-M., Rosser, E., & Reddy, M. A. (2018). A case of exudative vitreoretinopathy and chorioretinal coloboma associated with microcephaly in a female with contiguous Xp11.3-11.4 deletion. *Ophthalmic Genetics, 39*, 396–398.
116. Scott, A. L., Bortolato, M., Chen, K., & Shih, J. C. (2008). Novel monoamine oxidase A knockout mice with human-like spontaneous mutation. *Neuroreport, 19*, 739–743.
117. Sabol, S. Z., Hu, S., & Hamer, D. (1998). A functional polymorphism in the monoamine oxidase A gene promoter. *Human Genetics, 103*, 273–279.
118. Manuck, S. B., Flory, J. D., Ferrell, R. E., Mann, J. J., & Muldoon, M. F. (2000). A regulatory polymorphism of the monoamine oxidase-A gene may be associated with variability in aggression, impulsivity, and central nervous system serotonergic responsivity. *Psychiatry Research, 95*, 9–23.

119. Denson, T. F., Dobson-Stone, C., Ronay, R., von Hippel, W., & Schira, M. M. (2014). A functional polymorphism of the MAOA gene is associated with neural responses to induced anger control. *Journal of Cognitive Neuroscience, 26*, 1418–1427.
120. McDermott, R., Tingley, D., Cowden, J., Frazzetto, G., & Johnson, D. D. P. (2009). Monoamine oxidase A gene (MAOA) predicts behavioral aggression following provocation. *Proceedings of the National Academy of Sciences of the United States of America, 106*, 2118–2123.
121. Mandelli, L., Carli, V., Serretti, A., & Sarchiapone, M. (2015). Low-activity alleles of the MAOA gene are associated with measures of hostility. *Psychiatric Genetics, 25*, 215.
122. Foshee, V. A., et al. (2015). Self-regulatory failure and the perpetration of adolescent dating violence: Examining an alcohol use by gene explanation. *Aggressive Behavior, 41*, 189–203.
123. Lei, H., et al. (2014). A functional polymorphism of the MAOA gene modulates spontaneous brain activity in pons. *BioMed Research International, 2014*, 243280.
124. Cohen, I. L., et al. (2011). Autism severity is associated with child and maternal MAOA genotypes. *Clinical Genetics, 79*, 355–362.
125. Uršič, K., Zupanc, T., & Paska, A. V. (2018). Analysis of promoter polymorphism in monoamine oxidase A (MAOA) gene in completed suicide on Slovenian population. *Neuroscience Letters, 673*, 111–115.
126. Mertins, V., Schote, A. B., Hoffeld, W., Griessmair, M., & Meyer, J. (2011). Genetic susceptibility for individual cooperation preferences: The role of Monoamine Oxidase A Gene (MAOA) in the voluntary provision of public goods. *PLoS One, 6*, e20959.
127. Mueller, S. C., et al. (2014). Evidence of MAOA genotype involvement in spatial ability in males. *Behavioural Brain Research, 267*, 106–110.
128. Nikolac Perkovic, M., et al. (2016). Monoamine oxidase and agitation in psychiatric patients. *Progress in Neuro-Psychopharmacology & Biological Psychiatry, 69*, 131–146.
129. Kim, S. J., Kim, Y. S., Kim, S. Y., Lee, H. S., & Kim, C.-H. (2006). An association study of catechol-O-methyltransferase and monoamine oxidase A polymorphisms and personality traits in Koreans. *Neuroscience Letters, 401*, 154–158.
130. Yu, Y. W.-Y., et al. (2005). Association study of a functional MAOA-uVNTR gene polymorphism and personality traits in Chinese young females. *Neuropsychobiology, 52*, 118–121.
131. Ozen, F., et al. (2017). Lack of association between MAOA-uVNTR variants and excessive daytime sleepiness. *Neurological Sciences: Official Journal of the Italian Neurological Society and of the Italian Society of Clinical Neurophysiology, 38*, 769–774.
132. Hwang, I. W., Lim, M. H., Kwon, H. J., & Jin, H. J. (2018). Association of Monoamine Oxidase A (MAOA) gene uVNTR and rs6323 polymorphisms with attention deficit and hyperactivity disorder in Korean children. *Medicina (Kaunas, Lithuania), 54*(32), 1–12. https://doi.org/10.3390/medicina54030032.
133. Davis, L. K., et al. (2008). Cortical enlargement in autism is associated with a functional VNTR in the monoamine oxidase A gene. *American Journal of Medical Genetics. Part B, Neuropsychiatric Genetics: The Official Publication of the International Society of Psychiatric Genetics, 147B*, 1145–1151.
134. Lawson, D. C., et al. (2003). Association analysis of monoamine oxidase A and attention deficit hyperactivity disorder. *American Journal of Medical Genetics. Part B, Neuropsychiatric Genetics: The Official Publication of the International Society of Psychiatric Genetics, 116B*, 84–89.
135. Contini, V., Marques, F. Z. C., Garcia, C. E. D., Hutz, M. H., & Bau, C. H. D. (2006). MAOA-uVNTR polymorphism in a Brazilian sample: Further support for the association with impulsive behaviors and alcohol dependence. *American Journal of Medical Genetics. Part B, Neuropsychiatric Genetics: The Official Publication of the International Society of Psychiatric Genetics, 141B*, 305–308.
136. Ducci, F., et al. (2008). Interaction between a functional MAOA locus and childhood sexual abuse predicts alcoholism and antisocial personality disorder in adult women. *Molecular Psychiatry, 13*, 334–347.

137. Pérez de Castro, I., Ibáñez, A., Saiz-Ruiz, J., & Fernández-Piqueras, J. (2002). Concurrent positive association between pathological gambling and functional DNA polymorphisms at the MAO-A and the 5-HT transporter genes. *Molecular Psychiatry, 7*, 927–928.
138. Prom-Wormley, E. C., et al. (2009). Monoamine oxidase A and childhood adversity as risk factors for conduct disorder in females. *Psychological Medicine, 39*, 579–590.
139. Tassone, F., et al. (2011). MAOA, DBH, and SLC6A4 variants in CHARGE: A case-control study of autism spectrum disorders. *Autism Research: Official Journal of the International Society for Autism Research, 4*, 250–261.
140. Wang, C.-H., et al. (2018). Associations of serotonin transporter gene promoter polymorphisms and monoamine oxidase A gene polymorphisms with oppositional defiant disorder in a Chinese Han population. *Behavioral and Brain Functions: BBF, 14*, 15.
141. Plieger, T., et al. (2019). Moderator effects of life stress on the association between MAOA-uVNTR, depression, and burnout. *Neuropsychobiology, 78*, 86–94.
142. Hollerbach, P., et al. (2018). Main and interaction effects of childhood trauma and the MAOA uVNTR polymorphism on psychopathy. *Psychoneuroendocrinology, 95*, 106–112.
143. Deckert, J., et al. (1999). Excess of high activity monoamine oxidase A gene promoter alleles in female patients with panic disorder. *Human Molecular Genetics, 8*, 621–624.
144. Voltas, N., Aparicio, E., Arija, V., & Canals, J. (2015). Association study of monoamine oxidase-A gene promoter polymorphism (MAOA-uVNTR) with self-reported anxiety and other psychopathological symptoms in a community sample of early adolescents. *Journal of Anxiety Disorders, 31*, 65–72.
145. Vanyukov, M. M., et al. (2007). The MAOA promoter polymorphism, disruptive behavior disorders, and early onset substance use disorder: Gene-environment interaction. *Psychiatric Genetics, 17*, 323–332.
146. Wei, Y.-L., Li, C.-X., Li, S.-B., Liu, Y., & Hu, L. (2011). Association study of monoamine oxidase A/B genes and schizophrenia in Han Chinese. *Behavioral and Brain Functions: BBF, 7*, 42.
147. Cicchetti, D., Rogosch, F. A., & Thibodeau, E. L. (2012). The effects of child maltreatment on early signs of antisocial behavior: Genetic moderation by tryptophan hydroxylase, serotonin transporter, and monoamine oxidase A genes. *Development and Psychopathology, 24*, 907–928.
148. Fergusson, D. M., Boden, J. M., Horwood, L. J., Miller, A., & Kennedy, M. A. (2012). Moderating role of the MAOA genotype in antisocial behaviour. *The British Journal of Psychiatry: the Journal of Mental Science, 200*, 116–123.
149. Stetler, D. A., et al. (2014). Association of low-activity MAOA allelic variants with violent crime in incarcerated offenders. *Journal of Psychiatric Research, 58*, 69–75.
150. Armstrong, T. A., et al. (2014). Monoamine oxidase A genotype, childhood adversity, and criminal behavior in an incarcerated sample. *Psychiatric Genetics, 24*, 164–171.
151. Beaver, K. M., Barnes, J. C., & Boutwell, B. B. (2014). The 2-repeat allele of the MAOA gene confers an increased risk for shooting and stabbing behaviors. *The Psychiatric Quarterly, 85*, 257–265.
152. Cooke, E. M., et al. (2018). The relationship between the MAOA-uVNTR polymorphism, delinquent peer affiliation, and antisocial behavior with a consideration of sex differences. *The Psychiatric Quarterly, 89*, 841–853.
153. Tiihonen, J., et al. (2015). Genetic background of extreme violent behavior. *Molecular Psychiatry, 20*, 786–792.
154. Chester, D. S., et al. (2015). Monoamine oxidase A (MAOA) genotype predicts greater aggression through impulsive reactivity to negative affect. *Behavioural Brain Research, 283*, 97–101.
155. Haller, J., Makara, G. B., & Kruk, M. R. (1998). Catecholaminergic involvement in the control of aggression: Hormones, the peripheral sympathetic, and central noradrenergic systems. *Neuroscience and Biobehavioral Reviews, 22*, 85–97.

156. Nelson, R. J., & Chiavegatto, S. (2001). Molecular basis of aggression. *Trends in Neurosciences, 24*, 713–719.
157. Rosell, D. R., & Siever, L. J. (2015). The neurobiology of aggression and violence. *CNS Spectrums, 20*, 254–279.
158. Bonnet, U. (2003). Moclobemide: Therapeutic use and clinical studies. *CNS Drug Reviews, 9*, 97–140.
159. Noble, E. P., Blum, K., Ritchie, T., Montgomery, A., & Sheridan, P. J. (1991). Allelic association of the D2 dopamine receptor gene with receptor-binding characteristics in alcoholism. *Archives of General Psychiatry, 48*, 648–654.
160. Pohjalainen, T., et al. (1998). The A1 allele of the human D2 dopamine receptor gene predicts low D2 receptor availability in healthy volunteers. *Molecular Psychiatry, 3*, 256–260.
161. Berman, S. M., & Noble, E. P. (1995). Reduced visuospatial performance in children with the D2 dopamine receptor A1 allele. *Behavior Genetics, 25*, 45–58.
162. Asherson, P., & IMAGE Consortium. (2004). Attention-deficit hyperactivity disorder in the post-genomic era. *European Child & Adolescent Psychiatry, 13*(Suppl 1), I50–I70.
163. Missale, C., Nash, S. R., Robinson, S. W., Jaber, M., & Caron, M. G. (1998). Dopamine receptors: From structure to function. *Physiological Reviews, 78*, 189–225.
164. Preuss, U. W., et al. (2015). Serotonin and dopamine candidate gene variants and alcohol- and non-alcohol-related aggression. *Alcohol and Alcoholism (Oxford, Oxfordshire), 50*, 690–699.
165. Colzato, L. S., van den Wildenberg, W. P. M., Van der Does, A. J. W., & Hommel, B. (2010). Genetic markers of striatal dopamine predict individual differences in dysfunctional, but not functional impulsivity. *Neuroscience, 170*, 782–788.
166. Marino, C., et al. (2004). An assessment of transmission disequilibrium between quantitative measures of childhood problem behaviors and DRD2/Taql and DRD4/48bp-repeat polymorphisms. *Behavior Genetics, 34*, 495–502.
167. Ratsma, J. E., van der Stelt, O., Schoffelmeer, A. N., Westerveld, A., & Boudewijn Gunning, W. (2001). P3 event-related potential, dopamine D2 receptor A1 allele, and sensation-seeking in adult children of alcoholics. *Alcoholism: Clinical and Experimental Research, 25*, 960–967.
168. TJH, C., Blum, K., Mathews, D., & Cornings, D. E. (2007). Preliminary association of both the Dopamine D2 Receptor (DRD2) [Taq1 A1 Allele] and the Dopamine Transporter (DAT1) [480 bp Allele] genes with pathological aggressive behavior, a clinical subtype of Reward Deficiency Syndrome (RDS) in adolescents. *Gene Therapy and Molecular Biology, 11*, 93–112.
169. Eisenberg, D. T. A., et al. (2007). Examining impulsivity as an endophenotype using a behavioral approach: A DRD2 TaqI A and DRD4 48-bp VNTR association study. *Behavioral and Brain Functions: BBF, 3*, 2.
170. Comings, D. E., Muhleman, D., Ahn, C., Gysin, R., & Flanagan, S. D. (1994). The dopamine D2 receptor gene: A genetic risk factor in substance abuse. *Drug and Alcohol Dependence, 34*, 175–180.
171. Tsuchimine, S., et al. (2012). Association between the dopamine D2 receptor (DRD2) polymorphism and the personality traits of healthy Japanese participants. *Progress in Neuro-Psychopharmacology & Biological Psychiatry, 38*, 190–193.
172. Cherepkova, E. V., Maksimov, V. N., Kushnarev, A. P., Shakhmatov, I. I., & Aftanas, L. I. (2019). The polymorphism of dopamine receptor D4 (DRD4) and dopamine transporter (DAT) genes in the men with antisocial behaviour and mixed martial arts fighters. *The World Journal of Biological Psychiatry: The Official Journal of the World Federation of Societies of Biological Psychiatry, 20*, 402–415.
173. Hohmann, S., et al. (2009). Evidence for epistasis between the 5-HTTLPR and the dopamine D4 receptor polymorphisms in externalizing behavior among 15-year-olds. *Journal of Neural Transmission (Vienna, Austria: 1996), 116*, 1621–1629.

174. Dmitrieva, J., Chen, C., Greenberger, E., Ogunseitan, O., & Ding, Y.-C. (2011). Gender-specific expression of the DRD4 gene on adolescent delinquency, anger and thrill seeking. *Social Cognitive and Affective Neuroscience, 6*, 82–89.
175. Lu, R.-B., et al. (2012). Interaction between ALDH2*1*1 and DRD2/ANKK1 TaqI A1A1 genes may be associated with antisocial personality disorder not co-morbid with alcoholism. *Addiction Biology, 17*, 865–874.
176. Mota, N. R., et al. (2015). NCAM1-TTC12-ANKK1-DRD2 gene cluster and the clinical and genetic heterogeneity of adults with ADHD. *American Journal of Medical Genetics. Part B, Neuropsychiatric Genetics: The Official Publication of the International Society of Psychiatric Genetics, 168*, 433–444.
177. Waldman, I. D. (2007). Gene-environment interactions reexamined: Does mother's marital stability interact with the dopamine receptor D2 gene in the etiology of childhood attention-deficit/hyperactivity disorder? *Development and Psychopathology, 19*, 1117–1128.
178. Blum, K., et al. (1997). Association of polymorphisms of dopamine D2 receptor (DRD2), and dopamine transporter (DAT1) genes with schizoid/avoidant behaviors (SAB). *Molecular Psychiatry, 2*, 239–246.
179. Martel, M. M., Nikolas, M., Jernigan, K., Friderici, K., & Nigg, J. T. (2010). Personality mediation of genetic effects on attention-deficit/hyperactivity disorder. *Journal of Abnormal Child Psychology, 38*, 633–643.
180. Lee, S. H., et al. (2013). The association of DRD2 -141C and ANKK1 TaqIA polymorphisms with alcohol dependence in Korean population classified by the Lesch typology. *Alcohol and Alcoholism (Oxford, Oxfordshire), 48*, 426–432.
181. Dragan, W. Ł., & Oniszczenko, W. (2009). The association between dopamine D4 receptor exon III polymorphism and intensity of PTSD symptoms among flood survivors. *Anxiety, Stress, and Coping, 22*, 483–495.
182. Bocchetta, A., et al. (1999). Family-based association study between bipolar disorder and DRD2, DRD4, DAT, and SERT in Sardinia. *American Journal of Medical Genetics, 88*, 522–526.
183. Grady, D. L., et al. (2003). High prevalence of rare dopamine receptor D4 alleles in children diagnosed with attention-deficit hyperactivity disorder. *Molecular Psychiatry, 8*, 536–545.
184. Grady, D. L., et al. (2005). Sequence variants of the DRD4 gene in autism: Further evidence that rare DRD4 7R haplotypes are ADHD specific. *American Journal of Medical Genetics. Part B, Neuropsychiatric Genetics: The Official Publication of the International Society of Psychiatric Genetics, 136B*, 33–35.
185. Rowe, D. C., et al. (1999). The DRD2 TaqI polymorphism and symptoms of attention deficit hyperactivity disorder. *Molecular Psychiatry, 4*, 580–586.
186. Gervasini, G., et al. (2018). Effect of dopamine receptor D4 (DRD4) haplotypes on general psychopathology in patients with eating disorders. *Gene, 654*, 43–48.
187. Schwartz, J. A., & Beaver, K. M. (2014). Exploring whether genetic differences between siblings explain sibling differences in criminal justice outcomes. *Comprehensive Psychiatry, 55*, 93–103.
188. Jakubczyk, A., et al. (2017). Paraphilic sexual offenders do not differ from control subjects with respect to dopamine- and serotonin-related genetic polymorphisms. *The Journal of Sexual Medicine, 14*, 125–133.
189. Qadeer, M. I., Amar, A., Mann, J. J., & Hasnain, S. (2017). Polymorphisms in dopaminergic system genes; association with criminal behavior and self-reported aggression in violent prison inmates from Pakistan. *PLoS One, 12*, e0173571.
190. Vaske, J., Wright, J. P., & Beaver, K. M. (2011). A dopamine gene (DRD2) distinguishes between offenders who have and have not been violently victimized. *International Journal of Offender Therapy and Comparative Criminology, 55*, 251–267.
191. Boardman, J. D., et al. (2014). Genes in the dopaminergic system and delinquent behaviors across the life course: The role of social controls and risks. *Criminal Justice and Behavior, 41*, 713–731.

192. Beaver, K. M., Gibson, C. L., Jennings, W. G., & Ward, J. T. (2009). A gene X environment interaction between DRD2 and religiosity in the prediction of adolescent delinquent involvement in a sample of males. *Biodemography and Social Biology, 55*, 71–81.
193. Yun, I., Lee, J., & Kim, S.-G. (2015). Dopaminergic polymorphisms, academic achievement, and violent delinquency. *International Journal of Offender Therapy and Comparative Criminology, 59*, 1409–1428.
194. Guo, G., Roettger, M. E., & Shih, J. C. (2007). Contributions of the DAT1 and DRD2 genes to serious and violent delinquency among adolescents and young adults. *Human Genetics, 121*, 125–136.
195. Chhangur, R. R., et al. (2015). DRD4 and DRD2 genes, parenting, and adolescent delinquency: Longitudinal evidence for a gene by environment interaction. *Journal of Abnormal Psychology, 124*, 791–802.
196. Schwab-Reese, L. M., Parker, E. A., & Peek-Asa, C. (2017). The interaction of dopamine genes and financial stressors to predict adulthood intimate partner violence perpetration. *Journal of Interpersonal Violence, 35*, 1251. https://doi.org/10.1177/0886260517696841.
197. Kotler, M., et al. (1999). Homicidal behavior in schizophrenia associated with a genetic polymorphism determining low catechol O-methyltransferase (COMT) activity. *American Journal of Medical Genetics, 88*, 628–633.
198. Waddington, J. L., et al. (2001). The psychopharmacology-molecular biology interface: Exploring the behavioural roles of dopamine receptor subtypes using targeted gene deletion ('knockout'). *Progress in Neuro-Psychopharmacology & Biological Psychiatry, 25*, 925–964.
199. Kim, B., et al. (2018). Dopamine D2 receptor-mediated circuit from the central amygdala to the bed nucleus of the stria terminalis regulates impulsive behavior. *Proceedings of the National Academy of Sciences of the United States of America, 115*, E10730–E10739.
200. Linden, J., James, A. S., McDaniel, C., & Jentsch, J. D. (2018). Dopamine D2 receptors in dopaminergic neurons modulate performance in a reversal learning task in mice. *eNeuro, 5*(1), e0229-17.2018 1–1, 1–11. https://doi.org/10.1523/ENEURO.0229-17.2018.
201. Falzone, T. L., et al. (2002). Absence of dopamine D4 receptors results in enhanced reactivity to unconditioned, but not conditioned, fear. *The European Journal of Neuroscience, 15*, 158–164.
202. Thanos, P. K., et al. (2016). Dopamine D2 gene expression interacts with environmental enrichment to impact lifespan and behavior. *Oncotarget, 7*, 19111–19123.
203. Grady, D. L., et al. (2013). DRD4 genotype predicts longevity in mouse and human. *Journal of Neuroscience: The Official Journal of the Society for Neuroscience, 33*, 286–291.
204. Thibodeau, E. L., Cicchetti, D., & Rogosch, F. A. (2015). Child maltreatment, impulsivity, and antisocial behavior in African American children: Moderation effects from a cumulative dopaminergic gene index. *Development and Psychopathology, 27*, 1621–1636.
205. Comings, D. E., et al. (2000). Association between the adrenergic alpha 2A receptor gene (ADRA2A) and measures of irritability, hostility, impulsivity and memory in normal subjects. *Psychiatric Genetics, 10*, 39–42.
206. Kiive, E., Kurrikoff, T., Mäestu, J., & Harro, J. (2010). Effect of alpha2A-adrenoceptor C-1291G genotype and maltreatment on hyperactivity and inattention in adolescents. *Progress in Neuro-Psychopharmacology & Biological Psychiatry, 34*, 219–224.
207. Volavka, J., Bilder, R., & Nolan, K. (2004). Catecholamines and aggression: The role of COMT and MAO polymorphisms. *Annals of the New York Academy of Sciences, 1036*, 393–398.
208. Vevera, J., et al. (2009). COMT polymorphisms in impulsively violent offenders with antisocial personality disorder. *Neuro Endocrinology Letters, 30*, 753–756.
209. Asselmann, E., et al. (2018). Interplay between COMT Val158Met, childhood adversities and sex in predicting panic pathology: Findings from a general population sample. *Journal of Affective Disorders, 234*, 290–296.

210. Roy, A., et al. (2018). Family environment interacts with CRHR1 rs17689918 to predict mental health and behavioral outcomes. *Progress in Neuro-Psychopharmacology & Biological Psychiatry, 86*, 45–51.
211. Pawlak, J., et al. (2016). Suicide behavior as a quantitative trait and its genetic background. *Journal of Affective Disorders, 206*, 241–250.
212. Chen, B., et al. (2014). The CRHR1 gene contributes to genetic susceptibility of aggressive behavior towards others in Chinese Southwest Han population. *Journal of Molecular Neuroscience: MN, 52*, 481–486.
213. Zhou, Y., et al. (2014). Ventral midbrain correlation between genetic variation and expression of the dopamine transporter gene in cocaine-abusing versus non-abusing subjects. *Addiction Biology, 19*, 122–131.
214. Chen, T. J. H., et al. (2005). Are dopaminergic genes involved in a predisposition to pathological aggression? Hypothesizing the importance of 'super normal controls' in psychiatric-genetic research of complex behavioral disorders. *Medical Hypotheses, 65*, 703–707.
215. Cómbita, L. M., Voelker, P., Abundis-Gutiérrez, A., Pozuelos, J. P., & Rueda, M. R. (2017). Influence of the SLC6A3-DAT1 gene on multifaceted measures of self-regulation in preschool children. *Frontiers in Psychology, 8*, 26.
216. Comings, D. E., et al. (1997). Studies of the potential role of the dopamine D1 receptor gene in addictive behaviors. *Molecular Psychiatry, 2*, 44–56.
217. Holmes, C., et al. (2001). Psychosis and aggression in Alzheimer's disease: The effect of dopamine receptor gene variation. *Journal of Neurology, Neurosurgery, and Psychiatry, 71*, 777–779.
218. Corrales, E., Navarro, A., Cuenca, P., & Campos, D. (2016). Candidate gene study reveals DRD1 and DRD2 as putative interacting risk factors for youth depression. *Psychiatry Research, 244*, 71–77.
219. Pardini, M., et al. (2014). Aggression, DRD1 polymorphism, and lesion location in penetrating traumatic brain injury. *CNS Spectrums, 19*, 382–390.
220. Trucco, E. M., Villafuerte, S., Heitzeg, M. M., Burmeister, M., & Zucker, R. A. (2016). Susceptibility effects of GABA receptor subunit alpha-2 (GABRA2) variants and parental monitoring on externalizing behavior trajectories: Risk and protection conveyed by the minor allele. *Development and Psychopathology, 28*, 15–26.
221. Bauer, L. O., Covault, J., & Gelernter, J. (2012). GABRA2 and KIBRA genotypes predict early relapse to substance use. *Drug and Alcohol Dependence, 123*, 154–159.
222. Villafuerte, S., Trucco, E. M., Heitzeg, M. M., Burmeister, M., & Zucker, R. A. (2014). Genetic variation in GABRA2 moderates peer influence on externalizing behavior in adolescents. *Brain and Behavior: A Cognitive Neuroscience Perspective, 4*, 833–840.
223. Trucco, E. M., Villafuerte, S., Heitzeg, M. M., Burmeister, M., & Zucker, R. A. (2014). Rule breaking mediates the developmental association between GABRA2 and adolescent substance abuse. *Journal of Child Psychology and Psychiatry, 55*, 1372–1379.
224. Nelson, E. C., et al. (2009). Association of childhood trauma exposure and GABRA2 polymorphisms with risk of posttraumatic stress disorder in adults. *Molecular Psychiatry, 14*, 234–235.
225. Svob Strac, D., et al. (2019). The association between HTR1B gene rs13212041 polymorphism and onset of alcohol abuse. *Neuropsychiatric Disease and Treatment, 15*, 339–347.
226. Hakulinen, C., et al. (2013). Serotonin receptor 1B genotype and hostility, anger and aggressive behavior through the lifespan: The Young Finns study. *Journal of Behavioral Medicine, 36*, 583–590.
227. Hou, Y.-W., et al. (2018). Association of serotonin receptors with attention deficit hyperactivity disorder: A systematic review and meta-analysis. *Current Medical Science, 38*, 538–551.
228. Jensen, K. P., et al. (2009). A common polymorphism in serotonin receptor 1B mRNA moderates regulation by miR-96 and associates with aggressive human behaviors. *Molecular Psychiatry, 14*, 381–389.

229. Moul, C., Dobson-Stone, C., Brennan, J., Hawes, D., & Dadds, M. (2013). An exploration of the serotonin system in antisocial boys with high levels of callous-unemotional traits. *PLoS One, 8*, e56619.
230. Lappalainen, J., et al. (1998). Linkage of antisocial alcoholism to the serotonin 5-HT1B receptor gene in 2 populations. *Archives of General Psychiatry, 55*, 989–994.
231. Shinozaki, G., Romanowicz, M., Mrazek, D. A., & Kung, S. (2013). HTR2A gene-child abuse interaction and association with a history of suicide attempt among Caucasian depressed psychiatric inpatients. *Journal of Affective Disorders, 150*, 1200–1203.
232. Banlaki, Z., et al. (2015). Polymorphism in the serotonin receptor 2a (HTR2A) gene as possible predisposal factor for aggressive traits. *PLoS One, 10*, e0117792.
233. Zalsman, G., et al. (2011). Association of polymorphisms of the serotonergic pathways with clinical traits of impulsive-aggression and suicidality in adolescents: A multi-center study. *The World Journal of Biological Psychiatry: The Official Journal of the World Federation of Societies of Biological Psychiatry, 12*, 33–41.
234. Toshchakova, V. A., et al. (2017). Association of polymorphisms of serotonin transporter (5HTTLPR) and 5-HT2C receptor genes with criminal behavior in Russian criminal offenders. *Neuropsychobiology, 75*, 200–210.
235. Paes, L. A., et al. (2018). Association between serotonin 2C receptor gene (HTR2C) polymorphisms and psychopathological symptoms in children and adolescents. *Brazilian Journal of Medical and Biological Research = Revista brasileira de pesquisas médicas e biológicas, 51*, e7252.
236. Grzesiak, M., et al. (2017). Serotonin-related gene variants in patients with irritable bowel syndrome and depressive or anxiety disorders. *Gastroenterology Research and Practice, 2017*, 4290430.
237. Weissmann, D., et al. (2016). Region-specific alterations of A-to-I RNA editing of serotonin 2c receptor in the cortex of suicides with major depression. *Translational Psychiatry, 6*, e878.
238. Avery, B. M., & Vrshek-Schallhorn, S. (2016). Nonsynonymous HTR2C polymorphism predicts cortisol response to psychosocial stress I: Effects in males and females. *Psychoneuroendocrinology, 70*, 134–141.
239. Fortier, M.-È., et al. (2013). Genetic evidence for the association of the hypothalamic-pituitary-adrenal (HPA) axis with ADHD and methylphenidate treatment response. *Neuromolecular Medicine, 15*, 122–132.
240. Li, J., et al. (2017). Genetic associations and interactions between the NR3C1 (GR) and NR3C2 (MR) genes and aggressive behavior in a Central South Chinese Han Population. *Genetic Testing and Molecular Biomarkers, 21*, 497–505.
241. Plieger, T., Felten, A., Splittgerber, H., Duke, É., & Reuter, M. (2018). The role of genetic variation in the glucocorticoid receptor (NR3C1) and mineralocorticoid receptor (NR3C2) in the association between cortisol response and cognition under acute stress. *Psychoneuroendocrinology, 87*, 173–180.
242. Hartling, C., et al. (2019). Interaction of HPA axis genetics and early life stress shapes emotion recognition in healthy adults. *Psychoneuroendocrinology, 99*, 28–37.
243. Zheng, Y., et al. (2018). Glucocorticoid receptor (NR3C1) gene polymorphism moderate intervention effects on the developmental trajectory of African-American Adolescent Alcohol Abuse. *Prevention Science: The Official Journal of the Society for Prevention Research, 19*, 79–89.
244. Starr, L. R., & Huang, M. (2018). HPA-axis multilocus genetic variation moderates associations between environmental stress and depressive symptoms among adolescents. *Development and Psychopathology, 31*, 1339. https://doi.org/10.1017/S0954579418000779.
245. Gerra, G., et al. (2004). Association between low-activity serotonin transporter genotype and heroin dependence: Behavioral and personality correlates. *American Journal of Medical Genetics. Part B, Neuropsychiatric Genetics: The Official Publication of the International Society of Psychiatric Genetics, 126B*, 37–42.

246. Hallikainen, T., et al. (1999). Association between low activity serotonin transporter promoter genotype and early onset alcoholism with habitual impulsive violent behavior. *Molecular Psychiatry, 4*, 385–388.
247. Craig, I. W. (2007). The importance of stress and genetic variation in human aggression. *BioEssays: News and Reviews in Molecular, Cellular and Developmental Biology, 29*, 227–236.
248. Virkkunen, M., Goldman, D., Nielsen, D. A., & Linnoila, M. (1995). Low brain serotonin turnover rate (low CSF 5-HIAA) and impulsive violence. *Journal of Psychiatry & Neuroscience: JPN, 20*, 271–275.
249. Antypa, N., Serretti, A., & Rujescu, D. (2013). Serotonergic genes and suicide: A systematic review. *European Neuropsychopharmacology: The Journal of the European College of Neuropsychopharmacology, 23*, 1125–1142.
250. Brummett, B. H., et al. (2014). A putatively functional polymorphism in the HTR2C gene is associated with depressive symptoms in white females reporting significant life stress. *PLoS One, 9*, e114451.
251. Liu, R., et al. (2016). Early postnatal stress suppresses the developmental trajectory of hippocampal pyramidal neurons: The role of CRHR1. *Brain Structure & Function, 221*, 4525–4536.
252. Gonzalez-Nunez, V. (2015). Role of gabra2, GABAA receptor alpha-2 subunit, in CNS development. *Biochemistry and Biophysics Reports, 3*, 190–201.
253. Tucci, V., Lassi, G., & Kas, M. J. (2012). Current understanding of the interplay between catechol-O-methyltransferase genetic variants, sleep, brain development and cognitive performance in schizophrenia. *CNS & Neurological Disorders Drug Targets, 11*, 292–298.
254. Reed, J. L., et al. (2018). Interaction of childhood urbanicity and variation in dopamine genes alters adult prefrontal function as measured by functional magnetic resonance imaging (fMRI). *PLoS One, 13*, e0195189.
255. Chau, C. M. Y., et al. (2019). Hippocampus, amygdala, and thalamus volumes in very preterm children at 8 years: Neonatal pain and genetic variation. *Frontiers in Behavioral Neuroscience, 13*, 51.
256. Batalla, A., et al. (2018). The influence of DAT1, COMT, and BDNF genetic polymorphisms on total and subregional hippocampal volumes in early onset heavy cannabis users. *Cannabis and Cannabinoid Research, 3*, 1–10.
257. Pagliaccio, D., et al. (2015). Amygdala functional connectivity, HPA axis genetic variation, and life stress in children and relations to anxiety and emotion regulation. *Journal of Abnormal Psychology, 124*, 817–833.
258. Pratelli, M., & Pasqualetti, M. (2019). Serotonergic neurotransmission manipulation for the understanding of brain development and function: Learning from Tph2 genetic models. *Biochimie, 161*, 3–14.
259. Giegling, I., et al. (2010). Influence of neuronal cell adhesion molecule (NCAM1) variants on suicidal behaviour and correlated traits. *Psychiatry Research, 179*, 222–225.
260. Hawi, Z., et al. (2018). The role of cadherin genes in five major psychiatric disorders: A literature update. *American Journal of Medical Genetics. Part B, Neuropsychiatric Genetics: The Official Publication of the International Society of Psychiatric Genetics, 177*, 168–180.
261. Stork, O., et al. (2000). Recovery of emotional behaviour in neural cell adhesion molecule (NCAM) null mutant mice through transgenic expression of NCAM180. *The European Journal of Neuroscience, 12*, 3291–3306.
262. Scheiffele, P., Fan, J., Choih, J., Fetter, R., & Serafini, T. (2000). Neuroligin expressed in nonneuronal cells triggers presynaptic development in contacting axons. *Cell, 101*, 657–669.
263. Kohl, C., et al. (2013). Hippocampal neuroligin-2 overexpression leads to reduced aggression and inhibited novelty reactivity in rats. *PLoS One, 8*, e56871.
264. Kohl, C., et al. (2015). Hippocampal neuroligin-2 links early-life stress with impaired social recognition and increased aggression in adult mice. *Psychoneuroendocrinology, 55*, 128–143.

265. van der Kooij, M. A., et al. (2014). Impaired hippocampal neuroligin-2 function by chronic stress or synthetic peptide treatment is linked to social deficits and increased aggression. *Neuropsychopharmacology: Official Publication of the American College of Neuropsychopharmacology, 39*, 1148–1158.
266. Burrows, E. L., et al. (2015). A neuroligin-3 mutation implicated in autism causes abnormal aggression and increases repetitive behavior in mice. *Molecular Autism, 6*, 62.
267. Alimperti, S., & Andreadis, S. T. (2015). CDH2 and CDH11 act as regulators of stem cell fate decisions. *Stem Cell Research, 14*, 270–282.
268. Rivero, O., et al. (2013). Impact of the ADHD-susceptibility gene CDH13 on development and function of brain networks. *European Neuropsychopharmacology: The Journal of the European College of Neuropsychopharmacology, 23*, 492–507.
269. Scheinin, M., Sallinen, J., & Haapalinna, A. (2001). Evaluation of the alpha2C-adrenoceptor as a neuropsychiatric drug target studies in transgenic mouse models. *Life Sciences, 68*, 2277–2285.
270. Gogos, J. A., et al. (1998). Catechol-O-methyltransferase-deficient mice exhibit sexually dimorphic changes in catecholamine levels and behavior. *Proceedings of the National Academy of Sciences, 95*, 9991–9996.
271. Papaleo, F., Erickson, L., Liu, G., Chen, J., & Weinberger, D. R. (2012). Effects of sex and COMT genotype on environmentally modulated cognitive control in mice. *Proceedings of the National Academy of Sciences of the United States of America, 109*, 20160–20165.
272. Müller, M. B., et al. (2003). Limbic corticotropin-releasing hormone receptor 1 mediates anxiety-related behavior and hormonal adaptation to stress. *Nature Neuroscience, 6*, 1100–1107.
273. Molander, A., et al. (2012). Brain-specific inactivation of the Crhr1 gene inhibits post-dependent and stress-induced alcohol intake, but does not affect relapse-like drinking. *Neuropsychopharmacology: Official Publication of the American College of Neuropsychopharmacology, 37*, 1047–1056.
274. Rodriguiz, R. M., Chu, R., Caron, M. G., & Wetsel, W. C. (2004). Aberrant responses in social interaction of dopamine transporter knockout mice. *Behavioural Brain Research, 148*, 185–198.
275. Duka, T., et al. (2015). Motivational effects of methylphenidate are associated with GABRA2 variants conferring addiction risk. *Frontiers in Behavioral Neuroscience, 9*, 304.
276. Dixon, C. I., Walker, S. E., King, S. L., & Stephens, D. N. (2012). Deletion of the gabra2 gene results in hypersensitivity to the acute effects of ethanol but does not alter ethanol self administration. *PLoS One, 7*, e47135.
277. Dixon, C. I., Rosahl, T. W., & Stephens, D. N. (2008). Targeted deletion of the GABRA2 gene encoding alpha2-subunits of GABA(A) receptors facilitates performance of a conditioned emotional response, and abolishes anxiolytic effects of benzodiazepines and barbiturates. *Pharmacology, Biochemistry, and Behavior, 90*, 1–8.
278. Joshi, R. S., Quadros, R., Drumm, M., Ain, R., & Panicker, M. M. (2017). Sedative effect of Clozapine is a function of 5-HT2A and environmental novelty. *European Neuropsychopharmacology: The Journal of the European College of Neuropsychopharmacology, 27*, 70–81.
279. Han, S., et al. (2014). Impaired extinction of learned contextual fear memory in early growth response 1 knockout mice. *Molecules and Cells, 37*, 24–30.
280. Séjourné, J., Llaneza, D., Kuti, O. J., & Page, D. T. (2015). Social behavioral deficits coincide with the onset of seizure susceptibility in mice lacking serotonin receptor 2c. *PLoS One, 10*, e0136494.
281. Godar, S. C., et al. (2011). Maladaptive defensive behaviours in monoamine oxidase A-deficient mice. *The International Journal of Neuropsychopharmacology, 14*, 1195–1207.
282. Bortolato, M., et al. (2011). Social deficits and perseverative behaviors, but not overt aggression, in MAO-A hypomorphic mice. *Neuropsychopharmacology: Official Publication of the American College of Neuropsychopharmacology, 36*, 2674–2688.

283. Holmes, A., Murphy, D. L., & Crawley, J. N. (2002). Reduced aggression in mice lacking the serotonin transporter. *Psychopharmacology, 161*, 160–167.
284. Bischoff, S. C., et al. (2009). Role of serotonin in intestinal inflammation: Knockout of serotonin reuptake transporter exacerbates 2,4,6-trinitrobenzene sulfonic acid colitis in mice. *American Journal of Physiology. Gastrointestinal and Liver Physiology, 296*, G685–G695.
285. Igari, M., et al. (2015). Attenuated methamphetamine-induced locomotor sensitization in serotonin transporter knockout mice is restored by serotonin 1B receptor antagonist treatment. *Behavioural Pharmacology, 26*, 167–179.
286. Gutknecht, L., et al. (2015). Interaction of brain 5-HT synthesis deficiency, chronic stress and sex differentially impact emotional behavior in Tph2 knockout mice. *Psychopharmacology, 232*, 2429–2441.
287. Matosin, N., Frank, E., Engel, M., Lum, J. S., & Newell, K. A. (2014). Negativity towards negative results: A discussion of the disconnect between scientific worth and scientific culture. *Disease Models & Mechanisms, 7*, 171–173.
288. Teixeira da Silva, J. A. (2015). Negative results: Negative perceptions limit their potential for increasing reproducibility. *Journal of Negative Results in BioMedicine, 14*, 12.
289. Manolio, T. A., et al. (2009). Finding the missing heritability of complex diseases. *Nature, 461*, 747–753.
290. Barabási, A.-L., Gulbahce, N., & Loscalzo, J. (2011). Network medicine: A network-based approach to human disease. *Nature Reviews. Genetics, 12*, 56–68.
291. Huang, S., Ernberg, I., & Kauffman, S. (2009). Cancer attractors: A systems view of tumors from a gene network dynamics and developmental perspective. *Seminars in Cell & Developmental Biology, 20*, 869–876.
292. Rosvall, K. A. (2013). Proximate perspectives on the evolution of female aggression: Good for the gander, good for the goose? *Philosophical Transactions of the Royal Society of London. Series B, Biological Sciences, 368*, 20130083.
293. Manfredini, F., Brown, M. J. F., & Toth, A. L. (2018). Candidate genes for cooperation and aggression in the social wasp Polistes dominula. *Journal of Comparative Physiology. A, Neuroethology, Sensory, Neural, and Behavioral Physiology, 204*, 449–463.
294. Buades-Rotger, M., & Gallardo-Pujol, D. (2014). The role of the monoamine oxidase A gene in moderating the response to adversity and associated antisocial behavior: A review. *Psychology Research and Behavior Management, 7*, 185–200.

Chapter 4
Social Factors of Biological Change

Introduction

The previous chapter led to the conclusion that abnormal animal and human aggressions are unlikely to be due solely to genetic polymorphisms. Genetic backgrounds may only create vulnerabilities that are "exploited" and amplified by environmental insults. This association of factors is commonly called the gene x environment interaction and implicates stress hormones as both mediators of environmental influences and motors of the ensuing neural changes. Before evaluating the role of stress and stress hormones in aggression, however, we review here the most common environmental factors that can disturb development, particularly those social conditions and events that are assumed to underlie the emergence of both psychopathologies and violent crime. These are the social factors that induce behavioral changes which on their turn lead to altered mental states and functions. We will begin with criminological theories of crime that are reluctant to incorporate biological mechanisms, despite that at research level, these are readily studied by those who are interested in violent crime as shown in the previous and will be shown in the following chapter. Criminological theories will be followed by a brief overview of the social factors known to be involved in the emergence of criminal behavior. The chapter will end by the presentation of the various-number "hit" hypotheses that are believed to lead to mental disorders but may at the same time underlie violent crime.

J. Haller, *Neurobiopsychosocial Perspectives on Aggression and Violence*,
Advances in Preventing and Treating Violence and Aggression,
https://doi.org/10.1007/978-3-030-46331-1_4

4.1 Society and Crime

4.1.1 Criminological Theories of Crime

Out of the many theories of crime, we will address below the most important six, which will be presented in an alphabetic order. We will pay attention to the historic backgrounds of concepts by referring to pioneering publications but will also cite much newer work to demonstrate the present-day acceptance of these theories.

The *conflict theory* [1, 2] understands crime as a competition between social groups for limited resources, an idea that some historians trace back to the work of Marx, but which is also compatible with the biological approach to aggression. Recent versions have the following basic principles: (1) Society is made up of groups, each with its own social norms and interests. (2) Individuals who make up a group act in their self-interest, and this is reflected in the behavior of the group to which they belong. (3) The more power a group has, the more likely it is to conflict with the general norms and values of society. (4) "Bureaucracy" (including the police) will suppress those with the least power to minimize their investment and maximize their success, and therefore (5) the official crime statistics of the groups will be inversely proportional to their own political and economic power.

The *crime opportunity theory* [3] is in fact a variant of the rational choice theory (see below) but focuses on opportunity rather than on rational choice. It assumes that there are three premises that make perpetration likely: a motivated offender, a suitable target, and an opportunity, i.e., a set of conditions that make crime possible. Examples of such opportunities are general social breakdown and inadequate policing [4, 5].

The *rational choice theory* has its origins in the nineteenth century, but its modern form can be attributed to Becker [6]. The theory is still in use today [7, 8], and in addition to explaining crime, it is assumed to help crime prevention as well [9]. The theory posits that humans are reasoning actors who become perpetrators consciously by their own choice. One commits crime when this is advantageous, that is, when there is a hope for profit. Perpetrators are assumed to consider risks and benefits when deciding to commit crime. The perception of risk depends on social learning, e.g., on the summation of past and current experience with crime and arrest and on information from peers. Such risks are evaluated in conjunction with subjective reward expectations in terms of financial, psychological (excitement), and social (status) gains as well as the perception of opportunities.

The *social control theory* [10, 11] is perhaps the only criminological theory that focuses not on the factors that cause crime but on those that prevent it. Its key concept is social learning, which enforces self-restraint, which discourages someone from carrying out antisocial acts. Refraining from crime critically depends on the regularity of punishment of wrongful behavior and on rewards for compliance by family and authoritative figures.

The *social learning theory* [12, 13] is the opposite of social control as social learning focuses on the learning of criminal behavior. It hypothesizes that social learning consists of two components: an imitation component, that is, copying the behavior of others and a so-called operant conditioning component caused by the positive consequences of the act. Simply put, if a child observes a behavior – in this context crime – integrates the pattern of that behavior into his or her behavioral repertoire, but only if its outcome proves to be favorable. This explanation suggests that crime is in fact an adaptive response.

The *strain or anomie theory* was developed in 1938 by Merton [14], revised by the end of the last century by Agnew [15], and still serves as a framework for understanding crime [16]. The essence of the theory is that crime is committed under social pressure, i.e., the individual is constrained by circumstances into offender behavior. Constraints (strains) can be divided into three groups: (1) frustrating factors that make desired life goals unattainable; (2) threatening factors that may deprive the potential offender of the values she/he has already acquired; and (3) incapacitating factors that in some way disable the potential offender, e.g., she/he lacks appropriate education. The strain arouses emotions, primarily anger either because the individual lacks the skills to handle the situation or because it is objectively impossible to solve a life problem, e.g., there is no way to move out of the countryside that does not suit the individual. Because there is no legal way to prevent or counteract disadvantages, there is a high risk that the individual will move in the direction of lawlessness. Early theories focused primarily on young people, but recent versions have extended to adults who are exposed to strains such as unemployment. New concepts have been integrated into theory, such as conditioning, which creates an "automatic" connection between a particular situation and crime (crime becomes a "routine").

One can divide these theories into two groups. The strain, conflict, and opportunity theories emphasize the role of the society, whereas the other three, rational choice, social control, and social learning theories, emphasize the role of the individual. Demarcation lines, however, are not strict as a rational choice to commit crime may be motivated by social constraints; exploiting crime opportunities may be favored by inefficient social control; and the strain and opportunity theories complement each other, etc. In principle, however, criminological theories attribute crime to two major factors, which will be briefly reviewed below to provide a framework for understanding the biological – post-heritability – factors of violent crime.

4.1.2 Macrostructural Social Factors

These factors are called macrostructural because they affect major parts of the society – sometimes the whole society – and the conflicts are imbedded in its structure to a large extent.

4.1.2.1 Social Injustice

One of the very typical and critical social tensions is economic in nature and separates those who live under poor conditions, i.e., experience inequality or perceive their situation as such. Of course, inequality cannot be characterized by the absolute value of income. The income that can be a source of tension in a rich country can be a source of satisfaction in a poor one. To overcome this problem, a metric has been developed, the so-called Gini index [17], which aims to measure inequality by taking into account the way in which society's total income is distributed among its members. This metric lies between two extremes: its value is 0 if incomes are distributed equally between the members of the society and 100 if the income comes in the hands of a single person. These are obviously theoretical extremes; real Gini indices are somewhere between 25 and 60. To examine the relationship between the Gini index and crime, we conducted a mini study for this chapter, by associating the crime statistics [18] and Gini indices [19] of 32 European countries for which data were available. Results are shown in Fig. 4.1 (panel A).

The mini study shows that in Europe, violent crime – surprisingly – is inversely proportional to the Gini index. This finding, to say the least, does not support the strain theory; however, our sample was made up of countries that have relatively low Gini indices, and economic inequalities are not linearly related to the social tensions they cause [20]. To a certain extent, inequalities are well tolerated by members of society; problems emerge when the Gini index reaches a value close to or above 40. If the sample includes countries with such high values, we get the expected correlation: the higher the Gini index, the higher the crime rate (Fig. 4.1, panel B) [21]. These and a host of other findings show that economic inequality has no clear

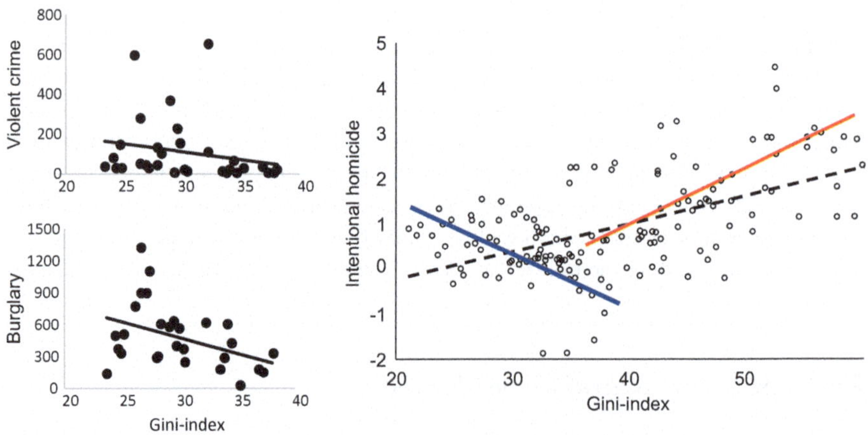

Fig. 4.1 Inequality and crime. *Left-hand panel.* The findings of the mini research performed for this chapter. The number of perpetrated violent crimes and burglaries, respectively, was correlated with the Gini indices in a total of 32 European countries based on open-source statistics as shown in text. Each closed circle represents a country. Both negative correlations were significant at $p < 0.05$ level. *Right-hand panel.* The correlation between intentional homicides and Gini indices in more than 100 countries based on published data as shown in text. The dashed black line shows the correlation evidenced by the publication. The blue and red correlation lines were inserted by the author. Note that the blue line reproduced the findings of the study shown on the left. Overall, these studies show that inequalities increase crime rates only when they transform into injustice (i.e., the Gini index is very high). It is difficult to explain at present why the correlation was negative at low Gini index values

relation to crime rates, that is, it is not a very significant risk factor for crime. Poverty in itself is not a crime risk, and well-being does not relieve from risks as shown by the occasional criminal behavior of the social elite [22–24]. Crime risks increase, however, when inequality becomes injustice.

4.1.2.2 Social Division and Identity

Societies consists of countless smaller or larger groups whose interests and objectives are not necessarily the same but generally accept, at least in substance, the social contract [25] that holds the system together. In more modern interpretations, the members of society express their agreement with the metaphorical social contract by not rebelling against society [26]. Staying with this metaphor, the social contract is not accepted by everyone, which creates groups that perceive their identity to be contrary to society or to any of its subsystems. This is expressed, accepting the position of modern "contract interpreters," by some form of rebellion against the social contract.

In some cases, identity differences confront small social groups. For instance, extreme groups of football fans, due to their conflicting and hostile identities, develop strong emotional tensions, often colored by political or nationalist ones, which together can become a risk of a wide range of violent crimes ranging from hooliganism to attacks on police [27]. In more problematic cases, social divisions lead to the development of criminal identities, which appear in smaller and larger criminal groups [28], just as in organized crime [29] and terrorism [30]. The essence of these divisions is the collision of "we" with "you," where "we" is the quintessence of good, while the concept of "you" can be summarized by the words "enemy" and/or "easy prey." The former concept is mainly valid for radical social groups, the other for criminal groups. Thus, there often is a hostile divide within society, which is a serious risk of crime, especially if the law and social consensus become loose, as seen in unrest [5] and drug crime [31].

4.1.2.3 Cataclysms

As a result of tragic events in society (war, natural disasters, terrorist attacks), the order is disrupted, opening the way to crime. At one extreme, individuals take advantage of the temporary weakening of law to commit crimes, essentially for the sake of profit; at the other, law-abiding citizens, when prevented from satisfying their basic needs, resort to acts that are normally illegal [32]. Beyond natural disasters, the risk of crime is increased by civil wars, which create opportunities not only for regular criminals or citizens in need but also for peacekeeping forces and aid agencies [33]. Similarly, political and other forms of unrest create opportunities for criminals who have nothing to do with the social tension that caused the riot [34].

4.1.3 Microstructural Social Factors

Microstructural factors are essentially small-scale, sometimes individual, projections of macrostructural social tensions and affect small social units (e.g., the family) or the individual.

4.1.3.1 Prenatal Social Factors

The expectant mother is the smallest possible social group; she will be the starting point for our investigation. In principle, the relationship between the mother and the fetus is biological; yet, the mother carries her child as a member of another social group, the family, and is also subject to the greater social tensions we have dealt with in the previous section. This tension, through the biological connection between the mother and the fetus (e.g., by the ability of maternal stress hormones to pass the placental barrier), affects the development of the child and carries risks for future criminal behavior, as shown by several studies.

For instance, the risks for violent crime perpetration and arrests in later life were increased if the fetus was indirectly exposed to the negative consequences of maternal malnutrition [35] or if the mother suffered other socioeconomic disadvantages [36]. In the same vein, depression during pregnancy, which indicates high levels of maternal stress, increased the risk of delinquency in the child [37]. Similarly, smoking by the pregnant mother [38] or the consumption of alcohol and other drugs [39] forecasted violent behavior and law infringements by the child when she/he grew up.

The issue is unquestionably understudied, yet the available findings may be sufficient to state that intrauterine life affects later criminal risks if pregnancy was disturbed by unfavorable conditions.

4.1.3.2 The Child's Social Environment

At the preschool age, society is reduced to the family for the child, or at least she/he has very little contact with the rest of the society. Ideally, the child is surrounded by loving care, but this is not always the case, primarily for social reasons. There are three factors that can interfere with the development of children and their risks of developing aggression problems later in life: early social neglect, stressful upbringing, and trauma.

The term "early social neglect" denotes a multicomponent condition [40]. The neglected child lacks emotional parental support, is insufficiently fed and dressed – which is especially problematic in the cold seasons – and is in the want of elementary hygiene. This state would be identified as poverty in adults as the child cannot adequately meet his/her basic needs. This may directly result from the socioeconomic status of parents but also from subjective factors (see below), which, however, may also have a social background. Early social neglect is consequential for adult life if at least two factors, physical neglect and lack of affection, occur together. Such multicomponent neglect leads to a range of mental disorders [41] and neurodevelopmental deficits [42] in adulthood, including a predisposition to violence.

Stressful childhoods often result from disrupted family life, the parents' alcoholism, and their abusive behavior. Although it occurs at family level, child abuse has essentially social causes; for example, it has been shown that children are most often abused in poor neighborhoods where police presence is high due to the high crime rates in the area [43]. Early stressors and victimization often result in abusive personalities, the consequences of which are felt not only by the social partners (victims) of the perpetrator but even by the next generation through the so-called cycle of violence – i.e., by the abusive behavior of those who were themselves abused in childhood [44]. In addition to adult intrafamilial conflicts that emerge from stressful nurturing, such experiences also increase the risk of violent offending [45] especially if early development takes place in impoverished neighborhoods [46]. Thus, economic inequalities and familial problems interact in increasing the risks of adult violence [47].

Finally, there are children who are traumatized, for example, those that experience a stressful crisis in which their existence or life is in danger, without any hope for help. Some of the traumas are not of social origin; a traumatic experience can be, for example, a fire or an earthquake. War, which is traumatic for children and adults alike, is created by society. In addition, a child may be traumatized if he or she is not simply abused but subjected to brutal violence or is sexually molested. An early traumatic experience has immediate psychological and occasionally psychiatric consequences but also constitutes a risk of adult crime [48], including murder [48] and serial killing [49], likely due to the development of an unstable personality, prone to both reactive and proactive aggression, and insensitive to the suffering of others, i.e., who carries psychopathic traits [50].

4.1.3.3 Society and Adolescence

Sometime during adolescence, the young person starts to lead a dual life by being subject to both familial and societal influences. As a result of emotional storms, the adolescent is almost inevitably in conflict with parents, who have to decide how to handle the situation. One line of research suggests that lenient education decreases the risks of becoming a criminal, whereas harsh parenting style increases it [51]. It was suggested that adolescents undergoing "hard" education are alienated from the family and may become more open to other influences. Cultural factors, however, must play a role here; as in contrast to American families, the liberal education is the one that poses a risk for crime in Latin American adolescents [52]. Irrespective to cultural differences, which will be reviewed below, it is clear that the attitude of the family and parents towards the adolescent is an important risk factor for crime. If adolescents do not receive what is appropriate for their development, a thread that binds them to the law-abiding society may be broken.

The second important social group to which the adolescent is attached is the school, which has two basic requirements: educational attainment and social integration. If adolescents fail in one or both, another strand that connects them to society may be broken. A number of studies have shown that poor schooling is a significant risk of crime [53], and data suggest that education is a protective factor [54]. Failure may compel the adolescent to turn against the school, especially his/her classmates, and to become a school bully who terrorizes his companions, which is a risk for both current problems with rules and for the most serious crimes, e.g., school shootings [55] prospectively. In short, if the adolescent fails in school, another obstacle to social integration occurs.

Finally, during adolescence, the individual becomes increasingly involved in the life of the society. Social rejection by the immediate social environment (the neighborhood) [56] or by the society as a whole [57] is also a crime risk.

As the threads that bind the adolescents to the law-abiding society start to break, the attractions of crime increase. They can relieve the frustration of rejection by joining groups (hardcore fans or gangs), to identify with them, to conform to their norms, to become cohesive, and to strive to acquire group goals such as status [58]. Adolescents may also join militant groups merely to seek a receptive community [59] or may participate in riots to experience the social acceptance of anger and aggression [34]. All these may be perceived as rational choices, but in fact decisions are taken under the influence of compelling social influences, and despite acquiring surrogate social acceptance, the new social groups are new sources of stress.

4.1.3.4 The Culture of Violence

Violence and crime can also be transmitted culturally as another criminological theory – suggestively called the "culture of violence theory" – posits [60]. It is generally believed that the culture of violence has gradually been overshadowed over the years and that, as a result, violence is rarely accepted today as a legitimate way of resolving conflicts. Areas of social attitudes where the culture of violence has allegedly not yet been broken down are sexual violence against women where the crime is often passed onto the victim [61], domestic violence where violence is still often seen as a legitimate manifestation of male dominance [62], and the glorification of physical violence in the media. Many believe that media violence influences young people in particular and that this has an impact on violent crime [63]. Although the relationship is debated [64], there is no doubt that media violence is a revealing expression of the culture of violence.

One form of the culture of violence is the so-called culture of honor whereby the stain on honor is washed away by force, even in schools [65]. Regional cultures of violence also seem to exist; for instance, men in the Southern United States appear to be more violent than those in the northern states [66], and overall, national differences in the frequency of violent crime as well as the conflicts between countries are sometimes also viewed in terms of the culture of violence [67]. This may especially be damaging in social groups that are marginalized by social conditions and where it may enhance the criminological effects of other macro- and microstructural factors.

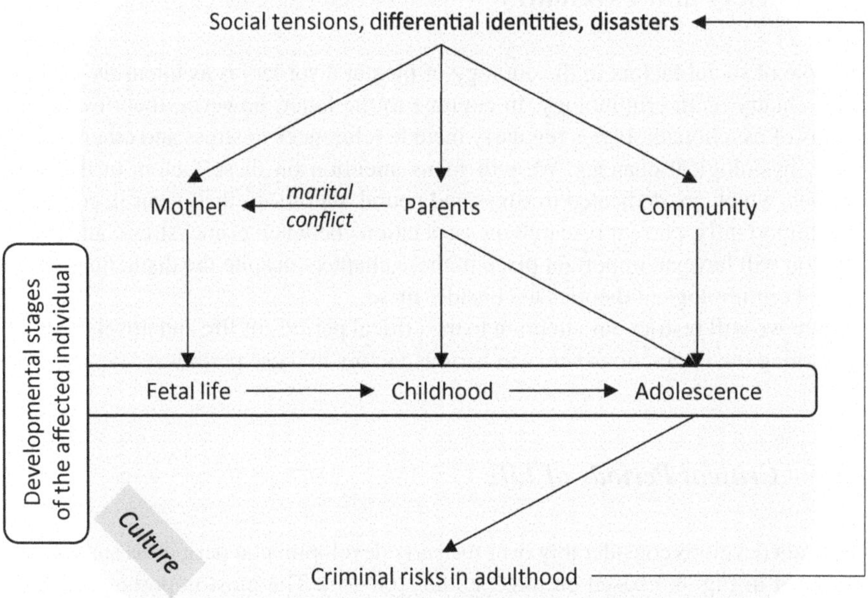

Fig. 4.2 The web of stressors affecting the developing individual. The arrows show the directional hierarchical structure of stressors that affect the individual at different stages of life to increase the risk of aggression problems and violent crime. The feedback-like loop symbolizes the cycle of violence. For other explanations see text

4.1.4 Overview and Outlook

The findings reviewed above are strong arguments in favor of criminological theories, by showing how social dynamics and individual developmental trajectories lead to crime under unfortunate conditions. The theories themselves may contradict each other – the social strain theory, for instance, attributes crime to social constraints, whereas the rational choice theory to personal preferences – yet each theory can find its place in the mosaic of interconnected social factors. While neither seems to explain alone crime, together they appear to cover causes to a fairly large extent. Yet all seem to miss an important aspect.

From a biomedical viewpoint, social factors of crime seem to constitute a hierarchical system of stressors (Fig. 4.2), which in addition to influencing sociopsychological aspects of personality also have a large impact on the development of the brain. This reluctance of criminological theories to consider factors other than social is not shared by psychiatric models.

4.2 Society and Psychiatry

The role of social factors in the etiology of mental disorders is as intensely studied in psychiatry as in criminology. In contrast to the latter, however, theories on the origins of psychopathologies regularly include references to stress and other underlying physiological changes. We will focus attention on these factors in the next sections, which are dedicated to stress and neural alterations that occur in conjunction. Importantly, current research on associations between crime, stress, and brain function will have an important place in these chapters despite the disinclination of general criminological theories to consider these.

Here we will restrict our attention to the critical periods of life and novel theories concerning the interactions between various factors in these periods.

4.2.1 Critical Periods of Life

The brain develops considerably over the early developmental periods as summarily presented in Fig. 4.3 based on three studies [68–70]. The most important changes can be grouped into two periods: early childhood and adolescence.

After birth, the arborization of neurons increases dramatically up to the age of 2 years, followed by a simplification that stabilizes sometime around age 6 years (upper panel), but only temporarily until adolescence when a second wave of restructuring takes place (middle panel). Importantly, epigenetic changes, which determine the plasticity of the brain in response to environmental influences, are also markedly increased in these two periods. Without going into further detail, early childhood and adolescence are periods, when the brain undergoes important changes within a short period. The magnitude of changes in these two periods of life is comparable except for the amygdala (the "home" of emotional control), the functional responsiveness of which culminates in adolescence, which may be responsible for the emotional storms typical to this life period. Finally, the forebrain develops after adolescence, around the age of 20–25 years. As a result, frontal brain connectivity increases, whereas the connectivity of more posterior regions decreases over time (lower panel). Note that the development of the prefrontal cortex – although peaks late – is strongly influenced by earlier changes, particularly those occurring in adolescence because these have influences on subsequent events.

This brief section was naturally not intended to overview brain development in detail but to show that this is not continuous but has two critical periods when neural changes are not only intense but are easily influenced by the environment. This explains why theories on psychopathology focus on these two life periods.

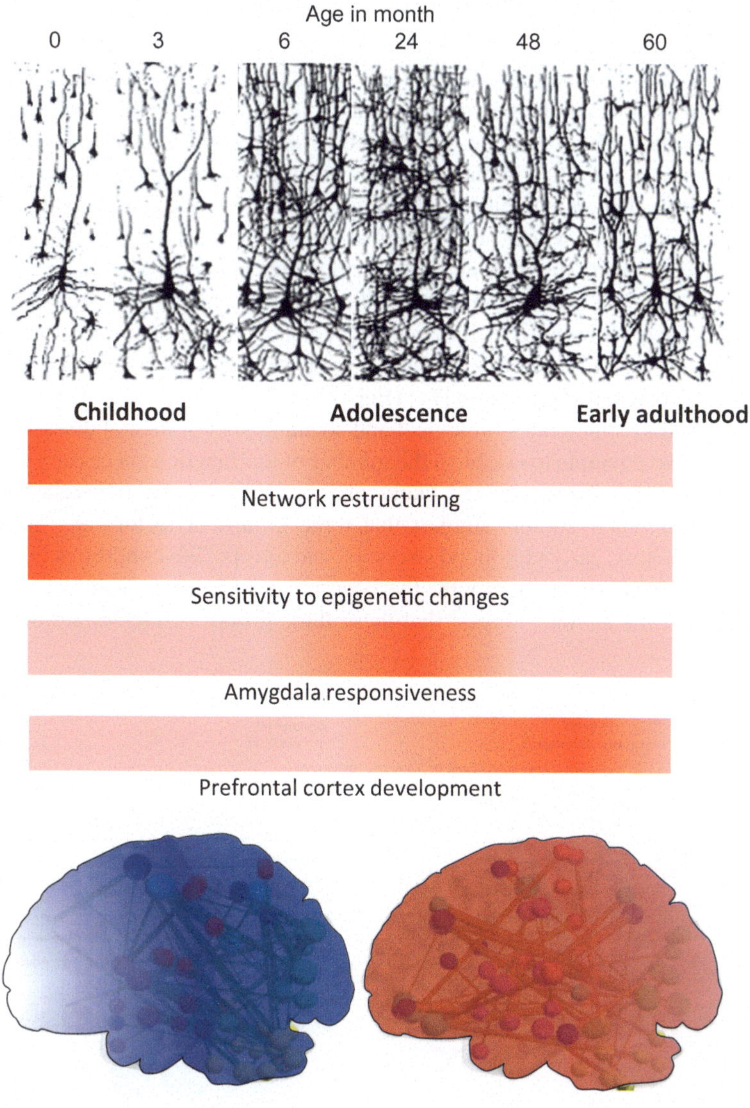

Fig. 4.3 Sensitive periods of brain development. *Upper panel*. Network restructuring in the first 5 years of life (based on Conel [68]). Similar changes occur in adolescence as shown in the first row of the next panel. *Middle panel*. The critical periods of change in epigenetic sensitivity, amygdala responsiveness, and prefrontal development, relevant for sensitivity to environmental influences, emotional instability, and cognitive development, respectively (based on Ganzel [70]). *Lower panel*. From age 7–35, connectivity decreases in posterior regions of the brain (blue) but increases in frontal regions (red) (based on Qin [69]). This may indicate a shift from a dominance of ancient brain structures to a dominance of frontal regions that host a series of important features including the ability for moral judgment

4.2.2 The Three-Hit Hypothesis of Psychopathology

Mental disorders can be explained by purely genetic factors, but the number of genetic "errors" that can be perceived as causal is extremely small as shown in the previous chapter. Minor genetic defects, however, become important when their consequences are amplified by the environment – e.g., by social factors that are very similar to those that are perceived to be linked to crime. These factors are believed to constitute stressors which, as etiological factors of mental disorders, result in altered psychological functioning. The relationship between genetic factors and stressors, however, is poorly understood. Therefore, psychiatrists seek explanations of how risk factors combine such to make a person ill, while others who also carry risk factors are exempted from this. One of the psychiatric explanations is summarized in the "three-hit" hypothesis [71] (Fig. 4.4).

This hypothesis integrates biological and social factors of mental disease, but in addition, it also attempts to establish the number of malfunctions necessary to make the emergence of disorders very likely and outlines the putative relationships between them. Their authors suggest that three groups of factors are "needed": genetic risk factors, early childhood stressors, and adverse life conditions in adolescence. If all three affect the youth, the occurrence of mental disorders is rather likely. In fact, the authors suggest that these three groups of factors are the mini-

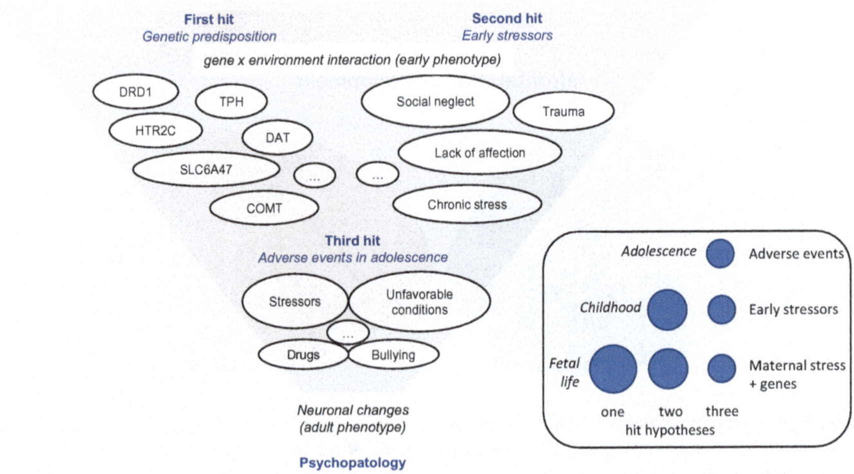

Fig. 4.4 The three-hit hypothesis of psychopathology. *Main panel.* The hypothesis posits that a mental disorder results from three categories of factors: *genetic polymorphisms* that make the individual sensitive to *early environmental insults* to form together the early phenotype, as well as additional *stressors suffered in adolescence* that aggravate the effects of the former and further increase the likelihood of mental disorders. The gene codes shown in the figure include several aggression-related genes. Circles with three dots indicate that the list is not complete. *Insert.* The proposed relationship between the strength of the hit and the number of hits "necessary" for the development of a mental disorder. The size of circles symbolizes the "strength" of the hit

mum: if one is missing, the onset of mental disorders becomes unlikely. The authors of the theory supported their ideas with a wealth of research evidence. However, this is general evidence that refers to a "general," often unnamed or merely exemplified psychiatric disorders, without a deep analysis. Since then, however, as it becomes more popular, the theory has been used to study a number of specific mental disorders [72, 73]. These cannot be reviewed here because they are irrelevant from the point of view of aggressiveness; nevertheless, such studies show that the theory is applicable in practice.

Although the new approach appears to answer important questions regarding the etiology of psychopathologies, it should be noted that children are not free from psychiatric problems [74], yet they could not suffer the third hit because of their age. The question, then, is how to reconcile an attractive three-hit hypothesis with an "inconvenient" fact. In the search for an answer, one should consider that certain disorders, e.g., autism, might be caused by single rare mutations with large clinical effect or a unique combination of two mutations with less robust effects when alone [75]. Albeit this was claimed by the authors of the study to be a two-hit phenomenon, actually both deficits were genetic and, as such, appear more eligible to be called a single-hit event. Consequently, "hits" at one single notably the genetic level might be enough to result in mental disorders, if the impact of genetic polymorphism was large. Furthermore, there is a two-hit hypothesis proposing that the combination of genetic predisposition and environmental insults during critical periods of development can lead to significant behavioral problems in adulthood [76]. The "first hit" (genetic factor) makes the brain vulnerable to insults such that when the "second hit" (environmental factor) comes, the onset of the disorder is triggered as shown primarily in schizophrenia [77].

We propose that the number of hits the individual suffers before developing a disorder depends to a large extent on the strength of the hit (Fig. 4.4 insert). In rare cases, the genetic deficit alone may be sufficient, while in other cases, the genetic deficit leads to the disorder only if its effects are supported by a stressor suffered in one critical period of life. Finally, even minor genetic deficits can become risk factors, if their risks are amplified by early and adolescent stressors. Independently, however, of the number of hits and their distribution over life periods, stress seems to be an important contributor of psychopathology risks. This will be discussed in the next chapter.

References

1. Black, P. (2014). Conflict theory of crime. In J. S. Albanese (Ed.), *The Encyclopedia of criminology and criminal justice* (1st ed., pp. 1–6). Hoboken: Wiley Blackwell.
2. Sellin, J. T. (1937). *Research memorandum on crime in the depression*. New York: Social Science Research Council.
3. Wilcox, P., & Cullen, F. T. (2018). Situational opportunity theories of crime. *Annual Review of Criminology, 1*, 123–148.

4. Useem, B. (1998). Breakdown theories of collective action. *Annual Review of Sociology, 24*, 215–238.
5. Slater, T. (2011). From 'criminality' to marginality: Rioting against a broken state. *Human Geography, 4*, 106–115.
6. Becker, G. S. (1968). Crime and punishment: An economic approach. *Journal of Political Economy, 76*, 169–217.
7. Toth, A. G., & Mitchell, O. (2018). A qualitative examination of the effects of international counter-drug interdictions. *The International Journal on Drug Policy, 55*, 70–76.
8. Matsueda, R. L., Huizinga, D., & Kreager, D. A. (2006). Deterring delinquents: A rational choice model of theft and violence. *American Sociological Review, 71*, 95–122.
9. Clarke, R. V. (1995). Situational crime prevention. *Crime and Justice, 19*, 91–150.
10. Hirschi, T. (1969). *Causes of delinquency*. Berkeley: University of California Press.
11. Kempf-Leonard, K., & Morris, N. A. (2012). Social control theory. In B. M. Huebner (Ed.), *Criminology*. New York: Oxford University Press.
12. Akers, R. L., Krohn, M. D., Lanza-Kaduce, L., & Radosevich, M. (1979). Social learning and deviant behavior: A specific test of a general theory. *American Sociological Review, 44*, 636–655.
13. Yarbrough, A., Jones, S., Sullivan, C., Sellers, C., & Cochran, J. (2012). Social learning and self-control: Assessing the moderating potential of criminal propensity. *International Journal of Offender Therapy and Comparative Criminology, 56*, 191–202.
14. Merton, R., & Social, K. (1938). Structure and anomie. *American Sociological Review, 3*, 672–682.
15. Agnew, R. (1992). Foundation for a general strain theory of crime and delinquency. *Criminology, 30*, 47–87.
16. McKenna, N. C., Golladay, K. A., & Holtfreter, K. (2019). Integrating general strain theory and trauma-informed principles into the study of older adult victimization. *Journal of Trauma and Dissociation, 21*, 187. https://doi.org/10.1080/15299732.2020.1692410.
17. Gini, C. (1909). Concentration and dependency ratios (English translation). *Rivista di Politica Economica, 87*, 769–789.
18. Crime statistics in European countries. (2018). http://ec.europa.eu/eurostat/statistics-explained/index.php/Crime_and_criminal_justice_statistics
19. GINI indexes of European countries. (2018). http://appsso.eurostat.ec.europa.eu/nui/show.do?dataset=ilc_di12
20. Rawls' fairness, income distribution and alarming level of Gini coefficient – Economics E-Journal. http://www.economics-ejournal.org/economics/discussionpapers/2017-67
21. Fajnzylber, P., Lederman, D., & Loayza, N. (2002). Inequality and violent crime. *Journal of Law and Economics, 45*, 1–39.
22. Haywood, T. W., Kravitz, H. M., Wasyliw, O. E., Goldberg, J., & Cavanaugh, J. L. (1996). Cycle of abuse and psychopathology in cleric and noncleric molesters of children and adolescents. *Child Abuse & Neglect, 20*, 1233–1243.
23. Sundquist, V. H. (2010). Political terrorism: An historical case study of the Italian red brigades. *Journal of Strategic Security, 3*, 53–67.
24. Beauregard, E., Rossmo, D. K., & Proulx, J. (2007). A descriptive model of the hunting process of serial sex offenders: A rational choice perspective. *Journal of Family Violence, 22*, 449–463.
25. Rousseau, J. J. (1895). *The social contract*. London: Swan Sonnenschein.
26. Pettit, P. (1999). *Republicanism: A theory of freedom and government*. Oxford: Oxford University Press.
27. Hiel, A. V., Hautman, L., Cornelis, I., & Clercq, B. D. (2007). Football hooliganism: Comparing self-awareness and social identity theory explanations. *Journal of Community and Applied Social Psychology, 17*, 169–186.

28. Hennigan, K., & Spanovic, M. (2012). Gang dynamics through the lens of social identity theory. In F.-A. Esbensen & C. L. Maxson (Eds.), *Youth gangs in international perspective. Results from the Eurogang perspective* (pp. 127–149). New York: Springer.
29. Travaglino, G. A., Abrams, D., Randsley de Moura, G., & Russo, G. (2014). Organized crime and group-based ideology: The association between masculine honor and collective opposition against criminal organizations. *Group Processes and Intergroup Relations, 17*, 799–812.
30. Arena, M. P., & Arrigo, B. A. (2005). Social psychology, terrorism, and identity: A preliminary re-examination of theory, culture, self, and society. *Behavioral Sciences & the Law, 23*, 485–506.
31. Afghanistan Opium Survey. (2017). Challenges to sustainable development, peace and security (May 2018) – Afghanistan. *ReliefWeb.* https://reliefweb.int/report/afghanistan/afghanistan-opium-survey-2017-challenges-sustainable-development-peace-and
32. Green, S. (2007). Looting, law, and lawlessness. *Tulane Law Review, 81*, 1–50.
33. Marsh, M., Purdin, S., & Navani, S. (2006). Addressing sexual violence in humanitarian emergencies. *Global Public Health, 1*, 133–146.
34. Claasen, C. (2014). Who participates in communal violence? Survey evidence from South Africa. *Research and Politics, 1*, 1–8.
35. Liu, J., & Wuerker, A. (2005). Biosocial bases of aggressive and violent behavior—Implications for nursing studies. *International Journal of Nursing Studies, 42*, 229–241.
36. Savolainen, J., et al. (2018). Socioeconomic disadvantage and psychological deficits: Pathways from early cumulative risk to late-adolescent criminal conviction. *Journal of Adolescence, 65*, 16–24.
37. Gentile, S. (2017). Untreated depression during pregnancy: Short- and long-term effects in offspring. A systematic review. *Neuroscience, 342*, 154–166.
38. Salatino-Oliveira, A., et al. (2016). COMT and prenatal maternal smoking in associations with conduct problems and crime: The Pelotas 1993 birth cohort study. *Scientific Reports, 6*, 29900.
39. Kleinhaus, K., et al. (2013). Prenatal stress and affective disorders in a population birth cohort. *Bipolar Disorders, 15*, 92–99.
40. Cowen, P. S. (1999). Child neglect: Injuries of omission. *Pediatric Nursing, 25*(401–405), 409–418.
41. Naughton, A. M., et al. (2013). Emotional, behavioral, and developmental features indicative of neglect or emotional abuse in preschool children: A systematic review. *JAMA Pediatrics, 167*, 769–775.
42. McLaughlin, K. A., Sheridan, M. A., & Nelson, C. A. (2017). Neglect as a violation of species-expectant experience: Neurodevelopmental consequences. *Biological Psychiatry, 82*, 462–471.
43. Gracia, E., López-Quílez, A., Marco, M., & Lila, M. (2017). Mapping child maltreatment risk: A 12-year spatio-temporal analysis of neighborhood influences. *International Journal of Health Geographics, 16*, 38.
44. Wright, K. A., Turanovic, J. J., O'Neal, E. N., Morse, S. J., & Booth, E. T. (2016). The cycle of violence revisited: Childhood victimization, resilience, and future violence. *Journal of Interpersonal Violence, 34*, 1261. https://doi.org/10.1177/0886260516651090.
45. Forsman, M., & Långström, N. (2012). Child maltreatment and adult violent offending: Population-based twin study addressing the 'cycle of violence' hypothesis. *Psychological Medicine, 42*, 1977–1983.
46. Hinsberger, M., et al. (2016). Perpetuating the cycle of violence in South African low-income communities: Attraction to violence in young men exposed to continuous threat. *European Journal of Psychotraumatology, 7*, 29099.
47. Wright, E. M., & Fagan, A. A. (2013). The cycle of violence in context: Exploring the moderating roles of neighborhood disadvantage and cultural norms. *Criminology: An Interdisciplinary Journal, 51*, 217–249.

48. Wolff, N., & Shi, J. (2012). Childhood and adult trauma experiences of incarcerated persons and their relationship to adult behavioral health problems and treatment. *International Journal of Environmental Research and Public Health, 9*, 1908–1926.
49. Allely, C. S., Minnis, H., Thompson, L., Wilson, P., & Gillberg, C. (2014). Neurodevelopmental and psychosocial risk factors in serial killers and mass murderers. *Aggression and Violent Behavior, 19*, 288–301.
50. Marshall, L. A., & Cooke, D. J. (1999). The childhood experiences of psychopaths: A retrospective study of familial and societal factors. *Journal of Personality Disorders, 13*, 211–225.
51. Patterson, G. R. (1986). Performance models for antisocial boys. *The American Psychologist, 41*, 432–444.
52. Estrada-Martínez, L. M., Padilla, M. B., Caldwell, C. H., & Schulz, A. J. (2011). Examining the influence of family environments on youth violence: A comparison of Mexican, Puerto Rican, Cuban, non-Latino Black, and non-Latino White adolescents. *Journal of Youth and Adolescence, 40*, 1039–1051.
53. Herrenkohl, T. L., Hawkins, J. D., Chung, I., Hill, K. G., & Battin-Pearson, S. (2001). School and community risk factors and interventions. In R. Loeber & D. P. Farrington (Eds.), *Child delinquents: Development, intervention, and service needs* (pp. 211–246). Thousand Oaks: Sage.
54. Hjalmarsson, R., & Lochner, L. (2012). The impact of education on crime: International evidence. *CESifo DICE Report, 10*, 49–55.
55. Leary, M. R., Kowalski, R. M., Smith, L., & Phillips, S. (2003). Teasing, rejection, and violence: Case studies of the school shootings. *Aggressive Behavior, 29*, 202–214.
56. Oberwittler, D. (2005). Social exclusion and youth crime in Europe – The spatial dimension: Do disadvantaged neighbourhoods cause adolescents to become more delinquent? In K. Aromaa (Ed.), *Penal policy, justice reform, and social exclusion* (pp. 27–44). Helsinki: European Institute for Crime Prevention and Control.
57. Lévay, M. (2005). 'Social exclusion': A thriving concept in contemporary criminology; social exclusion and crime in Central and Eastern Europe. In K. Aromaa (Ed.), *Penal policy, justice reform, and social exclusion* (pp. 27–44). Helsinki: European Institute for Crime Prevention and Control.
58. Wood, J. L. (2014). Understanding gang membership: The significance of group processes. *Group Processes and Intergroup Relations, 17*, 710–729.
59. Sraker, J. (1992). *Faces in the revolution*. Cape Town: David Philip.
60. Galtung, J. (2016). Cultural violence. *Journal of Peace Research, 27*, 291–305.
61. Kahlor, L. A., & Eastin, M. S. (2011). Television's role in the culture of violence toward women: A study of television viewing and the cultivation of rape myth acceptance in the United States. *Journal of Broadcasting & Electronic Media, 55*, 215–231.
62. Pan, A., et al. (2006). Understanding the role of culture in domestic violence: The Ahimsa Project for Safe Families. *Journal of Immigrant and Minority Health, 8*, 35–43.
63. Anderson, C. A., et al. (2003). The influence of media violence on youth. *Psychological Science in the Public Interest, 4*, 81–110.
64. Ferguson, C. J., & Kilburn, J. (2009). The public health risks of media violence: A meta-analytic review. *The Journal of Pediatrics, 154*, 759–763.
65. Brown, R. P., Osterman, L. L., & Barnes, C. D. (2009). School violence and the culture of honor. *Psychological Science, 20*, 1400–1405.
66. Nisbett, R. E. (1993). Violence and U.S. regional culture. *American Psychologist, 48*, 441–449.
67. Staub, E. (2003). Notes on the cultures of violence, cultures of caring and peace and the fulfillment of basic human needs. *Political Psychology, 24*, 1–21.
68. Conel, J. L. (1959). *The postnatal development of the human cerebral cortex*. Cambridge: Harvard University Press.
69. Qin, J., et al. (2015). Predicting individual brain maturity using dynamic functional connectivity. *Frontiers in Human Neuroscience, 9*, 418.

70. Ganzel, B. L., & Morris, P. A. (2011). Allostasis and the developing human brain: Explicit consideration of implicit models. *Development and Psychopathology, 23*, 955–974.
71. Daskalakis, N. P., Bagot, R. C., Parker, K. J., Vinkers, C. H., & de Kloet, E. R. (2013). The three-hit concept of vulnerability and resilience: Toward understanding adaptation to early-life adversity outcome. *Psychoneuroendocrinology, 38*, 1858–1873.
72. Walther, A., Rice, T., Kufert, Y., & Ehlert, U. (2016). Neuroendocrinology of a male-specific pattern for depression linked to alcohol use disorder and suicidal behavior. *Frontiers in Psychiatry, 7*, 206.
73. Rao, C. V., Farooqui, M., Asch, A. S., & Yamada, H. Y. (2018). Critical role of mitosis in spontaneous late-onset Alzheimer's disease; from a Shugoshin 1 cohesinopathy mouse model. *Cell cycle (Georgetown, Tex.), 17*, 2321–2334.
74. Zeanah, C. H., & Lieberman, A. (2016). Defining relational pathology in early childhood: The diagnostic classification of mental health and developmental disorders of infancy and early childhood DC:0-5 approach. *Infant Mental Health Journal, 37*, 509–520.
75. Gau, S. S.-F., Liao, H.-M., Hong, C.-C., Chien, W.-H., & Chen, C.-H. (2012). Identification of two inherited copy number variants in a male with autism supports two-hit and compound heterozygosity models of autism. *American Journal of Medical Genetics Part B: Neuropsychiatric Genetics, 159B*, 710–717.
76. Klug, M., et al. (2012). Long-term behavioral and NMDA receptor effects of young-adult corticosterone treatment in BDNF heterozygous mice. *Neurobiology of Disease, 46*, 722–731.
77. Bayer, T. A., Falkai, P., & Maier, W. (1999). Genetic and non-genetic vulnerability factors in schizophrenia: The basis of the 'two hit hypothesis'. *Journal of Psychiatric Research, 33*, 543–548.

Chapter 5
The Biology of Glucocorticoids: Normal and Abnormal Aggression

Introduction

Glucocorticoid stress responses affect neural functions and behavior on an extremely wide time scale that ranges from minutes to lifetime. Mechanisms mediating their effects range from rapid and direct influences on cellular, such as neural functions, to lasting or sometimes quasi-permanent modification of the genes themselves by epigenetic phenomena. These genetic alterations do not affect nucleotide sequences but influence gene function and expression and may even be heritable [1] as such, the effects of glucocorticoids may span generations.

All glucocorticoid effects influence aggressiveness in animals and are also associated with aggression-related psychopathologies and violent crime as shown later. The impact of glucocorticoids, however, depends to a large extent on the mechanisms activated, which on their turn depend on glucocorticoid secretion profiles and a series of other circumstances, for which the same observed phenomenon, for example, high levels of the hormone in blood, may have opposite effects on behavior and aggressiveness. To account for these intricacies, we will present the roles of glucocorticoids along the mechanisms they activate. Roughly, these can be divided into three categories: rapid, non-genomic glucocorticoid effects activated by stressors acutely, the long-term modulation of gene expression by the well-known genomic mechanisms of glucocorticoids, and brain programming by glucocorticoid epigenetics also known as toxic stress. The aim of this chapter is to clarify the basic biological phenomena that link glucocorticoids to aggression. This will serve as a basis for understanding stress-related processes underlying human aggression, aggression-related mental disorders, and violent crime, which will be discussed in the next chapter.

J. Haller, *Neurobiopsychosocial Perspectives on Aggression and Violence*, Advances in Preventing and Treating Violence and Aggression,
https://doi.org/10.1007/978-3-030-46331-1_5

5.1 Acute Stress: The Stimulation of Aggression

5.1.1 Background

5.1.1.1 A Brief History of Non-genomic Glucocorticoid Effects

In the early years of research, the interaction of glucocorticoids with the genetic apparatus was unknown; therefore, the time scale of effects was of no concern. The finding that locally applied corticosterone and its analogs (e.g., dexamethasone) can alter neuronal activity within several seconds [2, 3] or even milliseconds [4] raised no suspicion, and the hormone was granted with the ability of controlling brain function very rapidly. The discovery of genomic mechanisms [5, 6], however, cast some doubts on the validity of such findings, even on effects that developed within one or a few minutes [7, 8]. The reason was that the genomic mechanism is time-consuming and consists of a succession of events each requiring a considerable amount of time. The first event – after glucocorticoid secretion increased – is the penetration of the cell by glucocorticoids, where they bind to their cytoplasmic receptors, particularly the mineralocorticoid and glucocorticoid receptors. Thereafter, the ligand-receptor complex moves to the cell nucleus, where it binds to the DNA glucocorticoid recognition sites and affects transcription and ultimately protein synthesis. Finally, the effect becomes operational when the protein becomes functional and changes the functioning of the cell, for example, the neuron. A conservative estimate suggests that the duration of this sequence of events based on measurements concerning each step is probably about 30 minutes. Even calculating with the shortest lag times ever measured in any cell, the consequences might not be detectable within 15 min [9].

Yet, much faster effects were reported recurrently including effects on aggression [10] which strongly suggested the existence of non-genomic mechanisms of glucocorticoid action. The criteria for such mechanisms were established as follows [9]: (1) The effect develops considerably faster than 15 min (2). Effects are independent of cytoplasmic receptors, e.g., they can be observed when these were blocked. Alternatively, effects are elicited by glucocorticoids conjugated with proteins, such as bovine serum albumin, which cannot penetrate the cytoplasm where the genetically active receptors are located (3). Effects persist when protein synthesis was blocked, i.e., when the "genetic commands" cannot be carried out (4). Glucocorticoids bind to and affect the function of proteins other than the cytoplasmic receptors. Any of the criteria 2–3 are sufficient to prove the non-genomic mechanism of action especially when combined with criterion 1. When criterion 4 is fulfilled, it may indicate the subcellular mechanisms that mediate non-genomic effects. A rather early review of the findings available at that time suggested that many behavioral effects of glucocorticoids, including effects on aggression, are mediated non-genomically according these criteria [11].

We note that in this chapter, glucocorticoids will be named as such, because animals may secrete corticosterone, cortisol, or both depending on the species. For simplicity, the generic term glucocorticoids will be used throughout.

5.1.1.2 Mechanisms of Action

The molecular mechanisms of non-genomic effects were reviewed a relatively long time ago, and it was shown that glucocorticoids are able to affect membrane lipids nonspecifically (by altering membrane fluidity) and specifically by binding to glucocorticoid receptors located on the cellular membrane or to non-glucocorticoid receptors (e.g., the acetylcholine, kappa opioid, and other neurotransmitter receptors). Glucocorticoids are also able to directly affect calcium trafficking within the neuron and the voltage-dependent calcium channel in the synapse and may directly control a series of intracellular signaling pathways [9, 12]. These assumptions were mainly based on molecular biological findings, and the behavioral consequences of such mechanisms were assumed rather than proven. Subsequent studies grouped non-genomic effects differently and evidenced variants of the effects listed above; in some cases, specific mechanisms operating in nonbehavioral areas of functioning were hypothesized [13, 14]. Over the last decade, however, little progress has been made in this field. For instance, no particular non-genomic glucocorticoid mechanism was associated with a particular behavioral function. In other words, researchers continued to assume this mechanism based on indirect molecular evidence. More progress seems to be achieved in a related area, specifically the non-genomic effects of estrogens, which appear to be expressed in conjunction with non-genomic glucocorticoid effects [15]; yet, question marks also frequently remain in this area. As such, the field seems to be stuck at the level of assumptions as it regards the mechanisms, but the mere existence of non-genomic effects can be considered proven.

5.1.1.3 Non-genomic Mechanisms and the Stress Responses

Rapid, non-genomic mechanisms appear to be associated with acute stress responses, which consist of a rapid surge of glucocorticoid synthesis often associated with the term "eustress," a term that was introduced by Selye [16]. Such acute stressors elicit a transient increase in glucocorticoid synthesis, which is overall behavior-activating in nature, and contribute to the efficient handling of the stress-eliciting situation such as interpersonal conflict [17]. Findings suggest that even within the brief acute stress response, non-genomic mechanisms are responsible for behavioral aggressive responses for a few minutes only, their role being taken over by the early genomic mechanisms relatively rapidly (see below).

5.1.2 Acute Stress and Aggression

5.1.2.1 The Positive Feedback Between Stress and Aggression

Social challenges and the ensuing conflict rapidly activate glucocorticoid production in a variety of taxa, e.g., fish [18], lizards [19], birds [20], and mammals, as shown first in mice [21] and thereafter in rats [22]. Subsequent research demonstrated that this surge is different in the winners and losers of the conflict and is consequential for the status of the individual. These consequences, however, develop over a longer time scale than the acute stress response. This will be discussed in the next section.

The first question related to the acute impact of glucocorticoids on ongoing aggression concerns the timing of glucocorticoid synthesis. An increase in plasma glucocorticoids is detectable 3–5 min after the occurrence of the stressor with a peak after 30 min which limits the time window of glucocorticoid involvement in ongoing behavior. The mere sensory contact with potential opponents, however, is stressful [23] and increases plasma corticosterone in rats [24]. Similar findings were also obtained in feral animals [25]. Since most aggressive encounters are preceded by a series of nonsocial and nonaggressive social behaviors that can be perceived as preparations for and anticipations of fights, this finding demonstrates that glucocorticoids increase before the actual fights begin.

Concerning the role of glucocorticoids, the inhibition of their synthesis dramatically reduced aggressiveness [26], but aggressiveness was restored when the effects of the corticosterone synthesis inhibition were counteracted by corticosterone injections administered just before the social encounter [27]. Protein synthesis blockade did not influence the immediate effects of corticosterone on aggression (time frame ~2 min) but abolished those that were expressed more slowly (~20 min), demonstrating that at the beginning of the encounter glucocorticoids promoted aggressiveness non-genomically but the role of genomic mechanisms was overtaken shortly by genomic ones, which also promoted aggressiveness. A subsequent study employing a combination of endocrine, electrophysiological, and behavioral techniques demonstrated the existence of a fast, positive feedback loop between aggression and glucocorticoid secretion; glucocorticoid secretion and aggression reciprocally facilitated each other [28].

Taken together, these findings show that (i) the HPA-axis is activated by encounters with unfamiliar individuals, even before the actual fights start; (ii) glucocorticoids secreted in response to the encounter rapidly promote aggressiveness; (iii) the execution of aggression increases glucocorticoid secretion further (positive feedback); and (iv) in the early and late phases of the encounter, glucocorticoids promote aggressiveness by non-genomic and genomic mechanisms, respectively. In one sentence, aggressiveness is expressed concomitantly with and under the supportive contribution of the acute glucocorticoid stress response.

5.1.2.2 Aggression-Unrelated Glucocorticoid Surges

The positive feedback loop between social challenge-induced acute stress responses and the execution of aggressive behaviors raises questions regarding the role of extrinsic glucocorticoid surges such as those that are not triggered by social challenges. Would an acute stress response increase aggression if it was followed by a social challenge and would the "innocent" suffer from a mere coincidence of an extrinsic stress and a social encounter?

The simplest situation of this kind does not even require a stress response as glucocorticoid secretion shows natural variations called ultradian and diurnal rhythms. These are unrelated to external influences. The ultradian rhythm has a phase length of about 60–90 min, whereas the diurnal rhythm separates the dark and light phase of the day; glucocorticoid secretion is considerably larger in the active phase (which is the dark phase of the day in the rat) [29, 30]. Blood glucocorticoid levels at the zeniths of these rhythms are around two times higher than at the nadirs, and these differences in glucocorticoid levels are paralleled by changes in aggressiveness [31–33]. Specifically, rats were significantly more aggressive in the increasing phase of their corticosterone fluctuation than in the decreasing phase. Moreover, glucocorticoid enhancement-induced aggressiveness was normalized when the natural increase in glucocorticoid secretion was counteracted by glucocorticoid synthesis blockade. Taken together, these findings show that the "innocent" would indeed suffer if they accidentally met an opponent in the increasing phase of its natural glucocorticoid synthesis rhythm.

Aggression is also increased by social stressors, a phenomenon called attack priming [34]. If an animal was aggressively aroused by an encounter with an unfamiliar individual, a second social partner – the "innocent" – will be attacked more rapidly and more intensely than the first one. The effects of aggressive arousal disappear within 90 but not 30 min [35], which is in line with the time course of acute glucocorticoid stress responses that peak at around 30 min but vanish within 90 min.

Nonsocial stressors also increase aggression; for instance, handling and transportation rapidly increases aggressiveness in catfish [36]; similarly, brief stressors (e.g., immobilization for 15 min or the omission of a scheduled reward) enhance aggression in laboratory rodents [37–40]. This is in agreement with Cannon's fight-flight concept of acute stress responses which posits that brief acute stressors mobilize physiological and behavioral resources to cope with the situation [41].

Surprisingly, however, the aggression-facilitating role of glucocorticoids and stress subsides within less than 2 hours to give way to aggression-inhibiting effects. Laboratory rodents which submitted to restraint stress for 2 or more hours show a dramatic reduction in aggression [42, 43], an effect that persists for at least 24 hours [44]. This suggests that the aggression-enhancing effects of acute glucocorticoid surges are only temporary and rapidly transform into aggression-suppressing effects that are characteristic to chronic stressors.

5.1.3 Overview: Consequences for Brain and Body

The rapidity of the effect and their resistance to protein synthesis inhibition suggest that in early phases of the aggressive encounter the challenge-induced increase in glucocorticoid secretion promotes aggression non-genomically within a few minutes. The glucose supply of muscles is also augmented by non-genomic mechanisms, a phenomenon that is important for endurance [45]. The non-genomic phase of aggression control, however, is rapid – within about 20 min – followed by a brief genomic phase of glucocorticoid action that also promotes aggressiveness. This in turn seems to subside and give way to other, presumably also genomic mechanisms that dramatically decrease aggressiveness within approximately 2 hours.

The hormonal and behavioral changes presented above were associated with a series of neural changes, including alterations in serotonin and dopamine neurotransmission [39, 42], and functional changes in a variety of brain areas, including several regions of the amygdala [34, 46], hypothalamus [40], hippocampus [38], and various other brain regions [47]. Such findings outline important neural consequences of glucocorticoid action and stress exposure and demonstrate that glucocorticoids rapidly affect the functioning of neurotransmitter systems and brain areas of the aggression circuitry, which will be detailed in subsequent chapters. Concomitantly, glucocorticoids and the adrenaline stress response contribute to the fueling of the energy-consuming aggressive behavior by liberating energy substrates and generating glucose supply for brain and body [48, 49]. Thus, acute surges in glucocorticoids promote aggressiveness via both neural and bodily effects.

The acute impact of glucocorticoids on aggression undergoes a rapid succession of different mechanisms and behavioral outcomes. The precise neural and molecular mechanisms underlying these remain poorly understood, although their elucidation would not only increase our understanding of the initial phases of aggressive encounters but may substantiate speculations on the therapeutic and drug developmental potential of non-genomic mechanisms [50]. Nevertheless, the findings briefly reviewed above show that the acute glucocorticoid stress response is elicited by and supports aggressive behaviors in a positive feedback-like process (see Fig. 5.1).

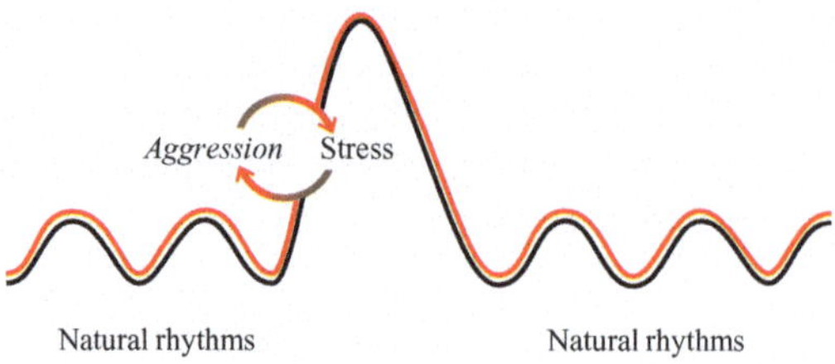

Fig. 5.1 *Acute interactions between glucocorticoids and aggression in animals.* The propensity to respond aggressively (red line) to challenges follows the ultradian and diurnal rhythms of glucocorticoid secretion (black line). The positive feedback between social challenge-induced glucocorticoid stress responses and aggressive behavior occurs under the effect of acute stressors only. Winning restores glucocorticoid secretion rapidly and normalizes behavior: the intense aggressive behavior characteristic to the conflict subsides after the opponent submits. Inhibition and stimulation studies suggest that the glucocorticoid-aggression relationship is causal. Prolonged stressors that exceed 2 h may decrease aggression as shown in the next section

5.2 Chronic Stress: The Inhibition of Aggression

5.2.1 Background

5.2.1.1 Molecular Mechanisms

Persistent stressors increase plasma glucocorticoid levels durably, which exert their effects by the "classical" genomic way of action. This involves the following six steps: [5, 6, 51]

1. The chronic stressor elicits a rise in plasma glucocorticoids that reaches a peak within 30 min and remains high for the duration of the stressor, also having an impact on the diurnal variation in glucocorticoid secretion [52, 53].
2. Glucocorticoids bind to their cytoplasmic receptors (the mineralocorticoid and glucocorticoid receptors, also known as glucocorticoid I and II receptors). Chronic stress increases the occupancy of these receptors considerably. Note that the basal (stress-independent) occupancy of mineralocorticoid and glucocorticoid receptors is largely different, but this does not affect the basics of the process.
3. The ligand-receptor complex moves to the cell nucleus and binds to glucocorticoid-responsive elements. Due to increased receptor occupancy, this generates a quasi-constant genomic impact.
4. Transcription is altered, with secondary consequences for protein synthesis. This might also be altered posttranscriptionally via glucocorticoid-responsive elements on messenger RNAs [54].
5. The altered protein machinery induces functional changes in the cell, which is consequential for the functioning of the whole organism including the brain.
6. Neural and bodily changes have behavioral consequences including but not restricted to changes in aggressiveness.

The number of genomic glucocorticoid-responsive elements is very high (estimates range from several hundreds to thousands of DNA loci). Glucocorticoid binding appears dynamic in the meaning that it depends on the duration of glucocorticoid action and the target cell type [55, 56]. Functional changes in gene expression are relatively modest, mostly in the range of 10–30%. Yet, this results in significant changes in a series of cellular and molecular processes including energy metabolism, signal transduction, neurotransmitter catabolism, neurotrophic factors, cell adhesion, etc., all of which have implications for aggression control. These effects are expressed after a variable lag time, some genomic effects becoming detectable within an hour, while others need days, weeks, and even months of chronic stress [57].

5.2.1.2 Allostasis

Chronic stress modifies the set point of homeostasis, a phenomenon called allostasis [58]. Homeostasis maintains physiological and biochemical conditions within the organism between certain limits, often by the active contribution of the neural system. Under the pressure exerted by chronic stressors, these limits are altered; for instance, the set point of plasma glucocorticoid regulation is increased, resulting in increased daily averages and higher nadirs and zeniths of secretion rhythms [52]. Sometimes secretion rhythms are flattened, whereas averages remain high. As such, the chronic increase in plasma glucocorticoids is an allostatic phenomenon: high levels result from a shift in the homeostatic set point. There are a series of similar changes in the organism, some of which lead to the emergence of diseases [59].

The behavioral consequences of chronic stress may also be interpreted in terms of allostasis, although the phrase is rarely used in this context. Behavioral activity from exploration [60] through aggression [61] to sexual behavior [62] is reduced, which increases the chances of survival that are jeopardized by chronic stress. By limiting activity, the animal avoids unnecessary losses of energy and the danger of harm until conditions become more favorable [11]. In addition, limited behavioral activity may protect from diseases [63]. One may hypothesize that allostatic load by chronic stress decreases the set point of behavioral activity, with obvious advantages for survival.

Importantly, chronic glucocorticoid effects are reversible, meaning that once the chronic stressor vanishes for one reason or another, the organism recovers. More durable effects – that persist after the stressor vanished – will be discussed in the next section, which will focus on "toxic stress."

5.2.2 Chronic Defeat Stress and Aggression

In dominants, the acute glucocorticoid stress response is a typical example of eustress: [16] It is transient and contributes to the solution of the "problem," i.e., the social confrontation. The stress response behaves differently in the losers of the conflict in which the stress response persists after the termination of the conflict as shown in a variety of taxa, e.g., fish [64], reptiles [65], birds [66], laboratory rodents [22, 67], and free-ranging monkeys [68]. Such changes in plasma glucocorticoids do not depend on the prefight status of individuals but only on the results of the conflict. For example, residents defeated by intruders show chronic glucocorticoid stress, whereas plasma corticosterone decreases in intruders if they won the conflict [69].

The behavioral significance of defeat-induced chronic glucocorticoid stress responses is evidenced by the phenomenon of conditioned defeat [70]. Animals exposed to a series of defeats respond by submissive behavior even to non-aggressive opponents without engaging in fights. Although mostly studied in hamsters, the phenomenon is present in other laboratory rodents [71, 72], and the so-called psychosocial stress model [73] shows that it is present in tree shrews. Defeated animals submit to any opponent, even to those that did not defeat them earlier [74]; thus, the phenomenon is not attributable to social recognition. The behavioral consequences of repeated defeat extend to other functions. Animals show multiple deficits including anxiety- and depression-like behaviors and increased sensitivity to the rewarding effects of ethanol [75] and cocaine [76], etc.

Although often attributed to defeat-induced decreases in testosterone production [77], the suppression of agonistic behavior by chronic social stress is largely dependent on chronic increases in glucocorticoid production, as chronic treatments with glucocorticoids inhibit aggressiveness and promote submissive behaviors in new conflicts, as shown in fish [47], reptiles [78, 79], birds [80, 81], and mammals [10, 61]. The importance of glucocorticoids is also shown by a study where rats were injected with corticosterone after the encounter to mimic the defeat-induced persistence of the stress response. These animals showed submissiveness the next day irrespective to the outcome of the earlier fight [82].

Taken together, these findings show that defeat-induced chronic increases in glucocorticoid production or glucocorticoids suppress aggression just as reliably as acute increases of glucocorticoids promote it.

5.2.3 The Paradoxical Effects of Repeated Restraint Stress

As shown above, the exposure of animals to restraint stress for at least 2 hours suppresses aggression [42, 43, 83], which is consistent with the anti-aggressive effects of chronic stress, and was used above to delimit temporally the aggression-heightening and aggression-suppressing effects of glucocorticoids. Surprisingly, however, repeating the restraint procedure for about 10 days reinstates aggressive behavior; moreover, rats become more aggressive than non-treated controls.

This recurrent finding is at variance with the aggression-suppressing effects of chronic stress and may be explained by two related phenomena: habituation to homotypic [84] and sensitization to heterotypic stressors [85]. Habituation to homotypic stressors (stressors of the same type) means that the effects of stressors diminish over time. For instance, the glucocorticoid response to restraint stress gradually decreases over repeated exposures [86], which may occur as early as the fifth exposure [87]. This phenomenon may account for the loss of the anti-aggressive effect of repeated restraint stress. The increase in aggression on its turn may be explained by an increased responsiveness to heterotypic stressors. For instance, chronically restrained rats show elevated acute glucocorticoid responses to foot shocks or other stressors that are different from restraint [88, 89]. Although this was not investigated specifically for the succession of repeated restraint and acute social challenge (as a heterotypic stressor), one can hypothesize that the phenomenon holds true for this heterotypic stressor as well.

We hypothesize that repeated restraints – as repeated homotypic stressors – lose their ability to maintain a chronically elevated level of plasma glucocorticoids; as such, they lose the ability to suppress aggression. At the same time, heterotypic stressors, specifically social challenges, induce an intensified acute glucocorticoid stress response, which enhances aggressive responses. As will be shown below, a similar mechanism may be operational in depression which is often associated with outbursts of aggression called anger attacks [90].

5.2.4 Overview and Brain Mechanisms

Animals experiencing repeated defeats, other chronic stressors, or simply repeated chronic glucocorticoid injections reduce their activity level in various behavioral domains. When confronting a potential opponent, for instance, they refrain from fighting and readily submit.

This behavioral state is akin to anxiety and depression in humans. Not surprisingly, social stressors – a major component of which is defeat – are often used as laboratory models of anxiety [91], social phobia [92], and depression [93, 94]. In biology, however, changes in behavior are interpreted in terms of function and evolutionary significance. From this point of view, the behavioral consequences of chronic stress are usually considered adaptive. By refraining from activity as far as possible, the animal saves energy, avoids risks, and increases its own chances of survival under unfavorable social conditions. The dominant animal may move away, may get sick or old, or may die. On its turn, the subordinate (the socially stressed animal) may grow more competitive over time, e.g., by physical development. In other words, social relationships are temporary and can change even within a relatively short time. Surviving chronic stress preserves the potential of the individual to lead a more normal life later on and to leave descendants.

The myriad of genomic mechanisms activated by glucocorticoids make it difficult to explain the molecular processes underlying these effects. Glucocorticoids may bind to hundreds, possibly thousands of genomic sites; they can activate or inhibit gene expression (depending on the gene) and may also affect posttranscriptional events. Their genomic effects depend on the cell type and unfold over a variable time scale depending on the nature of the glucocorticoid-responsive element; moreover, there might be a complex interaction between chronic effects and those elicited by acute glucocorticoid surges, as shown by the paradoxical effects of repeated restraint. At present, one cannot identify the molecular genomic mechanisms of any of the behavioral effects of chronic stress.

In contrast to molecular events, the neural consequences of chronic stress and their relationship to behavior are easier to address. Chronic social stress alters the activity of the noradrenergic [95], dopaminergic [96], and serotonergic [97] systems and the social challenge-induced activity of most of the areas of the aggression circuitry [98]. Changes have a time course: single and repeated defeats affect the circuitry differently. We do not enter into detail here as the mechanisms of aggression will be discussed later in detail. It is worth noting, however, that social stress (e.g., defeat) gradually alters the functioning of the aggression circuitry, leading to a state when aggression is suppressed and submission is promoted (see Fig. 5.2).

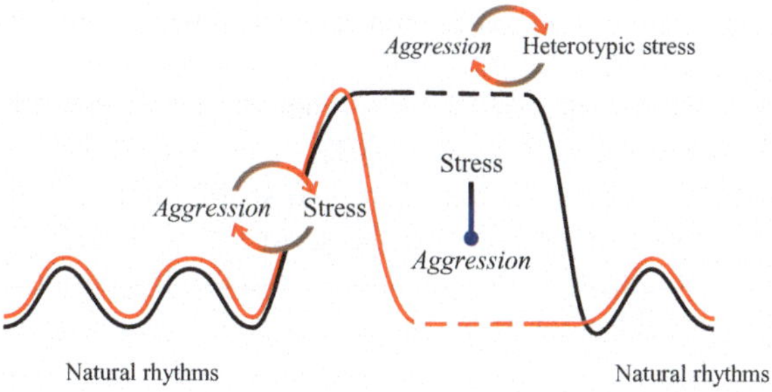

Fig. 5.2 *Chronic stress and aggression.* Glucocorticoid stress responses (black line) remain high if the animal was defeated, which decreases aggression (red line). The same happens if the animal was submitted to non-social stressors for more than 2 h and when it was treated chronically with glucocorticoids. The inhibition of aggression is just one symptom of a general inhibition of behavior, which promotes survival under unfavorable conditions. A strong heterotypic stressor may reactivate the positive feedback mechanism presented in the previous section as shown by repeated restraint stresses followed by a social challenge

5.3 Toxic Stress: Abnormal Aggression

5.3.1 Background

5.3.1.1 What Is Toxic Stress?

The chronic glucocorticoid stress response affects brain function and behavior as long as the occupancy of the cytoplasmic glucocorticoid receptors remains high, and the ligand-receptor complex binds in large numbers to glucocorticoid response elements in the genome. This implies that with the decrease of plasma glucocorticoid levels – when the stressor ceases to affect the organism – consequences fade away. Yet, there are a series of stressors, which affect brain function and behavior long after the glucocorticoid stress response vanished. These long-term effects were often attributed to changed development. For instance, chronic stress responses may change the development of the brain at early ages, and because such changes cannot be redressed later, consequences remain permanent. There are, however, a series of stressors that affect adults with fully developed neural systems, yet their effects overpass the period of enhanced glucocorticoid secretion. Such stresses will be collectively called in the following as "toxic stress."

The phrase "toxic stress" denotes stressors that leave a lasting signature on the organism long after the physiological/endocrine stress response ceased. The phrase is not new as it was used as early as 1958 [99]. At that time, however, the term "toxic" meant poisonous and referred to stress elicited by bacterial toxins, endotoxins, and environmental toxins like heavy metals, pesticides, etc. In the meaning adopted here, the phrase was first used rather recently. Initially it denoted the lifelong consequences of childhood stressors [100, 101] but was soon extended to cover stressors suffered by adolescents [102], young adults [103], adults [104], moreover, and elderly [105].

Today, the phrase has expanded and has gradually transformed into a concept. Some perceive it as a novel stress model [102]; others extend the notion to "toxic" social environments as sources of toxic stress to shape life trajectories [106], and web pages were created to explain the phrase to the public [107]. The concept becomes more and more fashionable, and not by chance. It identifies a stress action that is fundamentally different from those underlying acute and chronic stress responses.

5.3.1.2 Mechanisms: Epigenetics

One of the core mechanisms that underlie toxic stress is epigenetics, which consists in the remodeling of chromatin after birth, without affecting nucleotide sequences. The phenomenon was discovered in conjunction with viral infections and carcinogenesis more than 40 years ago [108, 109]. Subsequently it was discovered that epigenetics also governs cell differentiation and the maintenance of cell phenotypes during ontogeny [110, 111]; moreover, it mediates the effects of early stressors on adult disease susceptibility, including psychopathologies closely related to aggression [112].

In a previous book just 6 years old, we wrote "A PubMed search identified 11 studies that addressed the role of epigenetic phenomena in aggressive behavior; 5 were reviews and 6 were experimental studies" ([31], page 147). The same PubMed search today returned close to half thousand hits. The reason of this explosion of research output is the relevance of the phenomenon for aggressiveness, with special reference to abnormal aggression, psychopathology, and criminal violence.

Epigenetics essentially covers two phenomena: the methylation of nucleobases, which lowers the "readability" of genes, and the acetylation of histone proteins that may "close up" DNA segments. The former is analogous to those gene polymorphisms that hinder transcription, whereas the latter are like null mutations that make a gene dysfunctional. In other words, epigenetics may induce genetic changes after birth, which correspond to inherited genetic deficits as it regards their consequences for gene function. The involvement of glucocorticoid secretion in epigenetics and aggression is dual as follows:

1. The mechanisms that control the glucocorticoid stress response are subject to epigenetic changes themselves [113]. Subsequent to early stressors, three long-term changes in glucocorticoid secretion profiles were identified in humans: (i) elevated basal secretion and increased stress responses (11% of subjects); (ii) moderate basal secretions associated with low stress responses (26% of subjects); and (iii) low basal secretions with low stress responses (63% of subjects) [102]. One can hypothesize from the biological mechanisms alone (see above) that such changes alter aggressiveness. We will demonstrate below and in the following chapter that they are tightly associated with abnormal aggression in animals and psychopathological/criminal violence in humans.

2. Prolonged glucocorticoid stress responses are among the main engines of epigenetics [114, 115]. Naturally, glucocorticoids are neither the only stress-responsive elements in the organism nor the only mechanisms that trigger epigenetics. For instance, altered dopaminergic [116], noradrenergic [117], and serotonergic [118] neurotransmissions are also able to generate such phenomena. Notably, these systems also respond to environmental stressors, and their epigenetic effects may occur in conjunction with those of glucocorticoid stress responses [119]. At present, it is difficult to disentangle the relationships – possibly cascade-like interactions – between these systems. Yet, epigenetic changes in the brain are associated with various forms of aggression and violence suggesting a causal role of early toxic stress and adult aggressiveness [120].

5.3.1.3 Toxic Stress in Biology

Albeit the phrase was coined to describe human conditions, there is no reason to believe that toxic stress is missing from nature. One can rather confidently assume that human toxic stress is a species-specific case of a natural phenomenon, which operates throughout the animal kingdom. Not surprisingly, epigenetic alterations are present in free-ranging animals [121]; moreover, they may underlie certain forms of aggression [121]. Long-term alterations in glucocorticoid secretion patterns due to early environmental influences such as toxic stressors prepare the organism for predictable harsh circumstances and result in uncommon forms of aggression in adulthood [122]. Thus, aggression-related psychopathologies and rule-breaking (criminal) aggression may be human replicas of basic biological phenomena, which prepare the organism to endure and prevail in severe competition, which is predictable based on early experiences.

Considering the above, the aggression-related consequences of toxic stress can be considered adaptive. They serve successful competition under special circumstances and are in line with the biological approach to aggression. Unfortunately, the understanding of epigenetic processes in natural populations is limited. The area is expanding; yet, findings on aggression are sparse. In contrast, laboratory studies are more abundant and relevant to the topic. Therefore, the issue will be addressed in this context.

5.3.2 Toxic Stress: Abnormal Aggression Models

5.3.2.1 A Synopsis of the Findings

We will start this section by summarizing laboratory models of toxic stress and their long-term impact on both glucocorticoid secretion and social behavior including aggressiveness and abnormal forms of aggression (see Table 5.1). Note that the principles based on which aggression is deemed abnormal in laboratory models were presented in detail (see Table 1.2). Briefly, aggression is considered abnormal

Table 5.1 The effects of stressors suffered in critical periods of life on adult aggression

Model	Stress to	Effects in subjects at least one developmental stage later				
		Basal glucocorticoids	Stress response	Social behavior	Aggressive behavior	Abnormal aggression
Fetal (maternal) stress [123–126]	Mother	No change	Increased	Conflicting	Conflicting	**Absent**
Maternal separation [127–132]	Infant	No change	Increased	Conflicting	Conflicting	**Absent**
Post-weaning social isolation (PWSI) [135]	Juvenile	No change	Increased	Decreased	Increased	**Present**
Prepubertal subjugation (SUB) [133–137]	Juvenile	No change	Decreased	No change	Increased (conflicting)	**Present**
Peripubertal stress (PPS) [138–142]	Juvenile	No change	Decreased	Decreased	Increased	**Present**
ADXr* [143–147]	Adult	Decreased	Decreased	Decreased	No change	**Present**

Model	**Fulfilled criteria for abnormal aggression**
PWSI	Excessive, damaging, unpredictable, inappropriate context
SUB	Inappropriate targets (juveniles)
PPS	Excessive, damaging, unpredictable, inappropriate targets (females, etc.)
ADXr	Damaging, unpredictable

In most cases, the stressors employed are naturalistic and range from cat exposure, crowding, and confrontation with an unfamiliar male, in the case of maternal stress, through maternal separation in the case of infant stressors, to social isolation, social subjugation, and a series of non-social stressors administered to juveniles. The ADXr model was created experimentally to model glucocorticoid hypofunction seen in animals and humans experiencing stressors. Here, however, the hypo-glucocorticoid state is created by surgery rather than by stressors suffered at various periods of life.

if it involved a gross deviation from the evolutionary rules that limit the risks associated with aggression. The main symptoms are centered around dangerousness (damaging, potentially lethal attacks), unpredictability (poor social signaling), and inappropriate targets or contexts (attacks on females or pups, aggression in foreign territory, etc.).

The table depicts findings obtained in rodents. Monkey data obtained in semi-naturalistic environments will be presented later, because the timing, duration, and type of stress cannot be controlled well under such conditions. As such, the possible parallels between rodents and monkeys require some explanations.

The existence and transient nature of the glucocorticoid stress response that triggered the long-term alterations depicted in the table was documented for each early stressor. In all models, effects were investigated in at least one – frequently two or three – developmental stage later. For example, the effects of fetal stressors were investigated when subjects were juveniles (two developmental stages later) or adults (three developmental stages later).

A brief glance at the table reveals two important issues [1]. Early stressors have long-lasting effects on both glucocorticoid secretion patterns and behavior even though the triggering stressor was brief and terminated soon after the stressor was administered. This demonstrates that stressors suffered during critical periods of life are toxic in the meaning that they do not require high levels of glucocorticoids to maintain effects; moreover, these often develop on the background of persistently reduced glucocorticoid secretion patterns, which themselves are consequences of early toxic stress [2]. Effects are stressor- and developmental stage-dependent. Glucocorticoid production may be increased or decreased or may remain unaltered just like social behaviors (amiable or agonistic). We refrained from complicating the table by covering other physiological phenomena (e.g., adrenaline stress responses) or behavioral states (e.g., anxiety and depression), but it is worth noting that the effects of early stressors on these also depend on the timing and type of the toxic stressor.

Although abnormal aggression is a regular consequence of stressors administered in the juvenile period, its symptoms also depend on timing and type as shown in the lower part of the table.

5.3.2.2 The Particularities of the Main Models

Very early stressors (fetal stress and maternal separation) cannot be considered "good" aggression models, for two reasons. First, findings are rather conflicting. For instance, fetal stress decreased both social behavior and aggression in some studies [125], whereas social behavior was decreased but aggression was increased in others [123]. Similarly, maternal separation decreased aggression in some rat studies [127] but increased it in others [132]. Second, the increase in aggression was rather modest when it occurred and typically affected only one – often marginal – aggression variable. For instance, the latency to attack was reduced, or the time spent with offensive threats was increased, but bite counts remained unaltered [131, 132].

The effects of very early stressors seem more congruent in rhesus monkeys studied in captivity, where stress exposure in infancy regularly decreased social behavior and increased aggression [148–150]. In these studies, however, pups were separated because their mothers were reluctant to nurture them and were raised in peer groups. This type of maternal separation is quite different from the one studied in rodents, where the procedure involves the repeated separation of pups from their mother for several hours a day (typically 3) and the procedure was restricted to the lactating period. By contrast, peer rearing covered both infancy and adolescence in monkeys. As such, "maternal separation" in monkeys is in fact a mixed model of infant and juvenile stress, the latter affecting aggression more reliably in rodents as well.

While very early stressors are unreliable aggression models, they are good models of anxiety [151], depression [152], alcohol dependence [153], and drug abuse [154]. Moreover, early stressors affect learning [155] and some nonbehavioral functions like digestion in adulthood [156]. Taken together, these findings demonstrate that stressors suffered by the fetus or the infant are highly debilitating. Increases in aggression are weak symptoms of a wide array of much stronger dysfunctions. Further work with more adequately chosen stressors and time windows for stress application – important details from the point of view of delayed consequences [123, 125, 157] – may clarify many aspects of the early stress-aggression relationship, but the findings obtained so far make it unlikely that increased or abnormal aggression would emerge as a fundamental consequence of very early stress.

By contrast, stressors suffered during the peripubertal period have long-lasting effects on aggression. This is true for both social defeats and non-social stresses. Surprisingly, social defeats administered between postnatal days 28–42 have weaker effects than non-social stressors suffered within the same period.

Social defeats during the peripubertal period – called subjugation stress – have somewhat inconsistent effects on aggression. In hamsters it increased aggression against smaller but decreased it against larger opponents [158]; in rats, early subjugation increased aggression against "regular" (weight-matched) opponents [159]. Although abnormal features of aggression were not blatant, early subjugation accelerated the emergence of adult forms of aggression [160] and promoted attacks on juveniles [158, 161]. The former indicates that development was affected, whereas the latter is among the symptoms of abnormal aggression. Corticosterone was increased by subjugation in the juvenile stage, but this effect disappeared within 2 weeks [162], while behavioral effects emerged in adulthood and were persistent [159, 161]. Thus, the stressor was "toxic." Glucocorticoids administered in the peripubertal period had effects similar to those of subjugation [163] and were blocked by glucocorticoid receptor antagonists [164], demonstrating the causal involvement of the peripubertal glucocorticoid response in the delayed behavioral consequences of early subjugation.

Three non-social stressors, open field, fox odor, and elevated platform exposures administered around puberty affected adult aggression more dramatically than subjugations suffered during the same period. In adulthood, aggression increased dramatically [142]; rats readily attacked anaesthetized inoffensive opponents [140] and females [139]. In addition, attacks were damaging (targeted vulnerable body parts of opponents) and were poorly signaled socially [141]. Similar effects were observed in female rats [138]. As such, non-social peripubertal stress elicited the full spectrum of abnormal aggression symptoms, and its consequences were gender-independent. Noteworthy, the adult effects of peripubertal stressors were inhibited by glucocorticoid receptor blockers administered concurrently with the stressor to juveniles [165], demonstrating a causal relationship between juvenile glucocorticoid stress and adult behavioral modifications.

Abnormal aggressions were developed on the background of normal baseline glucocorticoids but blunted stress responses in the case of both peripubertal subjugation [161] and non-social stress [140, 141]. In the case of the latter, a downregulated glucocorticoid secretion was observed already in late puberty, when behavioral problems were not yet apparent [142, 165]. While the causal influence of juvenile glucocorticoid responses on adult aggressiveness was demonstrated in both cases (see above), the role of blunted glucocorticoid secretions in adulthood becomes obvious only when the findings of the ADXr model are also considered.

The development of this model was prompted by human observations demonstrating that some aggression-related psychopathologies, e.g., post-traumatic stress disorder [166] and criminal violence [167], develop on a downregulated glucocorticoid background. To mimic this condition, adult rats were adrenalectomized bilaterally (ADX) and were submitted to glucocorticoid replacement therapy (ADXr) by means of subcutaneous corticosterone pellets. The treatments ensured low basal levels of plasma glucocorticoids that did not react to stressors [143]. This procedure resulted in a wide spectrum of abnormal aggression symptoms without a quantitative change in aggressiveness [144, 146, 147]. In addition to the glucocorticoid component, these rats also showed decreased autonomic responses to social challenges [145]. Aggression-induced heart rate increases were not only lower than in controls, but the increase terminated before the aggressive encounter ended, which was in sharp contrast with controls, where heart rates remained high long after the termination of the aggressive encounter. Short-term inhibitions of glucocorticoid secretion had opposing effects on aggression (i.e., decreased it) [146], whereas repeated glucocorticoid injections abolished the effects of the long-term glucocorticoid inhibition [143], demonstrating that abnormal aggression observed in the ADXr model specifically develops on the background of a chronic decrease in glucocorticoids.

The findings briefly reviewed above strongly suggest that the blunted glucocorticoid stress responses seen in the early subjugation and peripubertal stress models are causally linked to the emergence of abnormal forms of aggression. Together with the lowered autonomic stress responses seen in the ADXr model, these findings lead to the hypoarousal theory of abnormal aggression [168, 169].

Increased stress reactivity can also make aggression abnormal. This conclusion is based on findings obtained with the post-weaning social isolation model. It was repeatedly shown that animals maintained in social isolation from weaning to early adulthood show increased aggression when confronted with conspecifics in adulthood. This was observed in rats [170, 171], guinea pigs [172], rhesus monkeys [173], and many other species. Later it was revealed that aggression elicited by post-weaning social isolation fulfills most requirements of abnormal aggression, is associated with a general behavioral agitation, and is developed on the background of markedly increased glucocorticoid and autonomic stress responses [134, 135]. Somewhat similar findings were obtained in rhesus monkeys [174]. The subjects of this primate study were peer-reared but for certain reasons were maintained in isolation for long periods when juveniles. Subsequent to this procedure, they occupied a low rank in the groups they were introduced later but displayed excessive aggressive responses when socially challenged. Aggression was so severe that they had to be isolated again to protect group mates from injuries. Thus, this post-weaning isolation-like procedure elicited the emergence of abnormal forms of aggression in monkeys like in rodents, where a "true" post-weaning social isolation model was employed.

Post-weaning social isolation is stressful for a couple of hours, but glucocorticoid production rapidly returns to normal and shows no deviations at any time point of the juvenile period [135]. Endocrine consequences become apparent only in adulthood, when animals are exposed to a social challenge. The behavioral, hormonal, and autonomic pattern is persistent and is resistant to social interventions, e.g., resocialization [136]. This strongly supports the toxic nature of the stress elicited by post-weaning social isolation; moreover, this appears to be the only model where the underlying epigenetic mechanisms were experimentally documented [175]. This model together with relevant human data leads to the development of the hyperarousal theory of abnormal aggression [176, 177].

5.3.3 Overview and Brain Mechanisms

The findings reviewed above derive from laboratory models and partly on the stressful experiences and behaviors of captive monkeys, which raises some questions regarding their validity for feral animals and possibly humans. It is worthwhile emphasizing, however, that the stressors employed in the laboratory are very similar to those experienced by free-ranging individuals. The exposure of pregnant females to crowding, dangerous social partners, etc. is frequent in both nature and society. After delivery, mothers often leave their offspring alone, because they need to feed themselves. Although losing contact with a mother is a daily experience, prolonged periods of maternal separation endanger survival and trigger stress responses in pups. Non-social stressors are probably also common in the peripubertal period, when the young start exploring the world beyond their home range. They may also meet aggressive males who defeat ("subjugate") them. Finally, abandoned or neglected offspring are not uncommon neither in nature nor in society. Briefly, laboratory models make use of naturalistic stressors, and their consequences are investigated by relevant behavioral tests.

Research performed so far reveals two basic developmental pathways elicited by early toxic stress. Stressors suffered in puberty elicit abnormal aggression on the background of downregulated arousal. Social isolation from weaning to early adulthood elicits abnormal aggression on the background of increased arousal (see Fig. 5.3). These two pathways are recognizable in humans as well (see below).

Beyond changes in brain function, all abnormal aggression – toxic stress – models elicit structural changes in the brain. For instance, post-weaning social isolation interfered with prefrontal development, which resulted in decreased cortical thickness, lowered glial density, and impoverished vascularization in this area [178]. Changes in prefrontal connectivity were also evident [175]. The peripubertal stress model of abnormal aggression resulted in white matter anomalies in the prefrontal cortex, amygdala, and hippocampal formation [142] and an altered expression of the MAOA gene and of synaptic adhesion molecules in the prefrontal cortex [140, 179]. Finally, the social subjugation model of abnormal aggression induced marked changes in the expression of genes related to neuronal plasticity [180] and altered vasopressinergic and serotonergic innervation in the hypothalamic attack area [158].

Structural deficits forecast the durability of the behavioral states produced by toxic stress, which in fact was demonstrated for these abnormal aggression models.

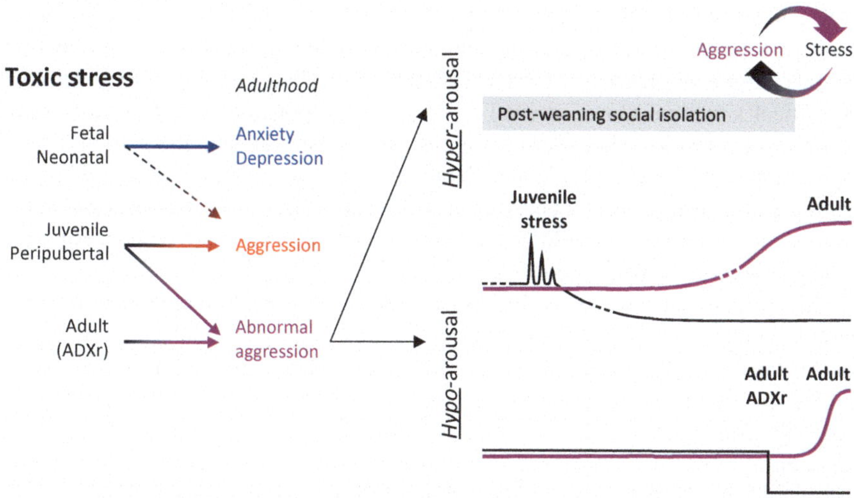

Fig. 5.3 *Toxic stress and aggression: abnormal aggression models. Left hand panel.* Very early stressors have massive effects on a variety of behavioral and somatic phenomena (exemplified here by anxiety and depression) but weak effects on aggression. By contrast, juvenile stressors robustly increase aggressiveness and lead to the emergence of abnormal aggression. Limiting plasma glucocorticoid levels and stress responses in adulthood (ADXr) leads to abnormal aggression. *Right hand panel.* Post-weaning social isolation does not affect glucocorticoid secretion during the isolation period but dramatically increases social challenge-induced glucocorticoid and autonomic stress responses, by this putatively exacerbating the positive feedback loop that connects glucocorticoid production and aggression (see Fig. 5.1). Stressors suffered in puberty downregulate glucocorticoid stress responses (black lines) and lead to the emergence of abnormal aggression (magenta). The behavioral change follows the endocrine one with a considerable delay and is causally linked to it. The same phenomenon is observed when glucocorticoid production is experimentally downregulated in adulthood (ADXr)

5.4 General Overview

One of the central concepts of biological sciences is that natural phenomena have functions and serve both the survival of the individual and the transmission of its genes to the next generation. The biological approach to aggression is in fact a typical example of this central concept (see Chap. 1). The glucocorticoid-aggression relationship is usually also viewed through this lens.

When development is not disturbed, challenges induce stress responses, which promote the appropriate response to the challenge. For instance, social challenges elicit glucocorticoid stress responses, which promote aggression. Aggression on its turn enhances the glucocorticoid stress response further, within the framework of a positive feedback loop. The mutual facilitation of the endocrine and behavioral stress responses ends when the challenge subsides. In the case of social challenges, this occurs when the conflict is won and the opponent submits.

When development is not disturbed, unsuccessful attempts to answer challenges result in a behavioral state akin to human depression: glucocorticoid production remains chronically high, and the individual limits its behavioral activity to survive the critical situation. Once survival is ensured, the potential to return to normal activity is preserved. This occurs, for instance, when an individual is defeated. Aggression is strongly inhibited, which prevents the unnecessary provocation of the victor, i.e., the useless loss of energies and the risks of injury. Submission promotes survival and preserves the ability of the individual to prevail in subsequent conflicts if the winner withdraws or weakens.

The critical contribution of glucocorticoids to behavioral changes was demonstrated in both cases. Hormonal effects are mediated by various subcellular components in the case of brief acute stressors collectively called non-genomic mechanisms and by the regulation of gene expression in the case of more durable stressors (genomic mechanisms). Behavioral effects are indirect consequences of the cellular – neural – processes influenced by glucocorticoids and are expressed until glucocorticoids bind to their subcellular targets. That is, changes are reversible.

In contrast, strong stressors suffered in critical periods of life – toxic stressors – disturb development and change life trajectories. This phenomenon is usually conceptualized as a preparation for harsh life conditions that were predicted by early experiences and is often viewed as an early programing of the brain. The critical contribution of glucocorticoids in the early programing of aggression was also demonstrated, but these consequences develop long after the glucocorticoid response to the early stressor vanished. Early stressors and adult consequences are linked by the phenomenon called epigenetics, the restructuring of the chromatin. Its consequences are comparable with those of genetic deficits and null mutations. Toxic stressors lead to structural changes in the brain; consequently, behavioral alterations are durable and rather resistant to interventions.

In response to toxic stress, abnormal forms of aggression emerge. These are damaging, poorly signaled socially, and unselective regarding social partners and locations. Although called abnormal for their human analogs (see below), such forms of aggression are likely effective and advantageous when social competition is severe. Abnormal aggression may be associated with both low and high glucocorticoid profiles or in more general terms with hypo- and hyperarousal. The former is triggered by stressors suffered around puberty, the latter by social isolation suffered by juveniles.

The impact of glucocorticoids on aggression was recently visualized by a U-shaped "dose-response curve," implying that high and abnormal aggression is associated with either very low or very high basal levels of glucocorticoids and/or glucocorticoid stress responses [181]. Such images, although suggestive, easily comprehensible, and memorable, remain somewhat one-sided because there is an inverted U-shaped curve in-between the one that visualizes the "normal" glucocorticoid-aggression relationship (see Fig. 5.4.)

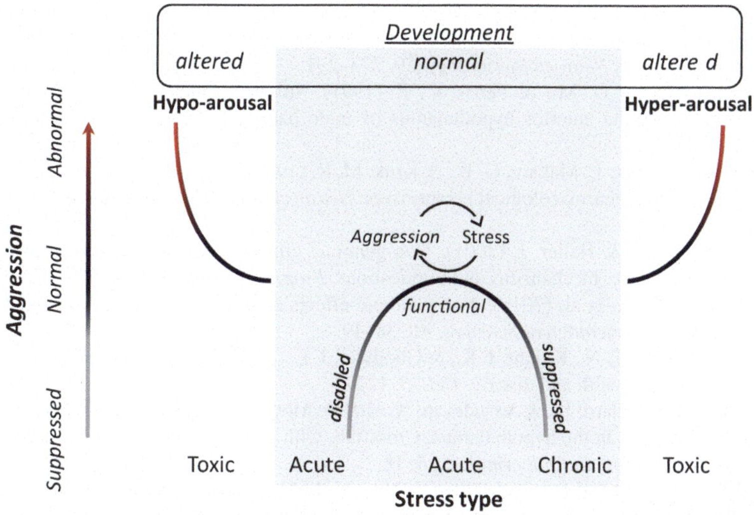

Fig. 5.4 *Glucocorticoids and aggression in normal and abnormal animal aggression: a general view.* The figure visualizes the glucocorticoid-aggression relationship in animals undergoing normal development (middle panel) and those with disturbed development (left and right panels). Note that words indicative of changes in aggressiveness were printed in italic. Inhibited stress responses disable, whereas chronically high glucocorticoid levels inhibit aggression under normal conditions. Analogous conditions engender high and abnormal forms of aggression when development was disturbed by early toxic stressors. Although a broader term – justified by analogous changes in autonomic stress responses – hypo- and hyperarousal also mean downregulated and upregulated glucocorticoid stress systems, respectively

References

1. Bird, A. (2007). Perceptions of epigenetics. *Nature, 447*, 396–398.
2. Ruf, K., & Steiner, F. A. (1967). Steroid-sensitive single neurons in rat hypothalamus and midbrain: Identification by microelectrophoresis. *Science, 156*, 667–669.
3. Steiner, F. A., Akert, K., & Ruf, K. (1969). Steroid-sensitive neurones in rat brain: Anatomical localization and responses to neurohumours and ACTH. *Brain Research, 12*, 74–85.
4. Saphier, D., & Feldman, S. (1988). Iontophoretic application of glucocorticoids inhibits identified neurones in the rat paraventricular nucleus. *Brain Research, 453*, 183–190.
5. McEwen, B. S., De Kloet, E. R., & Rostene, W. (1986). Adrenal steroid receptors and actions in the nervous system. *Physiological Reviews, 66*, 1121–1188.
6. Joëls, M., & de Kloet, E. R. (1992). Control of neuronal excitability by corticosteroid hormones. *Trends in Neurosciences, 15*, 25–30.
7. Avanzino, G. L., Celasco, G., Cogo, C. E., Ermirio, R., & Ruggeri, P. (1983). Actions of microelectrophoretically applied glucocorticoid hormones on reticular formation neurones in the rat. *Neuroscience Letters, 38*, 45–49.
8. Dubrovsky, B., Williams, D., & Kraulis, I. (1985). Effects of corticosterone and 5 alpha-dihydrocorticosterone on brain excitability in the rat. *Journal of Neuroscience Research, 14*, 117–128.

9. Haller, J., Mikics, E., & Makara, G. B. (2008). The effects of non-genomic glucocorticoid mechanisms on bodily functions and the central neural system. A critical evaluation of findings. *Frontiers in Neuroendocrinology, 29*, 273–291.
10. Hayden-Hixson, D. M., & Ferris, C. F. (1991). Steroid-specific regulation of agonistic responding in the anterior hypothalamus of male hamsters. *Physiology & Behavior, 50*, 793–799.
11. Haller, J., Halasz, J., Makara, G. B., & Kruk, M. R. (1998). Acute effects of glucocorticoids: Behavioral and pharmacological perspectives. *Neuroscience and Biobehavioral Reviews, 23*, 337–344.
12. Makara, G. B., & Haller, J. (2001). Non-genomic effects of glucocorticoids in the neural system. Evidence, mechanisms and implications. *Progress in Neurobiology, 65*, 367–390.
13. Panettieri, R. A., et al. (2019). Non-genomic effects of glucocorticoids: An updated view. *Trends in Pharmacological Sciences, 40*, 38–49.
14. Liu, B., Zhang, T.-N., Knight, J. K., & Goodwin, J. E. (2019). The glucocorticoid receptor in cardiovascular health and disease. *Cell, 8*, 1227.
15. Rainville, J., Pollard, K., & Vasudevan, N. (2015). Membrane-initiated non-genomic signaling by estrogens in the hypothalamus: Cross-talk with glucocorticoids with implications for behavior. *Frontiers in Endocrinology, 6*, 18.
16. Selye, H. (1974). *Stress without distress*. New York: The New American Library.
17. Haller, J. (2014). The glucocorticoid/aggression relationship in animals and humans: An analysis sensitive to behavioral characteristics, glucocorticoid secretion patterns, and neural mechanisms. *Current Topics in Behavioral Neurosciences, 17*, 73–109.
18. Earley, R. L., et al. (2006). Social interactions tune aggression and stress responsiveness in a territorial cichlid fish (Archocentrus nigrofasciatus). *Physiology & Behavior, 88*, 353–363.
19. Woodley, S. K., Matt, K. S., & Moore, M. C. (2000). Neuroendocrine responses in free-living female and male lizards after aggressive interactions. *Physiology & Behavior, 71*, 373–381.
20. Ramenofsky, M. (1985). Acute changes in plasma steroids and agonistic behavior in male Japanese quail. *General and Comparative Endocrinology, 60*, 116–128.
21. Bronson, F. H., & Eleftheriou, B. E. (1965). Adrenal response to fighting in mice: Separation of physical and psychological causes. *Science, 147*, 627–628.
22. Schuurman, T. (1980). Hormonal correlates of agonistic behavior in adult male rats. *Progress in Brain Research, 53*, 415–420.
23. Tornatzky, W., & Miczek, K. A. (1994). Behavioral and autonomic responses to intermittent social stress: Differential protection by clonidine and metoprolol. *Psychopharmacology, 116*, 346–356.
24. Haller, J., Barna, I., & Baranyi, M. (1995). Hormonal and metabolic responses during psychosocial stimulation in aggressive and nonaggressive rats. *Psychoneuroendocrinology, 20*, 65–74.
25. Landys, M. M., Goymann, W., Schwabl, I., Trapschuh, M., & Slagsvold, T. (2010). Impact of season and social challenge on testosterone and corticosterone levels in a year-round territorial bird. *Hormones and Behavior, 58*, 317–325.
26. Ruiz-Aizpurua, L., Buwalda, B., & De Boer, S. F. (2013). Acute and lasting effects of single mineralocorticoid antagonism on offensive aggressive behaviour in rats. *Behavioural Processes, 98*, 72–77.
27. Mikics, E., Kruk, M. R., & Haller, J. (2004). Genomic and non-genomic effects of glucocorticoids on aggressive behavior in male rats. *Psychoneuroendocrinology, 29*, 618–635.
28. Kruk, M. R., Halász, J., Meelis, W., & Haller, J. (2004). Fast positive feedback between the adrenocortical stress response and a brain mechanism involved in aggressive behavior. *Behavioral Neuroscience, 118*, 1062–1070.
29. Lightman, S. L., et al. (2008). The significance of glucocorticoid pulsatility. *European Journal of Pharmacology, 583*, 255–262.
30. Lightman, S. L., et al. (2002). Hypothalamic-pituitary-adrenal function. *Archives of Physiology and Biochemistry, 110*, 90–93.

31. Haller, J., Millar, S., & Kruk, M. R. (1998). Mineralocorticoid receptor blockade inhibits aggressive behaviour in male rats. *Stress (Amsterdam, Netherlands), 2*, 201–207.
32. Haller, J., Millar, S., van de Schraaf, J., de Kloet, R. E., & Kruk, M. R. (2000). The active phase-related increase in corticosterone and aggression are linked. *Journal of Neuroendocrinology, 12*, 431–436.
33. Haller, J., Halasz, J., Mikics, E., Kruk, M. R., & Makara, G. B. (2000). Ultradian corticosterone rhythm and the propensity to behave aggressively in male rats. *Journal of Neuroendocrinology, 12*, 937–940.
34. Potegal, M., Ferris, C. F., Hebert, M., Meyerhoff, J., & Skaredoff, L. (1996). Attack priming in female Syrian golden hamsters is associated with a c-fos-coupled process within the corticomedial amygdala. *Neuroscience, 75*, 869–880.
35. Potegal, M. (1992). Time course of aggressive arousal in female hamsters and male rats. *Behavioral and Neural Biology, 58*, 120–124.
36. Manuel, R., et al. (2016). Effects of acute stress on aggression and the cortisol response in the African sharptooth catfish Clarias gariepinus: Differences between day and night. *Journal of Fish Biology, 88*, 2175–2187.
37. Tonelli, L. H., Hoshino, A., Katz, M., & Postolache, T. T. (2008). Acute stress promotes aggressive-like behavior in rats made allergic to tree pollen. *International Journal of Child Health and Human Development, 1*, 305–312.
38. Chang, C.-H., & Gean, P.-W. (2019). The ventral hippocampus controls stress-provoked impulsive aggression through the ventromedial hypothalamus in post-weaning social isolation mice. *Cell Reports, 28*, 1195–1205.e3.
39. de Almeida, R. M. M., & Miczek, K. A. (2002). Aggression escalated by social instigation or by discontinuation of reinforcement ('frustration') in mice: Inhibition by anpirtoline: A 5-HT1B receptor agonist. *Neuropsychopharmacol, 27*, 171–181.
40. Takahashi, A., et al. (2012). Behavioral characterization of escalated aggression induced by GABA(B) receptor activation in the dorsal raphe nucleus. *Psychopharmacology, 224*, 155–166.
41. Cannon, W. B. (1915). *Bodily changes in pain, hunger, fear and rage: An account of recent researches into the function of emotional excitement.* D Appleton & Company. doi:https://doi.org/10.1037/10013-000.
42. Yohe, L. R., Suzuki, H., & Lucas, L. R. (2012). Aggression is suppressed by acute stress but induced by chronic stress: Immobilization effects on aggression, hormones, and cortical 5-HT(1B)/ striatal dopamine D(2) receptor density. *Cognitive, Affective, & Behavioral Neuroscience, 12*, 446–459.
43. Wood, G. E., Young, L. T., Reagan, L. P., & McEwen, B. S. (2003). Acute and chronic restraint stress alter the incidence of social conflict in male rats. *Hormones and Behavior, 43*, 205–213.
44. Albonetti, M. E., & Farabollini, F. (1993). Effects of single and repeated restraint on the social behavior of male rats. *Physiology & Behavior, 53*, 937–942.
45. Gong, H., et al. (2019). Corticosterone rapidly improves the endurance of high-intensity exercise (swimming) via nongenomic mechanisms in mice. *The Journal of Sports Medicine and Physical Fitness, 59*, 886–891.
46. den Boon, F. S., de Vries, T., Baelde, M., Joëls, M., & Karst, H. (2019). Circadian and Ultradian variations in corticosterone level influence functioning of the male mouse basolateral amygdala. *Endocrinology, 160*, 791–802.
47. Summers, C. H., et al. (2005). Glucocorticoid interaction with aggression in non-mammalian vertebrates: Reciprocal action. *European Journal of Pharmacology, 526*, 21–35.
48. Haller, J. (1993). Adrenomedullar catecholamine liberation and carbohydrate metabolism during the first 30 min of an aggressive encounter in rats. *Physiology & Behavior, 54*, 195–197.
49. Magomedova, L., & Cummins, C. L. (2016). Glucocorticoids and metabolic control. *Handbook of Experimental Pharmacology, 233*, 73–93.

50. Song, I.-H., & Buttgereit, F. (2006). Non-genomic glucocorticoid effects to provide the basis for new drug developments. *Molecular and Cellular Endocrinology, 246*, 142–146.
51. Nishi, M., & Kawata, M. (2007). Dynamics of glucocorticoid receptor and mineralocorticoid receptor: Implications from live cell imaging studies. *Neuroendocrinology, 85*, 186–192.
52. Lee, D. Y., Kim, E., & Choi, M. H. (2015). Technical and clinical aspects of cortisol as a biochemical marker of chronic stress. *BMB Reports, 48*, 209–216.
53. Adam, E. K., et al. (2017). Diurnal cortisol slopes and mental and physical health outcomes: A systematic review and meta-analysis. *Psychoneuroendocrinology, 83*, 25–41.
54. Ing, N. H. (2005). Steroid hormones regulate gene expression posttranscriptionally by altering the stabilities of messenger RNAs. *Biology of Reproduction, 72*, 1290–1296.
55. Datson, N. A., Morsink, M. C., Meijer, O. C., & de Kloet, E. R. (2008). Central corticosteroid actions: Search for gene targets. *European Journal of Pharmacology, 583*, 272–289.
56. Thormann, V., et al. (2019). Expanding the repertoire of glucocorticoid receptor target genes by engineering genomic response elements. *Life Science Alliance, 2*, e201800283.
57. de Kloet, E. R., Han, F., & Meijer, O. C. (2008). From the stalk to down under about brain glucocorticoid receptors, stress and development. *Neurochemical Research, 33*, 637–642.
58. McEwen, B. S. (1998). Stress, adaptation, and disease. Allostasis and allostatic load. *Annals of the New York Academy of Sciences, 840*, 33–44.
59. Korte, S. M., Koolhaas, J. M., Wingfield, J. C., & McEwen, B. S. (2005). The Darwinian concept of stress: Benefits of allostasis and costs of allostatic load and the trade-offs in health and disease. *Neuroscience and Biobehavioral Reviews, 29*, 3–38.
60. Płaźnik, A., Pałejko, W., Stefański, R., & Kostowski, W. (1993). Open field behavior of rats reared in different social conditions: The effects of stress and imipramine. *Polish Journal of Pharmacology, 45*, 243–252.
61. Leshner, A. I., Korn, S. J., Mixon, J. F., Rosenthal, C., & Besser, A. K. (1980). Effects of corticosterone on submissiveness in mice: Some temporal and theoretical considerations. *Physiology & Behavior, 24*, 283–288.
62. Pednekar, J. R., Mulgaonker, V. K., & Mascarenhas, J. F. (1993). Effect of intensity and duration of stress on male sexual behaviour. *Indian Journal of Experimental Biology, 31*, 638–640.
63. McEwen, B. S. (2005). Stressed or stressed out: What is the difference? *Journal of Psychiatry & Neuroscience, 30*, 315–318.
64. Höglund, E., Balm, P. H. M., & Winberg, S. (2002). Behavioural and neuroendocrine effects of environmental background colour and social interaction in Arctic charr (Salvelinus alpinus). *The Journal of Experimental Biology, 205*, 2535–2543.
65. Summers, C. H., et al. (2003). Temporal patterns of limbic monoamine and plasma corticosterone response during social stress. *Neuroscience, 116*, 553–563.
66. Carere, C., Welink, D., Drent, P. J., Koolhaas, J. M., & Groothuis, T. G. (2001). Effect of social defeat in a territorial bird (Parus major) selected for different coping styles. *Physiology & Behavior, 73*, 427–433.
67. Blanchard, D. C., et al. (1995). Visible burrow system as a model of chronic social stress: Behavioral and neuroendocrine correlates. *Psychoneuroendocrinology, 20*, 117–134.
68. Yodyingyuad, U., de la Riva, C., Abbott, D. H., Herbert, J., & Keverne, E. B. (1985). Relationship between dominance hierarchy, cerebrospinal fluid levels of amine transmitter metabolites (5-hydroxyindole acetic acid and homovanillic acid) and plasma cortisol in monkeys. *Neuroscience, 16*, 851–858.
69. Haller, J., Kiem, D. T., & Makara, G. B. (1996). The physiology of social conflict in rats: What is particularly stressful? *Behavioral Neuroscience, 110*, 353–359.
70. Potegal, M., Huhman, K., Moore, T., & Meyerhoff, J. (1993). Conditioned defeat in the Syrian golden hamster (Mesocricetus auratus). *Behavioral and Neural Biology, 60*, 93–102.
71. Siegfried, B., Frischknecht, H. R., & Waser, P. G. (1984). Defeat, learned submissiveness, and analgesia in mice: Effect of genotype. *Behavioral and Neural Biology, 42*, 91–97.

72. Hammack, S. E., Cooper, M. A., & Lezak, K. R. (2012). Overlapping neurobiology of learned helplessness and conditioned defeat: Implications for PTSD and mood disorders. *Neuropharmacology, 62*, 565–575.
73. van Kampen, M., Kramer, M., Hiemke, C., Flügge, G., & Fuchs, E. (2002). The chronic psychosocial stress paradigm in male tree shrews: Evaluation of a novel animal model for depressive disorders. *Stress (Amsterdam, Netherlands), 5*, 37–46.
74. McCann, K. E., & Huhman, K. L. (2012). The effect of escapable versus inescapable social defeat on conditioned defeat and social recognition in Syrian hamsters. *Physiology & Behavior, 105*, 493–497.
75. Macedo, G. C., et al. (2018). Consequences of continuous social defeat stress on anxiety- and depressive-like behaviors and ethanol reward in mice. *Hormones and Behavior, 97*, 154–161.
76. Ferrer-Pérez, C., Reguilón, M. D., Manzanedo, C., Miñarro, J., & Rodríguez-Arias, M. (2019). Social housing conditions modulate the long-lasting increase in cocaine reward induced by intermittent social defeat. *Frontiers in Behavioral Neuroscience, 13*, 148.
77. Solomon, M. B., et al. (2009). Gonadal hormones modulate the display of conditioned defeat in male Syrian hamsters. *Hormones and Behavior, 56*, 423–428.
78. DeNardo, D. F., & Sinervo, B. (1994). Effects of corticosterone on activity and home-range size of free-ranging male lizards. *Hormones and Behavior, 28*, 53–65.
79. Tokarz, R. R. (1987). Effects of corticosterone treatment on male aggressive behavior in a lizard (Anolis sagrei). *Hormones and Behavior, 21*, 358–370.
80. Meddle, S. L., et al. (2002). Steroid hormone interrelationships with territorial aggression in an Arctic-breeding songbird, Gambel's white-crowned sparrow, Zonotrichia leucophrys gambelii. *Hormones and Behavior, 42*, 212–221.
81. DiBattista, J. D., Anisman, H., Whitehead, M., & Gilmour, K. M. (2005). The effects of cortisol administration on social status and brain monoaminergic activity in rainbow trout Oncorhynchus mykiss. *The Journal of Experimental Biology, 208*, 2707–2718.
82. Timmer, M., & Sandi, C. (2010). A role for glucocorticoids in the long-term establishment of a social hierarchy. *Psychoneuroendocrinology, 35*, 1543–1552.
83. Corum, C. R., & Thurmond, J. B. (1977). Effects of acute exposure to stress on subsequent aggression and locomotion performance. *Psychosomatic Medicine, 39*, 436–443.
84. Armario, A., Vallès, A., Dal-Zotto, S., Márquez, C., & Belda, X. (2004). A single exposure to severe stressors causes long-term desensitisation of the physiological response to the homotypic stressor. *Stress (Amsterdam, Netherlands), 7*, 157–172.
85. Belda, X., Daviu, N., Nadal, R., & Armario, A. (2012). Acute stress-induced sensitization of the pituitary-adrenal response to heterotypic stressors: Independence of glucocorticoid release and activation of CRH1 receptors. *Hormones and Behavior, 62*, 515–524.
86. Babb, J. A., Masini, C. V., Day, H. E. W., & Campeau, S. (2014). Habituation of hypothalamic-pituitary-adrenocortical axis hormones to repeated homotypic stress and subsequent heterotypic stressor exposure in male and female rats. *Stress (Amsterdam, Netherlands), 17*, 224–234.
87. Kearns, R. R., & Spencer, R. L. (2013). An unexpected increase in restraint duration alters the expression of stress response habituation. *Physiology & Behavior, 122*, 193–200.
88. Belda, X., Nadal, R., & Armario, A. (2016). Critical features of acute stress-induced cross-sensitization identified through the hypothalamic-pituitary-adrenal axis output. *Scientific Reports, 6*, 31244.
89. Belda, X., Fuentes, S., Daviu, N., Nadal, R., & Armario, A. (2015). Stress-induced sensitization: The hypothalamic-pituitary-adrenal axis and beyond. *Stress (Amsterdam, Netherlands), 18*, 269–279.
90. Fava, M. (1998). Depression with anger attacks. *The Journal of Clinical Psychiatry, 59*(Suppl 18), 18–22.
91. Baranyi, J., Bakos, N., & Haller, J. (2005). Social instability in female rats: The relationship between stress-related and anxiety-like consequences. *Physiology & Behavior, 84*, 511–518.

92. Barsy, B., Leveleki, C., Zelena, D., & Haller, J. (2010). The context specificity of anxiety responses induced by chronic psychosocial stress in rats: A shift from anxiety to social phobia? *Stress (Amsterdam, Netherlands), 13*, 230–237.
93. Fuchs, E. (2005). Social stress in tree shrews as an animal model of depression: An example of a behavioral model of a CNS disorder. *CNS Spectrums, 10*, 182–190.
94. Larrieu, T., & Sandi, C. (2018). Stress-induced depression: Is social rank a predictive risk factor? *BioEssays: News and Reviews in Molecular, Cellular and Developmental Biology, 40*, e1800012.
95. Finnell, J. E., et al. (2019). The contribution of the locus coeruleus-norepinephrine system in the emergence of defeat-induced inflammatory priming. *Brain, Behavior, and Immunity, 79*, 102–113.
96. Kaufling, J. (2019). Alterations and adaptation of ventral tegmental area dopaminergic neurons in animal models of depression. *Cell and Tissue Research, 377*, 59–71.
97. Bartolomucci, A., et al. (2010). Increased vulnerability to psychosocial stress in heterozygous serotonin transporter knockout mice. *Disease Models & Mechanisms, 3*, 459–470.
98. Martinez, M., Calvo-Torrent, A., & Herbert, J. (2002). Mapping brain response to social stress in rodents with c-fos expression: A review. *Stress (Amsterdam, Netherlands), 5*, 3–13.
99. Gerwing, J. (1958). The effect of continued toxic stress on the activity of the thyroid gland in the rat and the guinea-pig. *The Journal of Physiology, 144*, 243–249.
100. Garner, A. S., Shonkoff, J. P., & Committee on Psychosocial Aspects of Child and Family Health, Committee on Early Childhood, Adoption, and Dependent Care & Section on Developmental and Behavioral Pediatrics. (2012). Early childhood adversity, toxic stress, and the role of the pediatrician: Translating developmental science into lifelong health. *Pediatrics, 129*, e224–e231.
101. Shonkoff, J. P., Garner, A. S., & Committee on Psychosocial Aspects of Child and Family Health, Committee on Early Childhood, Adoption, and Dependent Care & Section on Developmental and Behavioral Pediatrics. (2012). The lifelong effects of early childhood adversity and toxic stress. *Pediatrics, 129*, e232–e246.
102. Joos, C. M., McDonald, A., & Wadsworth, M. E. (2019). Extending the toxic stress model into adolescence: Profiles of cortisol reactivity. *Psychoneuroendocrinology, 107*, 46–58.
103. SmithBattle, L. (2019). Housing trajectories of teen mothers and their families over 28 years. *The American Journal of Orthopsychiatry, 89*, 258–267.
104. Sabri, B., & Granger, D. A. (2018). Gender-based violence and trauma in marginalized populations of women: Role of biological embedding and toxic stress. *Health Care for Women International, 39*, 1038–1055.
105. Andreescu, C., et al. (2008). Gray matter changes in late life depression–A structural MRI analysis. *Neuropsychopharmacol, 33*, 2566–2572.
106. McEwen, C. A., & McEwen, B. S. (2017). Social structure, adversity, toxic stress, and intergenerational poverty: An early childhood model. *Annual Review of Sociology, 43*, 445–472.
107. Toxic Stress. *Center on the Developing Child at Harvard University* https://developingchild.harvard.edu/science/key-concepts/toxic-stress/.
108. Chu, E. H., Trosko, J. E., & Chang, C. C. (1977). Mutational approaches to the study of carcinogenesis. *Journal of Toxicology and Environmental Health, 2*, 1317–1334.
109. Rubinstein, L. J. (1976). Current concepts in neuro-oncology. *Advances in Neurology, 15*, 1–25.
110. Blomen, V. A., & Boonstra, J. (2011). Stable transmission of reversible modifications: Maintenance of epigenetic information through the cell cycle. *Cellular and Molecular Life Sciences, 68*, 27–44.
111. Razin, A., & Riggs, A. D. (1980). DNA methylation and gene function. *Science, 210*, 604–610.
112. Seckl, J. R., & Meaney, M. J. (2006). Glucocorticoid 'programming' and PTSD risk. *Annals of the New York Academy of Sciences, 1071*, 351–378.

113. Meaney, M. J., & Szyf, M. (2005). Environmental programming of stress responses through DNA methylation: Life at the interface between a dynamic environment and a fixed genome. *Dialogues in Clinical Neuroscience, 7*, 103–123.
114. Reul, J. M. H. M., et al. (2015). Glucocorticoids, epigenetic control and stress resilience. *Neurobiology of Stress, 1*, 44–59.
115. Sasaki, A., & Matthews, S. G. (2019). Genome-wide epigenetic signatures of childhood adversity in early life: Opportunities and challenges. *Journal of Developmental Origins of Health and Disease, 10*, 65–72.
116. Limanaqi, F., Gambardella, S., Biagioni, F., Busceti, C. L., & Fornai, F. (2018). Epigenetic effects induced by methamphetamine and methamphetamine-dependent oxidative Stress. *Oxidative Medicine and Cellular Longevity, 2018*(4982453), 1.
117. Zhu, M.-Y., Raza, M. U., Zhan, Y., & Fan, Y. (2019). Norepinephrine upregulates the expression of tyrosine hydroxylase and protects dopaminergic neurons against 6-hydrodopamine toxicity. *Neurochemistry International, 131*, 104549.
118. Holloway, T., & González-Maeso, J. (2015). Epigenetic mechanisms of serotonin signaling. *ACS Chemical Neuroscience, 6*, 1099–1109.
119. Klengel, T., & Binder, E. B. (2015). Epigenetics of stress-related psychiatric disorders and gene × environment interactions. *Neuron, 86*, 1343–1357.
120. Waltes, R., Chiocchetti, A. G., & Freitag, C. M. (2016). The neurobiological basis of human aggression: A review on genetic and epigenetic mechanisms. *American Journal of Medical Genetics Part B Neuropsychiatric Genetics, 171*, 650–675.
121. Hu, J., & Barrett, R. D. H. (2017). Epigenetics in natural animal populations. *Journal of Evolutionary Biology, 30*, 1612–1632.
122. Van Lange, P. A. M., Rinderu, M. I., & Bushman, B. J. (2017). Aggression and violence around the world: A model of CLimate, Aggression, and Self-control in Humans (CLASH). *The Behavioral and Brain Sciences, 40*, e75.
123. Marchlewska-Koj, A., Kapusta, J., & Kruczek, M. (2003). Prenatal stress modifies behavior in offspring of bank voles (Clethrionomys glareolus). *Physiology & Behavior, 79*, 671–678.
124. Morley-Fletcher, S., Rea, M., Maccari, S., & Laviola, G. (2003). Environmental enrichment during adolescence reverses the effects of prenatal stress on play behaviour and HPA axis reactivity in rats. *The European Journal of Neuroscience, 18*, 3367–3374.
125. Patin, V., Lordi, B., Vincent, A., & Caston, J. (2005). Effects of prenatal stress on anxiety and social interactions in adult rats. *Brain Research. Developmental Brain Research, 160*, 265–274.
126. Schroeder, M., Sultany, T., & Weller, A. (2013). Prenatal stress effects on emotion regulation differ by genotype and sex in prepubertal rats. *Developmental Psychobiology, 55*, 176–192.
127. Boccia, M. L., & Pedersen, C. A. (2001). Brief vs. long maternal separations in infancy: Contrasting relationships with adult maternal behavior and lactation levels of aggression and anxiety. *Psychoneuroendocrinology, 26*, 657–672.
128. Hohmann, C. F., Hodges, A., Beard, N., & Aneni, J. (2013). Effects of brief stress exposure during early postnatal development in balb/CByJ mice: I. Behavioral characterization. *Developmental Psychobiology, 55*, 283–293.
129. Parfitt, D. B., et al. (2004). Differential early rearing environments can accentuate or attenuate the responses to stress in male C57BL/6 mice. *Brain Research, 1016*, 111–118.
130. Tsuda, M. C., Yamaguchi, N., & Ogawa, S. (2011). Early life stress disrupts peripubertal development of aggression in male mice. *Neuroreport, 22*, 259–263.
131. Veenema, A. H., Bredewold, R., & Neumann, I. D. (2007). Opposite effects of maternal separation on intermale and maternal aggression in C57BL/6 mice: Link to hypothalamic vasopressin and oxytocin immunoreactivity. *Psychoneuroendocrinology, 32*, 437–450.
132. Veenema, A. H., Blume, A., Niederle, D., Buwalda, B., & Neumann, I. D. (2006). Effects of early life stress on adult male aggression and hypothalamic vasopressin and serotonin. *The European Journal of Neuroscience, 24*, 1711–1720.

133. Bibancos, T., Jardim, D. L., Aneas, I., & Chiavegatto, S. (2007). Social isolation and expression of serotonergic neurotransmission-related genes in several brain areas of male mice. *Genes, Brain, and Behavior, 6*, 529–539.
134. Tóth, M., Halász, J., Mikics, E., Barsy, B., & Haller, J. (2008). Early social deprivation induces disturbed social communication and violent aggression in adulthood. *Behavioral Neuroscience, 122*, 849–854.
135. Toth, M., Mikics, E., Tulogdi, A., Aliczki, M., & Haller, J. (2011). Post-weaning social isolation induces abnormal forms of aggression in conjunction with increased glucocorticoid and autonomic stress responses. *Hormones and Behavior, 60*, 28–36.
136. Tulogdi, A., et al. (2014). Effects of resocialization on post-weaning social isolation-induced abnormal aggression and social deficits in rats. *Developmental Psychobiology, 56*, 49–57.
137. Wall, V. L., Fischer, E. K., & Bland, S. T. (2012). Isolation rearing attenuates social interaction-induced expression of immediate early gene protein products in the medial prefrontal cortex of male and female rats. *Physiology & Behavior, 107*, 440–450.
138. Cordero, M. I., Ansermet, F., & Sandi, C. (2013). Long-term programming of enhanced aggression by peripuberty stress in female rats. *Psychoneuroendocrinology, 38*, 2758–2769.
139. Cordero, M. I., et al. (2012). Evidence for biological roots in the transgenerational transmission of intimate partner violence. *Translational Psychiatry, 2*, e106.
140. Márquez, C., et al. (2013). Peripuberty stress leads to abnormal aggression, altered amygdala and orbitofrontal reactivity and increased prefrontal MAOA gene expression. *Translational Psychiatry, 3*, e216.
141. Papilloud, A., Guillot de Suduiraut, I., Zanoletti, O., Grosse, J., & Sandi, C. (2018). Peripubertal stress increases play fighting at adolescence and modulates nucleus accumbens CB1 receptor expression and mitochondrial function in the amygdala. *Translational Psychiatry, 8*, 156.
142. Walker, S. E., et al. (2018). Alterations in brain microstructure in rats that develop abnormal aggression following peripubertal stress. *The European Journal of Neuroscience, 48*, 1818–1832.
143. Haller, J., van de Schraaf, J., & Kruk, M. R. (2001). Deviant forms of aggression in glucocorticoid hyporeactive rats: A model for 'pathological' aggression? *Journal of Neuroendocrinology, 13*, 102–107.
144. Haller, J., Tóth, M., & Halász, J. (2005). The activation of raphe serotonergic neurons in normal and hypoarousal-driven aggression: A double labeling study in rats. *Behavioural Brain Research, 161*, 88–94.
145. Haller, J., Halász, J., Mikics, E., & Kruk, M. R. (2004). Chronic glucocorticoid deficiency-induced abnormal aggression, autonomic hypoarousal, and social deficit in rats. *Journal of Neuroendocrinology, 16*, 550–557.
146. Halasz, J., et al. (2008). The effect of neurokinin1 receptor blockade on territorial aggression and in a model of violent aggression. *Biological Psychiatry, 63*, 271–278.
147. Tulogdi, A., et al. (2010). Brain mechanisms involved in predatory aggression are activated in a laboratory model of violent intra-specific aggression. *The European Journal of Neuroscience, 32*, 1744–1753.
148. Feng, X., et al. (2011). Maternal separation produces lasting changes in cortisol and behavior in rhesus monkeys. *Proceedings of the National Academy of Sciences of the United States of America, 108*, 14312–14317.
149. Howell, B. R., et al. (2013). Brain white matter microstructure alterations in adolescent rhesus monkeys exposed to early life stress: Associations with high cortisol during infancy. *Biology of Mood & Anxiety Disorders, 3*, 21.
150. Winslow, J. T., Noble, P. L., Lyons, C. K., Sterk, S. M., & Insel, T. R. (2003). Rearing effects on cerebrospinal fluid oxytocin concentration and social buffering in rhesus monkeys. *Neuropsychopharmacol, 28*, 910–918.
151. Callaghan, B. L., & Richardson, R. (2013). Early experiences and the development of emotional learning systems in rats. *Biology of Mood & Anxiety Disorders, 3*, 8.

152. Andersen, S. L. (2015). Exposure to early adversity: Points of cross-species translation that can lead to improved understanding of depression. *Development and Psychopathology, 27*, 477–491.
153. Roman, E., & Nylander, I. (2005). The impact of emotional stress early in life on adult voluntary ethanol intake-results of maternal separation in rats. *Stress (Amsterdam, Netherlands), 8*, 157–174.
154. Moffett, M. C., et al. (2007). Maternal separation alters drug intake patterns in adulthood in rats. *Biochemical Pharmacology, 73*, 321–330.
155. Bonapersona, V., et al. (2019). The behavioral phenotype of early life adversity: A 3-level meta-analysis of rodent studies. *Neuroscience and Biobehavioral Reviews, 102*, 299–307.
156. O'Mahony, S. M., Hyland, N. P., Dinan, T. G., & Cryan, J. F. (2011). Maternal separation as a model of brain-gut axis dysfunction. *Psychopharmacology, 214*, 71–88.
157. Sánchez, M. M., Ladd, C. O., & Plotsky, P. M. (2001). Early adverse experience as a developmental risk factor for later psychopathology: Evidence from rodent and primate models. *Development and Psychopathology, 13*, 419–449.
158. Delville, Y., Melloni, R. H., & Ferris, C. F. (1998). Behavioral and neurobiological consequences of social subjugation during puberty in golden hamsters. *Journal of Neuroscience, 18*, 2667–2672.
159. Cunningham, R. L., & McGinnis, M. Y. (2008). Prepubertal social subjugation and anabolic androgenic steroid-induced aggression in male rats. *Journal of Neuroendocrinology, 20*, 997–1005.
160. Wommack, J. C., & Delville, Y. (2003). Repeated social stress and the development of agonistic behavior: Individual differences in coping responses in male golden hamsters. *Physiology & Behavior, 80*, 303–308.
161. Ferris, C. F., Messenger, T., & Sullivan, R. (2005). Behavioral and neuroendocrine consequences of social subjugation across adolescence and adulthood. *Frontiers in Zoology, 2*, 7.
162. Wommack, J. C., Salinas, A., Melloni, R. H., & Delville, Y. (2004). Behavioural and neuroendocrine adaptations to repeated stress during puberty in male golden hamsters. *Journal of Neuroendocrinology, 16*, 767–775.
163. Wommack, J. C., Salinas, A., & Delville, Y. (2005). Glucocorticoids and the development of agonistic behaviour during puberty in male golden hamsters. *Journal of Neuroendocrinology, 17*, 781–787.
164. Wommack, J. C., & Delville, Y. (2007). Cortisol controls the pubertal development of agonistic behavior in male golden hamsters via type II corticosteroid receptors. *Hormones and Behavior, 51*, 306–312.
165. Papilloud, A., et al. (2019). Peripubertal stress-induced heightened aggression: Modulation of the glucocorticoid receptor in the central amygdala and normalization by mifepristone treatment. *Neuropsychopharmacol, 44*, 674–682.
166. Yehuda, R., et al. (1990). Low urinary cortisol excretion in patients with posttraumatic stress disorder. *The Journal of Nervous and Mental Disease, 178*, 366–369.
167. Virkkunen, M. (1985). Urinary free cortisol secretion in habitually violent offenders. *Acta Psychiatrica Scandinavica, 72*, 40–44.
168. Haller, J., Mikics, E., Halász, J., & Tóth, M. (2005). Mechanisms differentiating normal from abnormal aggression: Glucocorticoids and serotonin. *European Journal of Pharmacology, 526*, 89–100.
169. Haller, J., & Kruk, M. R. (2006). Normal and abnormal aggression: Human disorders and novel laboratory models. *Neuroscience and Biobehavioral Reviews, 30*, 292–303.
170. Day, H. D., Seay, B. M., Hale, P., & Hendricks, D. (1982). Early social deprivation and the ontogeny of unrestricted social behavior in the laboratory rat. *Developmental Psychobiology, 15*, 47–59.
171. Potegal, M., & Einon, D. (1989). Aggressive behaviors in adult rats deprived of playfighting experience as juveniles. *Developmental Psychobiology, 22*, 159–172.

172. Sachser, N., Lick, C., & Stanzel, K. (1994). The environment, hormones, and aggressive behaviour: A 5-year-study in guinea pigs. *Psychoneuroendocrinology, 19*, 697–707.
173. Kempes, M. M., Gulickx, M. M. C., van Daalen, H. J. C., Louwerse, A. L., & Sterck, E. H. M. (2008). Social competence is reduced in socially deprived rhesus monkeys (Macaca mulatta). *Journal of Comparative Psychology, Washington, D.C., 1983*(122), 62–67.
174. Higley, J. D., Suomi, S. J., & Linnoila, M. (1996). A nonhuman primate model of type II alcoholism? Part 2. Diminished social competence and excessive aggression correlates with low cerebrospinal fluid 5-hydroxyindoleacetic acid concentrations. *Alcoholism: Clinical and Experimental Research, 20*, 643–650.
175. Mikics, É., et al. (2018). Social learning requires plasticity enhanced by fluoxetine through prefrontal Bdnf-TrkB signaling to limit aggression induced by post-weaning social isolation. *Neuropsychopharmacol, 43*, 235–245.
176. Haller, J. (2013). The neurobiology of abnormal manifestations of aggression--a review of hypothalamic mechanisms in cats, rodents, and humans. *Brain Research Bulletin, 93*, 97–109.
177. Haller, J. (2018). The role of central and medial amygdala in normal and abnormal aggression: A review of classical approaches. *Neuroscience and Biobehavioral Reviews, 85*, 34–43.
178. Biro, L., et al. (2017). Structural and functional alterations in the prefrontal cortex after post-weaning social isolation: Relationship with species-typical and deviant aggression. *Brain Structure & Function, 222*, 1861–1875.
179. Tzanoulinou, S., et al. (2016). Neuroligin-2 expression in the prefrontal cortex is involved in attention deficits induced by peripubertal stress. *Neuropsychopharmacol, 41*, 751–761.
180. Arendt, D. H., et al. (2012). Contrasting hippocampal and amygdalar expression of genes related to neural plasticity during escape from social aggression. *Physiology & Behavior, 107*, 670–679.
181. Walker, S. E., Papilloud, A., Huzard, D., & Sandi, C. (2018). The link between aberrant hypothalamic-pituitary-adrenal axis activity during development and the emergence of aggression-animal studies. *Neuroscience and Biobehavioral Reviews, 91*, 138–152.

Chapter 6
Glucocorticoids in Humans

Introduction

Glucocorticoids are believed to be crucial for understanding human aggression, psychopathologies, and crime because they can bridge adverse environmental events and the brain mechanisms of aggressive behavior, both acutely – i.e., while events unfold – and on the long run, by contributing to the epigenetic signature of toxic stressors over the lifetime. Yet, the role of glucocorticoids in human aggression is debated. There is one association that raises relatively little doubts; this is the one that links acute elevations in glucocorticoid secretion to aggressive responses, which indirectly supports the frustration–aggression hypothesis, one of the most popular psychological theories. Beyond its utility in psychology, this theory might also explain certain psychopathologies and emotional crime. The association of aggression with low glucocorticoid production by contrast is more disputed. Although demonstrated by many studies, the question remains open because the opposite association – high glucocorticoids–high aggression – is a similarly recurrent finding. It was suggested that contradictions may be solved by an approach sensitive to both the type of aggression and the psychopathology underlying aggression on one side and the glucocorticoid measures employed to study the phenomenon on the other [17, 83]. This chapter – already armed with the biological information presented in the previous one – aims at disentangling the intricate web of connections along this concept. The ultimate aim is to understand the acute and long-term alterations in glucocorticoid secretion in response to various types of stressors and the impact of the resulting glucocorticoid state on normal and abnormal human aggression. The neural consequences of altered glucocorticoid productions will also be addressed but briefly, because this will be dealt with in subsequent chapters.

J. Haller, *Neurobiopsychosocial Perspectives on Aggression and Violence*,
Advances in Preventing and Treating Violence and Aggression,
https://doi.org/10.1007/978-3-030-46331-1_6

6.1 A Brief History

The debate concerning the role of glucocorticoids in aggression derives from two apparently contradictory discoveries made about 50 years apart. The frustration theory of aggression – that implicitly involves the stress response – predicts that increases in glucocorticoids promote aggression, whereas the low glucocorticoid levels observed in habitually violent offenders suggest the opposite.

The association between frustration and aggression was first described by Dollars et al. in 1939 [1] and was formulated as a hypothesis on causal interrelationships by Miller in 1941 [2]. Presently this hypothesis is about 80 years old and can be considered one of the oldest psychological theories of aggression. The hypothesis was reformulated and adapted to current discoveries almost 50 years later by Berkowitz [3]. Biological concepts were incorporated into the theory later by Henry [4], who outlined the connection between frustration, stress hormones, and behavioral responses. The concept is still alive today and is continuously enriched by new findings concerning, for instance, the relationship between diurnal and momentary increases in glucocorticoids [5], the impact of frustration on aggression types [6], the neural mechanisms underlying behavioral responses [7], etc. The key points of this theory are the following. Frustration is elicited by a failure to reach desired goals due to an obstacle. Frustration emerges if the obstacle was either unavoidable or avoidable or if it was general, i.e., it affected many people not only the frustrated individual. The behavioral effects of frustration are mediated by a variety of biological responses, including glucocorticoid secretion, and are associated with an altered function of the neural circuitry of aggression.

The frustration–aggression hypothesis forecasted that increased glucocorticoids are associated with increased aggression. However, Virkkunen [8] demonstrated in 1985 that habitually violent offenders show markedly low levels of plasma glucocorticoids as compared to non-habitually violent offenders, non-violent offenders, and clinic personnel. However, opposite findings were published at the same time, which all suggested that high aggression is associated with high glucocorticoids [9–12]. The Public Health Report published in 1983 was especially influential, as it clearly attributed violence to stress. Consequently, Virkkunen's findings were almost unnoticed for a relatively long time. The paper was first cited by a review as late as 4 years later [13]; the first confirmatory study was published almost a decade later [14], and the first laboratory model for the endocrine condition and its impact on aggression was developed 15 years later [15]. The slow start of this milestone paper was likely due to the counterintuitive nature of its finding, because if interpreted mechanically, it contradicted the widely accepted frustration–aggression hypothesis by associating aggression with low glucocorticoids. Another important paper in this respect was published in the first year of this century [16] which showed that low glucocorticoid production precedes aggression problems in children by at least 2 years. This suggested that aggression problems can be predicted years ahead by simply measuring plasma glucocorticoids. The assumption that aggression is associated with low glucocorticoids is still current; moreover, it is among the most intensely studied phenomena in all four fields of aggression research, biology [17], psychology [18], psychiatry [19], and law enforcement [20].

In the followings, we will not try to solve the conflict by arguing for either the "high glucocorticoid" or the "low glucocorticoid" theory of aggression control. Evidence shows that both theories are true. In some people and under certain conditions, aggression is associated with high glucocorticoid secretion whereas in others with low glucocorticoid secretion. Instead of taking sides, we will try to answer questions related to "when" and "who," e.g., when and who becomes aggressive under the influence of acute glucocorticoid stress responses and when and who becomes aggressive under the influence of blunted stress responses.

Note that in contrast to animals, which may secrete either or both corticosterone and cortisol, humans secrete only the latter. Therefore, we will use in the followings the term cortisol to denote the main stress hormone.

6.2 Psychology

6.2.1 Background

Due to its focus on behavior when defining aggression, psychology uses the term aggression to cover behaviors as diverse as malicious gossip and manslaughter (see Chap. 1). As such, psychology covers all actors, be those everyday people, psychiatric patients, or violent criminals; moreover, it also covers animals if their behavior was viewed from the perspective of comparative psychology. To preserve the individuality of this section, we will review here studies performed in mentally healthy, non-criminal populations. These are generally identified as "healthy subjects," "general population," "community sample," and alike. The available studies are focused on acute cortisol–aggression relationships in the following three ways:

1. Participants were submitted to laboratory tests of aggression (see below), while cortisol was measured before, during, and after the test. These paradigms are similar to studies performed in animals which were submitted to aggression tests.
2. Aggression tests were run subsequent to treatments that increased plasma cortisol. These were either cortisol agonists – agents that stimulate cortisol receptors – or stressors. These procedures are akin to animal studies aimed at clarifying causal relationships between stress-induced glucocorticoid secretion and aggression.
3. Field studies, where diurnal changes in cortisol secretion were compared with aggressive behaviors that were studied in parallel. This procedure is analogous with animal studies where correlations between natural variations in glucocorticoid secretion patterns and aggression were studied. The difference was that extrinsic stressors were excluded experimentally in animals, whereas humans were studied under naturalistic settings; consequently, natural oscillations and daily hassles influenced cortisol secretion concurrently.

There are a series of other methodologies to study the role of cortisol in aggression. One can study the role of chronic stress or the impact of early traumatic events on long-term changes in cortisol secretion. In theory, such studies can be done in healthy subjects, because chronic and toxic stress may not inevitably lead to psychopathologies and crime. Practically, however, such studies are rarely if ever done in healthy subjects; therefore, they will be reviewed in the following sections.

6.2.1.1 Laboratory Tests of Human Aggressiveness

Studying aggression is easiest retrospectively, or with respect to life histories, because the behavior is expressed rarely and randomly and participants are uncooperative while aggressive and may be dangerous for their surroundings including the investigator. Consequently, psychologists are not in the comfortable position of those studying animals, which can easily be handled to suit the needs of the experimenter. To solve this problem, experimental psychologists developed a series of laboratory tests to study human aggression while it unfolds.

The Taylor Aggression Paradigm, developed more than 50 years ago [21], is probably among the first tests developed to this end. Participants play a competitive reaction time task against a fictional opponent. Losers receive punishments from the winners in the form of noise blasts or electric shocks. The fictional opponent delivers punishments of a preset level, whereas the participants are free to choose the level of punishment when they win. Two measures of aggression are deduced from the procedure: total punishment delivered and the escalation of punishment in response to increasing levels of punishment received from the opponent.

In the Point Subtraction Aggression Paradigm [22], players earn points convertible into money at the end of the trial. Participants may follow three strategies: They may strive at increasing own earnings, at protecting what they earned, or at decreasing the earnings of the opponent. The latter strategy is used as retaliation to the improper behavior of the opponent and offers a way to measure retaliatory aggression.

There are a series of somewhat more sophisticated aggression-monitoring games like the ultimatum game, where participants split money and unfair offer rejections are considered aggressive [23]. In the Game of Chickens, participants can chose cooperation or aggression in a situation where mutual aggression results in money loss, and mutual cooperation leads to moderate earnings, while aggression against cooperation is the most profitable tactics [24]. In the Survivor Contest, displaced aggression is measured in terms of money subtraction from innocent victims in response to provocation by others [25], etc. In the Articulated Thoughts in Simulated Situations, participants display behaviors that belong to the natural behavioral repertoire of humans, e.g., verbal aggression in response to a simulated conflict with spouse [26]. In the Rosenzweig Picture-Frustration paradigm [27], probably the oldest laboratory aggression test, aggression remains merely imaginary. In this test, participants are shown cartoon drawings that depict frustrating interpersonal situations and are asked to imagine themselves in the situation and tell how they would handle it. Violent video games offer new ways to study aggression. In contrast to other paradigms, the opponent is visible here, and game characters and their actions are highly realistic. The use of video games as experimental tools to monitor aggression is relatively new, and the possibility has been exploited mostly by neuroscientists [28]. Psychological studies – the first being almost 40 years old [29] – focused mostly on social worries triggered by playing violent games by youth.

All these paradigms are tightly related to the biological approach to aggression in both theoretical and practical terms. They model competitive situations and result in advantages to the perpetrator. As such, they measure the readiness of participants for resource competition by aggressive means, which is the essence of the biological approach. The procedures allow researchers to stage aggression as they wish without endangering participants or themselves. Moreover, participants can wear technology to sample blood or saliva for cortisol measurements before, during, or after an event. Thus, laboratory paradigms of human aggression show multiple similarities with the biological approach to aggression and to laboratory methods utilizing animals.

6.2.1.2 Field Studies

Another approach quite frequently employed is the establishment of correspondence between behaviors shown over the day with cortisol measurements made several times over the same period ("field studies"). This approach is easiest to perform in nurseries, kindergartens, and summer schools; therefore, participants are usually children or adolescents. Taking saliva samples for cortisol measurements is easy and noninvasive. Further, observing behavior is easy, as children and adolescents behave freely most of the time. Performing similar studies in workplaces poses much larger problems, for which adult participants are missing from this research area.

6.2.1.3 The Measurement of Cortisol

The experimental techniques described above require repeated cortisol measurements to correlate secretion changes with changes in aggressive behavior. The first time point in the series is usually called the "baseline," which term was correct if it meant the level from which changes started but was misleading if considered a measure of the individual's propensity to secrete cortisol. The reason is that cortisol levels vary over the day for multiple reasons and such variations are not synchronous in participants. The so-called baseline is in fact a momentary state influenced by a series of factors. For instance, cortisol may be high because it increased in the anticipation of being tested or due to various events the participant was faced with while traveling to the research site or simply because sampling was done when ultradian oscillations were in their increasing or decreasing phase – because ultradian and diurnal oscillations are just as typical in humans as in any other mammals.

Ideally, the first cortisol sample is taken after a 1 h long rest. This time may be used to fill in psychometric inventories or may be allowed to pass under calm and pleasant conditions, e.g., by listening to soft music. The impact of anticipatory or transient stressors vanishes within 1 h; moreover, the ultradian rhythm of cortisol secretion may be synchronized by the rest. Under such conditions, subjects exposed to laboratory tests of aggression show a bell-shaped cortisol response. If there was an association, the magnitude of the cortisol stress response and the level of aggression displayed during the test would correlate with each other. In studies where participants were not allowed to rest for a sufficient time, plasma cortisol often shows a steady decline over the trial, and the impact of aggression is captured as a lack of, or a delayed, decrease from the initial baseline value. In such cases, the baseline was inappropriate, because it reflected a pretest stress response rather than the resting level of hormone production. Cortisol levels may correlate with aggression in this case too, but the bell-shaped cortisol response will be observed only when the study was properly performed, i.e., the first sample was preceded by resting.

In three of the studies reviewed here, the cortisol awakening response was also studied. The phrase "awakening response" covers those 30–60 min which separate the inactive and active period of the day, during which plasma cortisol approximately doubles. Under normal conditions, e.g., when the night was relaxing and awakening was not stressful, the awakening response provides an estimate of the constitutive functioning of the stress system, i.e., its overall trend in cortisol production. The awakening response is synchronized, meaning that under normal conditions, cortisol rises in all people within the first 30–60 min of the day and is not compromised by momentary stressful experiences. To exclude accidental cortisol increases, the awakening response is usually averaged for a few days. The next section offers more information on the way cortisol can be measured and the significance and interpretation of each type of measurement.

6.2.2 Findings

Table 6.1 summarizes the findings obtained in 24 studies. Efforts were made to cover the topic as completely as possible. To this end, studies focusing on psychopathologies were also included by considering the findings obtained in healthy controls.

The relationship between acute cortisol stress responses and aggression appears clear from these findings; as disagreements are few and even in such cases, findings are not contradictory. A few authors failed to find associations, but their findings were not opposite to those of others. The overwhelming majority of findings show that aggression is coincident and correlates with increased cortisol secretion.

Table 6.1 Acute interactions between cortisol and aggression in healthy participants

Correlational studies			
Paradigm	**Awakening response ("Constitutive secretion")**	**Cortisol stress response**	**Participants**
Taylor [30]	↓	↑	Adults M & F
Taylor-like [31]	n.i.	↑	Adults F[a]
Point subtraction [32]	n.i.	↑	Adults M
Point subtraction [32]	n.i.	↑	Adults M
Point subtraction [33]	n.i.	↑	Adults M
Point subtraction [34]	n.i.	↑	Adults M
Point subtraction [35]	n.i.	↑	Adults M
Point subtraction [36]	n.i.	↑	Adults M
Point subtraction [37]	n.i.	→	Adults M
Point subtraction [38]	n.i.	→	Adults M & F
Ultimatum game [39]	n.i.	↑	Adults F
Violent video game [40]	n.i.	↑	Children M & F[c]
Violent video game [41]	n.i.	↑	Adults M[c]
Field studies [42]	n.i.	↑	Children M (~~F~~)
Field studies [43]	n.i.	↑	Children M & F
Field studies [44]	n.i.	↑	Children M & F
Field studies [45]	n.i.	↑	Children M (~~F~~)[d]
Field studies [5]	n.i.	↑	Adolescents M & F[d]
Field studies [46]	↑	↑	Adolescents F (~~M~~)[d]
Field studies [47]	↓	n.i.	Children M & F[b]
Effects of treatments administered before the aggression test			
Model	**Treatment**	**Change in aggression**	**Participants**
Taylor [48]	20 mg hydrocortisone (cortisol agonist)	⌂	Adults F (~~M~~)
Taylor-like [49]	Acute stressor	⌂	Adults M (~~F~~)
Taylor-like [50]	Acute stressor	⌂	Adults M (~~F~~)
Taylor-like [50]	Frustration	⌂	Adults M & F

Cortisol–aggression relationship: ↑, high aggression correlates with high cortisol; →, no association; ⌂, treatments increased aggression. *Other abbreviations*: *Taylor-like*, a variant of the Taylor Aggression Paradigm; *n.i.*, not investigated; *M*, males; *F*, females; ~~M~~ or ~~F~~, association not valid for the respective gender; [a] population rich in psychopathic traits but not at diagnostic level; [b] in this study, not the awakening response but the diurnal variation in cortisol was investigated. This is another measure of constitutive cortisol secretion as shown below; [c] violent video games increased plasma cortisol; correlations were not investigated; [d] association between cortisol on one side and high externalizing behavior or anger on the other (i.e., aggression was not investigated in these studies)

The causal involvement of cortisol in eliciting aggression was not as systematically investigated as in animals. The reasons might be ethical in nature: humans cannot be submitted to risky interventions as easily as animals, for instance, there is an ethical limit to glucocorticoid doses that can be administered. Glucocorticoid synthesis inhibitors and receptor antagonists also carry risks, whereas the administration of protein synthesis inhibitors – used to disentangle molecular mechanisms in animals – is not possible in human aggression research. Although one feels that more could be done, e.g., the use of the glucocorticoid secretion inhibitor metyrapone is likely acceptable ethically, the available findings, especially when combined with biological ones, support the assumption that acute increases in cortisol production promote aggression in humans. On their turn, field studies show that findings obtained in the laboratory are relevant to real life.

In contrast to acute cortisol stress responses, the role of individual differences in constitutive hypothalamic–pituitary–adrenal axis function remains unclear. There are only three studies addressing this issue, and their findings are contradictory.

6.2.3 Overview

The survey of the literature suggests that as it regards healthy humans, studies on the glucocorticoid–aggression relationship focus on acute interactions. The conclusions of the findings reviewed above can be formulated as follows: (1) social challenges increase both cortisol secretion and aggression; (2) the two responses correlate; and (3) cortisol administration and stressors promote aggression. These findings agree with both the role of acute glucocorticoid responses in animals and the frustration theory of human aggression.

Most human paradigms are built on retaliation. As such, they model reactive aggression, suggesting that acute increases in cortisol promote this type of aggression in humans. As exceptions, violent video games have a strong instrumental component, as players “fight” for rewards offered by the game and use skills and planning to reach their goal. As such, these games may model proactive aggression. Unfortunately, the level of aggression is difficult to measure in these games, as behaviors are predetermined by the software. Therefore, correlations between cortisol secretion and aggression were not studied so far in this paradigm. One variable of the Taylor Aggression Paradigm may also reflect the propensity of participants for proactive aggression, particularly the amount of punishment delivered under non-challenging situations. The studies reviewed above, however, focused on provocation-induced, i.e., reactive aggressive responses.

Thus, acute increases in cortisol production appear to enhance reactive aggression, whereas their effects on proactive forms remain obscure. The only finding suggesting a different involvement of cortisol in reactive and proactive aggression was obtained in a field study performed in children [43]. In this study, physical aggression, which was likely reactive under the given experimental setup, was associated with increased cortisol responses, whereas relational aggression, more likely

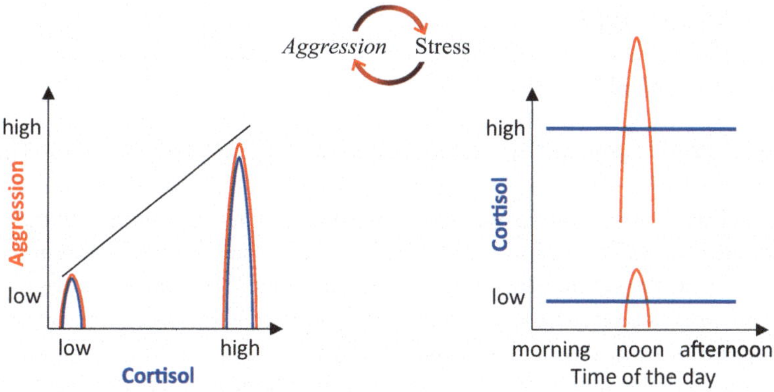

Fig. 6.1 Healthy humans: a graphical summary. *Left-hand panel*. In laboratory tests of aggression, cortisol plasma levels and aggressive behaviors correlate positively. This means that a small increase in cortisol (blue) is associated with low aggression (red) in the test and the other way around. *Right-hand panel*. When aggression was directly observed in groups of children or adolescents over the day, higher cortisol was observed in those participants who showed higher aggression. The temporal match between plasma cortisol and aggressive behaviors was not investigated so far. Usually, higher cortisol levels were observed in one or a few time points, which makes the presence of chronic stress unlikely. Aggression was characterized for the whole day by one figure usually. *Middle panel*. When corroborated with studies involving glucocorticoid administrations or the application of stressors, these findings suggest that the positive feedback loop between aggression and acute stress responses is present in humans

proactive, was associated by blunted stress responses. The issue clearly needs further studies.

Taken together, these findings show that in healthy humans, high stress responses correlate with and likely contribute to the expression of aggression under conditions of social challenge. A graphical summary of this section is presented in Fig. 6.1. This suggests that the available studies are congruent with findings obtained in animals submitted to acute social challenges, i.e., the role of glucocorticoids in aggression tests does not differentiate animal and human subjects.

6.3 Psychopathologies and Crime

Separating studies on mental disorders from those on violent crime is difficult for two reasons. First, certain psychopathologies (e.g., conduct, antisocial personality, and intermittent explosive disorders) include crime among their symptoms. Moreover, reference to the criminal behavior of participants was frequent even with disorders unrelated to crime directly. Second, law enforcement studies often refer to, moreover, quantify psychopathologies in their study participants. As such, a clear demarcation line cannot be drawn between the two areas. Here we presented findings in one section, with a separate subsection for those law enforcement studies where psychopathologies were not addressed or were only mentioned.

6.3.1 Background

6.3.1.1 Theoretical Framework

Current thinking attributes the development of psychopathologies and criminal behavior to strong and/or long-lasting stressors suffered in various – usually early – periods of life. The general assumption is that such events, depending on individual differences in stress susceptibility, alter brain structure and function with important consequences for psychological and social functioning. This state of the art encourages those interested in cortisol, because this hormone is believed to be among the main engines of brain development and function.

Stressors are followed by increased cortisol secretion, which is consequential for brain function until cortisol levels remain elevated. This phenomenon is called chronic stress, and out of the mental disorders addressed below is typical to depression. This disorder develops on the background of chronically elevated cortisol secretion and is often associated with outbursts of anger, and its symptoms vanish together with the amelioration of the disorder and the return of plasma cortisol levels to normal.

Stress, however, may leave a durable imprint on physiology and behavior long after the stressor and the associated cortisol response subsided. Long-term changes elicited by such toxic stressors include durable alterations in cortisol secretion patterns, which are often opposite to that elicited acutely. Most of the disorders discussed below fall into this category and are consequences of toxic stressors suffered in various – usually early – periods of life. Emerging evidence suggests that long-term alterations in cortisol secretion patterns are causally involved in the behavioral consequences of toxic stress. Therefore, understanding long-term alterations in cortisol production is crucial for understanding psychopathologies and crime.

6.3.1.2 Early Programming of Cortisol Production

Many studies demonstrate that adverse experiences qualifiable as toxic stressors lead to diminished cortisol secretion on the long run. One concept that explains such long-term changes was suggestively called "allostatic crash" and posits that severe stressors "burn out" the HPA axis, which subsequently fails to produce adequate amounts of cortisol in later stages of life [51]. The crash may result from allostatic loads that exceed the adaptive capacities of the HPA axis. In molecular mechanistic terms, the somewhat metaphoric "allostatic crash" concept may be rephrased as epigenetic alterations occurring in various genes that control the HPA axis. Although the epigenetics of such changes are poorly understood at present, important developments were recorded in recent years [52].

Adverse events leading to "allostatic crash" are diverse and may occur any time over the life span. They include pre-birth events like glucocorticoid treatments received by mothers to increase premature infant survival [53] and the maternal consumption of xenobiotics such as nicotine, alcohol, drugs, etc. [54, 55] In early childhood, long-term downregulation of cortisol secretion may be elicited by inconsistent discipline and poor parental monitoring [56, 57], institutional or orphanage care [58], and neglect and abuse [59]. Cortisol secretion may also be downregulated on the long run by traumatic experiences [60], including emotional [61], physical, and sexual abuse [62]. Similarly, bullying in schools [63], the proximity of pubs [64], and community violence in general [65] were all negatively associated with indices of HPA axis function in adulthood. Finally, traumatic experiences [66, 67], intimate partner violence [68], drug addiction [69], overwork leading to chronic fatigue syndrome [70], and psychotic illness [71] have similar effects in adolescents and adults. Indeed, many of these studies associated hypocortisolism with epigenetic changes and aggression.

Under certain conditions, however, adverse life experiences augment rather than downregulate the HPA axis. Moreover, factors leading to the lasting up- and downregulation of cortisol secretion are essentially similar [72–74], despite repeated trials to associate certain early stressors with particular HPA axis outcomes and to derive subsequent changes in aggression from such specific effects [75, 76]. Although traumatic experiences usually downregulate, whereas early neglect most likely upregulates cortisol secretion, this association is statistical only, and either event can lead to an atypical cortisol response in the long run. Opposite consequences of adverse life events may even develop in succession: An initial phase of HPA axis upregulation – which may last years – is in some cases followed by an extended period of downregulation [55, 77, 78]. An illustrative study [79] showed, for instance, that after an initial acute response, early stressors did not affect cortisol secretion till the age of 5 years, upregulated the HPA axis between 5 and 11 years, and downregulated it thereafter.

These findings point to the surprising conclusion that the same stressor may either upregulate or downregulate the stress system on the long run; moreover, it can elicit both responses in succession. The reasons for this variability are poorly known at present. The severity of the stressor [59], however, and the genetics of the individual together with subsequent life events [80] play important roles. Whatever the reason was, adverse experiences may result in both upregulated and downregulated HPA axis. In most cases, cortisol secretion is downregulated; however, a non-negligible minority undergoes the opposite long-term change [81, 82].

6.3.1.3 Ways to Monitor Cortisol: A Non-technical Note

We already mentioned above that measuring cortisol in relevant ways is not easy. The sections above focused on those issues which were important for studies performed in healthy people. Here we provide further details, because measurements are not important in technically terms only. The issue was reviewed repeatedly [83–85]; here we reiterate the main points.

When measuring cortisol, one may essentially ask two questions: (1) Are there constitutive changes in cortisol secretion? (2) Is there a change in stress responsiveness? The two questions are not necessarily related. A recent study found the following HPA axis functional states following early traumas: elevated basal secretion and increased stress responses, normal basal secretions associated with low stress responses, and low basal secretions with low stress responses [81]. In addition, normal basal secretion profiles may be associated with increased stress responses [86].

Constitutive changes in cortisol secretion can be investigated in several ways, including point measurements that are subject to high individual variation as shown above. As an example of this limitation, such measurements often failed to identify associations between cortisol and aggression as shown below. The situation is considerably improved by precautions (e.g., allowing participants to rest and requesting them to refrain from eating or drinking coffee and alcohol before the study), by high sample sizes, or by averaging point measurements over several days. These procedures minimize a good deal of the intrinsic variability of point measurements. Still, measuring cortisol several times over the day, i.e., grasping diurnal variations, appears to be a better approach, especially when the awakening cortisol response was included (see above). Cortisol may also be measured in urine or feces, which provides a clear picture of the amount of cortisol secreted within a certain period, because the hormone is not degraded in these excretions. Finally, cortisol may be measured in hair, by this obtaining overall information on secretion patterns for periods that cover month. Although rarely used, this procedure is reliable and can spare the work of sampling for cortisol repeatedly over prolonged periods of time.

The evaluation of stress responses is more straightforward and involves the measurement of plasma cortisol repeatedly. Minimally, one time point should precede the stress procedure to serve as a reference point; another should immediately follow it to see effects; and yet another should be taken 30–60 min later to check for the return of levels to reference values. The last time point carries important information, because response magnitudes may not differentiate groups due to a ceiling effect, but a slower recovery may still indicate upregulated stress responses.

In the following sections, we will refer to cortisol measurements as "constitutive," "point," and "responsive." The first term covers any of the procedures mentioned above except for point measurements, which will be presented separately due to their poorer reliability. In the case of stress responses, the stressor will be indicated. Further details will not be provided, mostly due to space constraints.

6.3.2 Findings: Concurrent Association Studies

Here we briefly overview associations between cortisol- and aggression-related disorders, which will be addressed based on the *Diagnostic and Statistical Manual of Mental Disorders* (DSM-5) [87] and the *Classification of Mental and Behavioral Disorders* (ICD-10) [88]. Diagnostic details will be provided at each subsection.

Regarding the cortisol–aggression relationship, there are several important gaps in knowledge, which complicate the evaluation of this relationship. For instance, our sustained efforts failed to identify relevant papers on intermittent explosive and disruptive mood dysregulation disorders, even though these are the only ones where symptoms include little else than aggression and where outbursts are usually elicited by provocations indicating an involvement of the stress response. The lack of studies means that two of the most important psychopathologies related to the cortisol–aggression relationship are missing from the records.

With other disorders, e.g., attention-deficit/hyperactivity disorder (ADHD), and major depressive disorders, the cortisol–aggression relationship was often addressed, even though aggression-related symptoms are entirely missing from the psychiatric description of the disorder. With yet other disorders where aggression was listed among the symptoms, e.g., posttraumatic stress disorder (PTSD), the cortisol–aggression relationship received little attention although cortisol production was frequently studied with respect to the disorder. Despite these deficiencies, the cortisol–aggression relationship seems to be well studied regarding mental disorders, and the available findings allow the drawing of important conclusions.

6.3.2.1 Attention-Deficit/Hyperactivity Disorder

Studies in this disorder are complicated by two of its characteristics. First, patients are not homogenous regarding their symptoms. Some are primarily inattentive, others are prevalently hyperactive-impulsive, and there also is a considerable subpopulation showing both types of symptoms ("composite" type). Second, those suffering from the disorder are at a high risk of developing conduct disorder in childhood and antisocial personality disorder (ASPD) in adulthood. They also are liable to substance abuse, law infringement, and incarceration. The predilection towards aggressiveness is also evident from the high prevalence of comorbidities with aggression-related disorders and violent crime [89], despite the lack of aggression-related symptoms.

In a subgroup of the studies reviewed below (see Table 6.2), neither subtypes nor comorbidities were studied, most likely because sample sizes were relatively low. Other studies not only mentioned disease subtypes and the range of comorbidities but specifically focused on differences observed along these lines. Therefore, the table was divided into two sections. The first section deals with studies addressing "pure" ADHD. The term does not mean that comorbidities were lacking but only that these were not studied. The second section covers studies that focused on patients with comorbid aggression-related psychopathologies. The disorder may also be associated with anxiety; this issue will be discussed later.

The table suggests that the relationship between the disorder and cortisol secretion is confusing. Some suggested that explanations should be sought along symptom differences, but the findings do not support this assumption. The same endocrine condition was associated with one subtype in some but with another in other studies. Moreover, there is a study where low stress responses were associated with both the inattentive and hyperactive, but not with the "composite" subtype. One cannot exclude that subtypes are important, but this still needs to be clarified. In contrast, comorbidities may indeed have an impact on the association with cortisol secretion. In the "pure" disorder, an upregulated stress response was observed in most cases. Some studies are at variance with this conclusion; the reason might be that partici-

Table 6.2 Cortisol secretion profiles in participants showing attention-deficit/hyperactivity disorder

Attention-deficit/hyperactivity disorder						
Experimental details			Cortisol measurement			
Subtype	Comorbidity	Participants	Constitutive	Point	Responsive	Stressor
"Pure" (scientific question unrelated to comorbidities)						
Not specified [90]	"Pure"	Children M & F	↓	→	↑	DST
Inattentive ~~(hyperactive, Combined)~~ [91]	"Pure"	Children M & F	n.i.	→	↑	PS
Combined [92]	"Pure"	Children M & F	n.i.	→	↑	CPT
Not specified [93]	"Pure"	Adults M & F	n.i.	→	↑	TSST
Not specified [94]	"Pure"	Adolescents M & F	n.i.	→	→	CPT
Combined ~~(inattentive, Hyperactive)~~ [91]	"Pure"	Children F	n.i.	→	↓	PS
Hyperactive (~~inattentive~~) [95]	"Pure"	Children M & F	n.i.	↓	↓	TCT
Studied with respect to comorbid conditions						
Not specified [96]	AGG	Children M	n.i.	→	n.i.	None
Not specified [97]	ODD	Children M & F	n.i.	↓	n.i.	None
Composite [98]	CD	Adolescents M & F	n.i.	↓	n.i.	None
Not specified [99]	CD	Adolescents M & F	n.i.	→	↓	PF
Not specified [100]	AGG	Children M & F	n.i.	→	↓	CPT
Not specified [101]	AGG, CD-CU	Children M	n.i.	→	↓	TSST
Inattentive (~~hyperactive~~) [102]	CD, ODD	Children M & F	→	→	↓	TSST
Inattentive and hyperactive (~~composite~~) [103]	DB	Children M	→	→	↓	BS-T
Not specified [104]	AGG	Children M & F	↓	→	↓	CPT

Comorbid conditions: *AGG*, aggressiveness; *CD*, conduct disorder; *CU*, callous–unemotional traits; DB, disruptive behavior; *ODD*, oppositional defiant disorder. *Gender of participants*: *M*, male; *F*, female. *Interaction with cortisol*: ↓, negative correlation (low cortisol associates with stronger symptoms); →, no association; ↑, positive correlation (high cortisol associates with stronger symptoms). *Stressors applied*: *BS-T* transport to the sampling facility and blood sampling, *PS* public speaking, *CPT* Continuous Performance Test, *TSST* Trier Social Stress Test, *DST* dexamethasone suppression test, *TCT* timed cognitive task, *PF* provocation and frustration. ~~Strikethrough~~, finding not valid for the respective condition

pants showed aggression-related comorbidities that were not studied. In contrast, all studies showed blunted stress responses when the disorder was comorbid with aggression-related psychopathologies. As conclusions, we suggest the following:

1. ADHD is associated with increased stress responses.
2. Comorbid conditions involving aggression and aggression-related psychopathologies are characterized by blunted stress responses.
3. Blunted stress responses are not due to the disorder but to aggression-related comorbidities.

Note that "pure" forms of the disorder may not always be devoid of aggression problems; the lack of comorbidities may simply mean that these do not reach levels sufficient for a comorbid diagnosis. As such, patients may show aggression on the background of both up- and downregulated cortisol secretions, more dramatic forms of aggression being associated with the latter.

6.3.2.2 Conduct Problems in Children and Adolescents

Aggression and conduct problems in youth were named and described in a variety of ways when their relationship with cortisol was investigated. Oppositional defiant and conduct disorders are at one end of the spectrum, because these are precisely defined in both DSM-5 and ICD-10. Without entering diagnostic detail, conduct-disordered children are in permanent conflict with rules and society, including most of their peers. Oppositional defiant behavior characterizes the child who clashes with authoritative figures, e.g., parents and teachers, but not necessarily with rules and society as whole. In contrast to these two disorders, children were often characterized as showing disruptive or externalizing behavior, which are not clinical diagnoses of their own right. For many researchers, disruptive behavior covers a mixture of conduct and oppositional defiant symptoms, which are sufficient to diagnose neither but are enough to make the child highly problematic. For others, the term describes children fulfilling either diagnosis but who are delinquents in addition. In yet others, disruptive behavior is identified in participants who scored above a cutoff score in various inventories with unclear links to diagnoses. Externalizing behavior on its turn was also frequently studied but was also defined inconsistently. In some studies, it covered defiance, impulsivity, inattention, hyperactivity, theft, and substance abuse as well as aggression, i.e., various symptoms of conduct, oppositional defiant, attention-deficit/hyperactivity, and substance use disorders. In other papers, externalizing behavior was used as a synonym of conduct disorder, an approach shared by ICD-10. Finally, some papers used terms like "antisocial behavior," "rule breaking," and "conduct problems," which might be replaced with almost any of the above.

Due to the above, separating childhood conduct and aggression problems into diagnostic or behavioral categories was difficult. In some instances, different terms were used to name highly similar participants; in other cases, the same term covered different participants. Therefore, childhood conduct and aggression problems will be addressed below together, but naturally, the term employed by authors will also be indicated. Findings were grouped according to cortisol measurements (see Table 6.3).

Table 6.3 Interactions between childhood aggression problems and cortisol measures

Disorder/condition			Cortisol measurement			
Primary	Secondary	Participants	Constitutive	Point	Response	Stressor
INT [105]		Children, M & F	↑			
INT [106]		Adolescents M & F	↑			
CD [107]		Adolescents M & F	↑			
CD [108]	CU, DELIN	Adolescents M & F	↑			
EXT [46]		Adolescents F	↑			
DB [109]		Children, M & F	→			
CD [110]	CU, DELIN	Adolescents, male	→			
EXT [106]		Adolescents M & F	→			
EXT [46]		Adolescents M	→			
INT [111]		Children, M & F	↓			
INT [112]		Children, M & F	↓			
EXT [105]		Children, M & F	↓			
EXT [111]		Children, M & F	↓			
EXT [112]		Children, M & F	↓			
DB [113]	Severe	Children, M	↓			
CD [114]	CU	Children, M	↓			
CD [115]	CU	Children, F	↓			
EXT [56]		Children M & F	↓			
ODD [116]	DB	Children M	↓			
DB [117]	DELIN	Adolescents, M	↓			
DB [118]	CU	Adolescents, M & F	↓			
CD [119]	AGG, DELIN	Adolescents, M & F	↓			
CD [120]		Adolescents F	↓			
CD [121]	AGG	Adolescents F	↓			
EXT [122]	AGG, CU	Adolescents M & F	↓			
CD [123]	AGG	Adolescent mothers		→		
INT [106]		Adolescents M & F		→		
CD [108]	CU, DELIN	Adolescents M & F		→		
EXT [106]		Adolescents M & F		→		
DB [124]	CU	Adolescents, M & ~~F~~		→		
DB [113]	Severe	Children, M		→		
DB [125]		Children, M & F		→		
DB [124]	AGG, DELIN	Adolescents, M & ~~F~~		↓		
DB [126]	AGG, DELIN	Adolescents, ~~M~~ & F		↓		
ODD [127]	EXT	Children M		↓		
CD [128]	Severe	Children, M		↓		
DB [129]	AGG	Children, M & F		↓		
INT [106]		Adolescents M & F			↑	CDP
DB [130]	AB, RB	Adolescents M & ~~F~~			↑	TSST
DB [126]	AGG, DELIN	Adolescents, ~~M~~ & F			↑	CDP
CP [131]	Severe	Children M & F			↑	EMC

(continued)

Table 6.3 (continued)

Disorder/condition			Cortisol measurement			
Primary	Secondary	Participants	Constitutive	Point	Response	Stressor
EXT [106]		Adolescents M & F			→	CDP
DB [132]	AB	Adolescent, M & ~~F~~			↓	GSST
CD [107]		Adolescents M & F			↓	FVG
DB [133]		Children M			↓	FVG
ODD [127]	EXT	Children M			↓	FVG
DB [134]	AGG, DELIN	Children, M			↓	DCT
DB [113]	Severe	Children, M			↓	FVG
DB [125]		Children, M & F			↓	FVG
ODD [135]	ADHD	Children, M & F			↓	PC
DB [136]	DELIN	Adolescents M			↓	PST
EXT [137]	AGG, RB	Adolescents, M & F			↓	TSST
Cortisol measure			*Constitutive*	*Point*	*Response*	
Association with cortisol % share of studies		Positive (increased cortisol)	20	0	26	
		No association	16	58	7	
		Negative (decreased cortisol)	64	42	67	

Associations with cortisol: ↑, condition associated with high cortisol; →, no association; ↓, condition associated with low cortisol. *Disorder/condition*: *AB* antisocial behavior, *ADHD* attention-deficit/hyperactivity disorder, *AGG* aggressiveness, *CD* conduct disorder, *CP* conduct problems, *CU* callous–unemotional traits, *DB* disruptive behavior, *DELIN* delinquency, *EXT* externalizing behavior, *INT* internalizing behavior, *ODD* oppositional-defiant disorder, *RB* rule breaking. *Gender: M* male, *F* female, ~~M~~ or ~~F~~ association not valid for the respective gender. *Stressors employed*: *CDP* Conflict Discussion Paradigm, *DCT* demanding cognitive task, *EMC* emotional memory challenge, *FVG* frustrating video game, *GSST* Groningen Social Stress Test, *PC* pharmacological challenge, *PST* public speaking task, *TSST* Trier Social Stress Test. Note that for clarity, we grouped findings based on the cortisol measurements. Studies employing several ways to measure cortisol secretion are referred to repeatedly in the table

Although not consistent, a clear trend is still apparent from the findings. About two-thirds of the studies suggest that aggression-related psychopathologies are associated with low cortisol production. As expected, point measurements provide the least clear information, as the share of “no association” studies was extremely high within this group of studies. In contrast, both the “constitutive secretion” and “stress response” studies point to the association of these diagnoses with diminished cortisol production. It should be emphasized, however, that a non-negligible minority of studies (20–30%) show the opposite. Note that conflicting findings cannot be explained by comorbidities, gender, or age. These may have an impact as suggested by some authors, but the totality of findings fails to confirm such assumptions.

As a general conclusion, it is about two to three times more likely that aggression-related psychopathologies develop under the influence of downregulated rather than upregulated cortisol production in youth. Answering scientific questions by likelihoods is naturally not entirely comforting. We will try to provide a more specific hypothesis after reviewing the reminder of psychopathologies.

6.3.2.3 Personality Disorders

There are two personality disorders which were frequently investigated with respect to their relationship with cortisol. Antisocial personality-disordered people fail to conform to social norms to a degree that brings about legal apprehension: are deceitful, impulsive, irritable and aggressive, reckless, and irresponsible; and lack remorse and empathy. As only three of these symptoms need to be present for a diagnosis, patients are not necessarily aggressive (see Chap. 1). They are, however, grossly overrepresented in violent and non-violent criminal populations [138]. Borderline patients are characterized by instability in relations and affect, identity disturbances, suicidality, inappropriate anger, paranoid ideations, and dissociative symptoms. Although aggressive behavior is mentioned by DSM-5 only in parentheses as "physical fights," many patients are violent, and the disorder is overrepresented in incarcerated populations [139]. The externalizing-like antisocial personality disorder is typical to males (gender ratio is 3:1 in their "favor") [140], whereas the internalizing-like borderline disorder is more frequent in females (male/female gender ratio 1:3) [141]. This explains the gender selection of the studies reviewed below.

A specific category in this section is psychopathy, which is not a diagnostic entity of its own right, because the term was replaced by "antisocial personality disorder" in DSM from around 1980 onwards [142], and currently, both diagnostic manuals consider the two terms synonyms. Yet, many studies "diagnosed" psychopathy, mainly based on the Hare Psychopathy Checklist [143]. Usually, however, patients did not reach the cutoff score for full-blown psychopathy, had no concurrent ASPD, and came from the general population. Such individuals will be characterized below by the phrase "psychopathic traits," meaning that they had no established psychopathology. In antisocial personality-disordered subjects, psychopathy (usually established based on the same checklist) was indicated as a comorbidity (Table 6.4.).

Psychopathic traits in individuals lacking a psychiatric diagnosis do not seem to associate with a typical cortisol profile, as the few available studies are contradictory. The reason might be that these study participants were essentially healthy and showed a variable and usually low level of psychopathic traits.

Although contradictions are not lacking in antisocial and borderline personality disorders, trends are easily recognizable. Over two-thirds of the studies recorded low constitutive cortisol secretion and blunted stress responses in ASPD, whereas the opposite was true in borderline patients. Similar to studies on early conduct problems, point measurements were rather inconclusive. The relevance of findings for aggression was obvious with ASPD because a related measure, including violent crime, was regularly investigated. In borderline patients, aggression was studied in one study only, and there were three studies where violent suicide attempts were a research target. These studies, combined with a few others where comorbidities make the presence of aggressiveness likely (e.g., PTSD), suggest that borderline patients are aggressive on the background of an upregulated cortisol secretion.

Table 6.4 Antisocial and borderline personality disorders and cortisol secretion profiles

Healthy controls with psychopathic traits						
Condition	*Comorbidity*	*Participants*	*Constitutive*	*Point*	*Response*	*Stressor*
Community [144]	PP traits	Adults M & F		↑T		
Community [145]	PP traits 2	Adults ~~M~~ & F		↑		
Community [146]	PP traits	Adults M & F		→		
Community [147]	PP traits	Adults M & F		→		
Community [145]	PP traits 1	Adults ~~M~~ & F		↓		
Community [147]	PP traits	Adults M & F			↓T	EMT + TSST
Community [146]	PP traits	Adults M & F			↓	SRST
Antisocial personality disorder						
Diagnosis	*Comorbidity*	*Participants*	*Constitutive*	*Point*	*Response*	*Stressor*
APD [148]	CRIM, PP	Adults, M	↑			
APD [149]	LowSoc	Adults, M & F	→			
APD [150]	AGG	Adults, M	↓			
APD [151]	CRIM, PP 1	Adults, M	↓			
APD [152]	AGG, ALC CRIM	Adults, M	↓			
APD [153]	AGG, ALC CRIM	Adults, M	↓			
APD [8]	AGG, CRIM	Adults, M	↓			
APD [154]	PP	Adults, M & F		↑ T		
APD [155]	PP	Adults, M		↑ AA		
APD [149]	LowSoc	Adults, M & F		→		
APD [150]	AGG	Adults, M		→		
APD [156]	CRIM, PP	Adults, M		→		
APD [157]	PP	Adults, M & ~~F~~		→		
PD [158]	AGG	Adults, M & F		→		
APD [150]	AGG	Adults, M			→	GCH
APD [155]	PP	Adults, M & ~~F~~			→	PS
APD [159]	* CD, COC	Adults, M			↓CD	TSST
APD [149]	LowSoc	Adults, M & F			↓	EMT + PS
APD [156]	CRIM, PP	Adults, M			↓	TSST
APD [157]	PP	Adults, M & ~~F~~			↓	TSST
PD [158]	AGG	Adults, M & F			↓	PHC

(continued)

Table 6.4 (continued)

Association with cortisol % share of studies		*Direction*	*Constitutive*	*Point*	*Response*	
		Positive (cortisol high)	14	28	0	
		No association	15	72	29	
		Negative (cortisol low)	71	0	71	
Borderline personality disorder						
Diagnosis	*Comorbidity*	*Participants*	*Constitutive*	*Point*	*Response*	*Stressor*
BPD [160]	AGG	Adults, ~~M~~ & F	↑			
BPD [161]	PTSD (weak)	Adults, F	↑			
BPD [162]	ABH, PTSD	Adults, F	↑			
BPD [163]	VSB	Adults, F	↑			
BPD [164]	DISS	Adults, F	→			
BPD [161]	MD	Adults, F	→			
BPD [164]	DISS	Adults, F		→		
BPD [165]		Adults, F		↑		
BPD [166]	DISS	Adults, F		↑		
BPD [167]	ABH, PTSD	Adults, F		↑		
BPD [164]	DISS	Adults, F			↑	TSST
BPD [165]		Adults, F			↑	TSST
BPD [166]	DISS	Adults, F			↑	DS
BPD [168]	n-IMP	Adults, F			↑	PHC
BPD [169]	MD	Adults, F			↑	DS
BPD [170]	PTSD	Adults, F			↑	DS
BPD [171]	ABH, PTSD	Adults, F			↑	DS
BPD [172]	IMP, SB	Adults, M & F			↑	DS
BPD [173]	VSB	Adults, F			↑	DS
BPD [174]	ABH, ATTA	Adults, F			→	TSST
Association with cortisol % share of studies		*Direction*	*Constitutive*	*Point*	*Response*	
		Positive (cortisol high)	67	75	89	
		No association	33	25	11	
		Negative (cortisol low)	0	0	0	

Associations with cortisol: ↑, high cortisol; ↑*T*, high testosterone and high cortisol; ↑*AA*, high alpha amylase activity and high cortisol; →, no association; ↓, low cortisol; ↓*T*, high testosterone and low cortisol; ↓*CD*, relationship valid for CD history not to current APD. *Disorders and conditions*: *ABH* abuse history, *AGG* aggressiveness, *ALC* alcoholism, *APD* antisocial personality disorder, *ATTA* strong attachment anxiety, *BPD* borderline personality disorder, *CD* conduct disorder history, *COC* cocaine addiction, *CRIM* criminal history, *DIS* strong dissociative symptoms, *IMP* impulsive, *LowSoc* low sociability, *MD* major depression, *nIMP* non-impulsive, *PD* several personality disorders in sample including both APD, *PP* psychopathy on the background of APD or CRIM, *PP traits* psychopathic traits in community samples with no evidence of ASPD, *PP traits 1* cold affect and manipulation, *PP traits 2* criminal tendencies and erratic lifestyle, *PTSD* post-traumatic stress disorder, *SB* suicidal behavior, *VSB* violent suicidal behavior. *Gender*: *M* male, *F*

(continued)

Table 6.4 (continued)

female, ~~M~~ or ~~F~~ association not valid for the respective gender. *Stressors administered*: *DS* dexamethasone suppression, *EMT* effortful mental task, *GCH* glucose challenge, *PHC* pharmacologic challenge, *PS* public speaking, *SRST* social rejection stress task, *TSST* Trier Social Stress Test. Note that we grouped findings based on the cortisol measurements. Studies employing several cortisol measures were referred to repeatedly

Overall, the findings suggest that aggressiveness is associated with hypocortisolism in antisocial but with hypercortisolism in borderline personality disorder. However, a non-negligible minority of studies suggests the opposite.

6.3.2.4 "Clinical Disorders"

Since the elimination of the so-called axes from DSM-5, the term quoted in the title is rarely used. Originally, it differentiated Axis I ("clinical") from Axis II disorders, i.e., personality disorders that develop early, potentially last a lifetime, do not involve disease awareness and are rather resistant to treatment. Clinical disorders may occur at any age; patients are aware of their condition and usually seek treatment which is often successful at symptomatic level at least. Here we cover three such psychopathologies (see Table 6.5). Major depression and bipolar disorder are characterized by lasting periods of depressed mood, low energy and self-esteem, feelings of hopelessness, diminished interest in pleasure, and cognitive impairments and suicidal ideations. In addition, manic episodes occur in bipolar disorder. These implicate inflated self-esteem, psychomotor agitation, and engagement in risky behaviors. The relationship of these disorders with aggression is like that seen in ADHD. Although diagnostic criteria are not indicative of aggression problems, about 25% of patients show severe outbursts of aggression sometimes reaching the level of criminal violence (major depression [205, 206]; bipolar disorder [207, 208]). Unfortunately, the studies reviewed below did not differentiate the two conditions, mostly because depression was evaluated by psychometric instruments insensitive in this respect.

In the second psychopathology reviewed, posttraumatic stress disorder is elicited by life-threatening situations, develops slowly, and lasts very long despite trials of treatment. For instance, some Vietnam veterans traumatized before 1975 still showed the disorder 40 years later [209]. Patients show a variety of disturbances including anxiety, depression, memory deficits, hostility, and psychosis [210]. In addition, posttraumatic stress-disordered patients are often aggressive and violent [211, 212].

We also included in the table studies where participants showed anxiety. The reason was that such comorbidities were suggested to reverse the cortisol correlates of aggression-related psychopathologies [213]. A direct evidence for this assumption comes from a study [103] that compared attention-deficit/hyperactivity patients comorbid either with disruptive behavior or with anxiety. The first group had blunted, whereas the latter heightened stress response. Anxiety is rarely associated

Table 6.5 Associations with cortisol: anxiety, depression, and posttraumatic stress disorder

Depression (DEP) and anxiety (ANX)						
Condition 1	*Condition 2*	*Participants*	*Constitutive*	*Point*	*Response*	*Stressor*
ANX [103]	ADHD	Children M	→			
DEP [116]		Children M	↑			
DEP [175]		Adolescents M & F	↑			
DEP [176]		Adults M & F	↑			
DEP [175]	ANX	Adolescents M & F	↑↑			
DEP [175]	AGG	Adolescents M & F	↑↑			
DEP [177]	AGG	Adults M & F	↑↑			
DEP [178]	EXT	Children M & F	↑			
DEP, ANX, DET [179]	AGG CRIM	Adults M		↑		
ANX [127]	ODD, EXT	Children M		↑		
ANX [103]	ADHD	Children M		→		
ANX [103]	ADHD	Children M			↑↑	BsT
ANX [127]	ODD, EXT	Children M			↑↑	FVG
ANX [133]	DB	Children M			↑↑	FVG
DEP [180]	AGG	Adults M & F			↑↑	Various
DEP [181]	AGG	Adults M & F			↑↑	Various
DEP [182]	AGG	Adults M & F			↑↑	PHC
DEP [169]	BPD	Adults F			↑↑	DS
DEP [183]	SB	Adolescents M & F			↑↑	DS
Association with cortisol % share of studies		*Direction*	*Constitutive*	*Point*	*Response*	
		Positive (high cortisol)	80	67	100	
		No association	20	33	0	
		Negative (low cortisol)	0	0	0	
Posttraumatic stress disorder (PTSD)						
Trauma	*Condition*	*Participants*	*Basal*	*Point*	*Response*	*Stressor*
IPV [184]		Adults F	↑			
P/FO [185]		Officers M & F	↑			
P/FO [186]		Officers M & F	↑			
IPV [187]	ANX, DEP	Adults F	↑			
WAR [188]	ANX, DEP	Adolescents F & M	↑			
VAR [189]	DEP	Adults M & F	↑			
IPV [190]	DEP	Adults F	↑			
IPV [191]	DEP	Adults F	↑			

(continued)

Table 6.5 (continued)

VAR [192]	HYPER	Adolescents ~~M~~ & F	↑			
WAR [193]		Adolescents F	→			
COM [194]		Adults M	→			
VAR [189]		Adults M & F	→			
HOL [195]		Adults M & ~~F~~	→			
VAR [196]		Adults F	→			
IpV [197]		Adults F	↓			
CV [198]		Children M & F	↓			
DISAS [199]		Adults M & F	↓			
HOL [67]		Adults M	↓			
HOL [200]		Adults M & F	↓			
IPV [68]	Severe	Adults F	↓			
IPV [201]	DISS	Adults F	↓			
HOL [202]	AVOID	Adults M & F	↓			
VAR [203]	HYPER	Adults M & F	↓			
P/FO [204]	HYPER	Officers M & F	↓			
IpV [197]		Adults F		↑		
P/FO [185]		Officers M & F		↑		
P/FO [204]	HYPER	Officers M & F		↑		
HOL [195]		Adults M & ~~F~~			↑	EMT
IpV [197]		Adults F			↓	ST
Association with cortisol % share of studies		*Direction*	*Constitutive*	*Point*	*Response*	
		Positive (high cortisol)	38	100	50	
		No association	21	0	0	
		Negative (low cortisol)	41	0	50	

Associations with cortisol: ↑, high cortisol; ↑↑, cortisol higher in aggressive than in nonaggressive depression patients; →, no association; ↓, low cortisol. *Traumatizing events and diagnoses*: *ADHD* attention-deficit/hyperactivity disorder, *AGG* aggression, *CRIM* crime, *ANX* anxiety, *AVOID* avoidance symptoms in PTSD, *BPD* borderline personality disorder, *COM* combat experience, *CV* community violence, *DB* disruptive behavior, *DEP* depression, *DET* addicts in detoxification program, *DISS* dissociative symptoms in PTSD, *DISAS* victims of disaster, *EXT* externalizing behavior, *HOL* holocaust survivor, *HYPER* hyperarousal symptoms in PTSD, *IPV* intimate partner violence, *IpV* interpersonal conflict, *ODD* oppositional-defiant disorder, *PTSD* posttraumatic stress disorder, *P/FO* police or firefighter operations, *SB* suicidal behavior, *VAR* various sources for PTSD in the sample, *WAR* non-combatant war victim. *Gender*: *M* male, *F* female, ~~M~~ or ~~F~~ association not valid for the respective gender. *Stressors administered*: *EMT* emotional memory stress, *ST* separation stress. *Gender*: *M* male, *F* female, ~~M~~ or ~~F~~, association not valid for the respective gender. Note that for clarity, we grouped findings based on the cortisol measurements. Studies employing several ways to measure cortisol secretion are referred to repeatedly in the table

with aggression; nevertheless, such reversals of cortisol correlates appear important for this chapter.

The findings confirm that anxiety reverses the cortisol correlates of aggression-related disorders (e.g., attention-deficit/hyperactivity and oppositional defiant disorders) and behaviors (e.g., externalizing and disruptive behaviors). If comorbid with anxiety, these disorders become associated with high cortisol production. There were no conflicting findings; the only study where no association was found for constitutive cortisol production did find an increased stress response.

The situation seems similarly clear with depression. This disorder is associated with increased cortisol production irrespective to age as shown in the first three rows of the table. The association of depression with aggression (or diagnoses associated with aggression) increases cortisol secretion even further as indicated by the double arrows. This is true for both constitutive cortisol secretion and stress responses. Virtually no conflicting findings were reported.

Findings in depression may indirectly be informative for intermittent explosive disorder, as the two conditions show high comorbidity [214], and aggression in intermittent explosive disorder is associated with a state called "micromania," which resembles manic episodes in bipolar disorder [215]. In addition, intermittent explosive disorder can be treated with antidepressants [216]. Although convincing arguments suggest that intermittent explosive disorder is a psychiatric entity of its own right [217], its cortisol background may be similar to that seen in depression associated with outbursts of aggression as suggested by behavioral similarities, high comorbidities, and shared effective treatments.

In contrast to anxiety and depression, findings in PTSD are conflicting. The first, highly influential study published by Yehuda [67] suggested that the disorder is associated with low cortisol secretion. Subsequent research, however, provided mixed findings, indicating that the disorder may be associated with either increased or decreased cortisol secretion. Contradictions cannot be resolved by considering the source of the trauma, because all traumatic events (including the Holocaust studied by Yehuda) have divergent consequences for cortisol secretion. Cortisol was not studied explicitly in conjunction with the aggressiveness so far, possibly because the basic phenomenon appears controversial. Indirectly, however, associations between hyperarousal symptoms and cortisol may be relevant in this respect because aggression in PTSD tightly correlates with this symptom [218]. However, this correlation was also bidirectional.

6.3.2.5 Violent and Non-violent Crime

Cortisol is relatively frequently investigated in criminal populations because of its potential usefulness for the assessment of criminological risks and recidivism [219, 220]. Delinquent and criminal populations were amply represented in Tables 6.2, 6.3, 6.4, and 6.5; to have a complete picture on crime, these findings were reiterated here and complemented with studies where psychiatric diagnoses were of no concern. The organizing principle for Table 6.6 was the nature of the crime – violent or

Table 6.6 Cortisol secretion profiles in participants with a criminal history

Crime type	Psychiatric condition	Study participants	Cortisol measurement			
			Constitutive	Point	Responsive	Stressor
Violent [221]	AGGt	Adults, M & F	↓			
Violent [222]	PP	Adults, M	↓ PP			
Violent [223]	Several	Adults, F	↓			
Violent [224]	AGG	Adolescents, M	↓ T			
Violent [119]	CD	Adolescents, M & F	↓			
Violent [151]	APD, PP	Adults, M	↓			
Violent [152]	APD	Adults, M	↓			
Violent [153]	APD	Adults, M	↓			
Violent [8]	APD	Adults, M	↓			
Violent [221]	AGGt	Adults, M & F		→		PSP
Violent [225]	AGG	Adults, M		→		SV
Violent [134]	DB	Children, M		→		DCT
Violent [124]	DB	Adolescents, M & F		↓		
Violent [221]	AGGt	Adults, M & F			↓	PSP
Violent [225]	AGG	Adults, M			↓	SV
Violent [134]	DB	Children, M			↓	DCT
Association with cortisol % share of studies		*Association*	*Constitutive*	*Point*	*Responsive*	
		Positive (high cortisol)	0	0	0	
		No association	0	75	0	
		Negative (low cortisol)	100	25	100	
Mixed [108]	CD-CU	Adolescents, M & F	↑			
Mixed [148]	APD	Adults, M	↑			
Mixed [110]	CD-CU	Adolescents, male	→			
Mixed [117]	DB	Adolescents, M	↓			
Mixed [226]	CU	Adolescents, M	↓			
Mixed [108]	CD-CU	Adolescents M & F		→		
Non-violent [227]	Several	Adults, M		→		
Non-violent [220]	APD	Adults, M		→		
Non-violent [228]	RT	Adolescents, M		→		
Mixed [156]	APD, PP	Adults, M		→		
Mixed [229]	PD	Adults, M		↓T		
Mixed [126]	DB	Adolescents, M & F		↓		

(continued)

Table 6.6 (continued)

Crime type	Psychiatric condition	Study participants	Cortisol measurement Constitutive	Point	Responsive	Stressor
Mixed [126]	DB	Adolescents, M & F			↑	CDP
Non-violent [227]	Several	Adults, M			↓	PS + DI
Non-violent [220]	APD	Adults, M			↓	DCT
Non-violent [228]	RT	Adolescents, M			↓	DCT
Mixed [136]	DB	Adolescents, M			↓	PS
Mixed [156]	APD, PP	Adults, M			↓	TSST
Association with cortisol % share of studies		*Association*	*Constitutive*	*Point*	*Responsive*	
		Positive (high cortisol)	40	0	17	
		No association	20	72	17	
		Negative (low cortisol)	40	28	66	

Associations with cortisol: ↓, low cortisol compared with non-criminals; ↓PP, low cortisol compared to criminals without psychopathy; ↓T, high testosterone/cortisol ratio compared to non-criminals; → no association. *Psychiatric condition*: *AGGt* high trait aggression, *APD* ASPD, *CD* conduct disorder, *CU* callous–unemotional traits, *DB* disruptive behavior, *several* a variety of psychiatric conditions not specifically investigated, *PD* a variety of personality disorders, *PP* psychopathy, *RT* risk-taking behaviors. *Gender*: *M* male, *F* female. *Stressors administered*: *CDP* conflict discussion paradigm, *DCT* demanding cognitive task, *DI* dating interview, *PS* public speaking, *PSP* point subtraction paradigm, *SV* stressful video, *TSST* Trier Social Stress Test. *Notes*: For clarity, we grouped findings based on the cortisol measurements. Studies employing several ways to measure cortisol secretion were referred to repeatedly in the table. Studies on mental disorders were reiterated here if they were performed in criminal populations

non-violent. There are several studies where the study population committed both types of crimes without these being separated; in their case, the crime type was termed "mixed."

Violent criminals detach from all the other study populations by their exclusive association with low cortisol secretion profiles. This is equally true for constitutive cortisol secretion and stress responses. There is some variance regarding point measurements, but in all cases where the point measurement failed to evidence associations, stress responses were reduced. The lack of divergent findings may be changed by subsequent studies, but for the time being, committing violent crime is the only condition whit a unison low cortisol association.

The picture is more varied with non-violent crime, where findings on constitutive cortisol secretion are conflicting; nevertheless, most findings show that stress responses are blunted in this case too.

6.3.3 Findings: Prospective Association Studies

In the studies reviewed here, associations were investigated prospectively. The question asked was whether low cortisol at one time point would predict the emergence of conduct problems several years later. Typically, study participants did not show conduct problems when the first trial was run; at this time point, however, considerable differences were observed in cortisol secretion patterns.

We showed above that at least in some cases, adverse life events (toxic stress) may lead to a succession of changes in cortisol secretion: an initial upregulation may be followed by a long-term downregulation. Therefore, we grouped studies according to the age when the cortisol measurement was performed (Table 6.7).

In infants, subsequent aggression problems may be predicted by both increased and decreased cortisol secretion but more likely by the former. These findings are at variance with those obtained at more advanced ages and may be related to the biphasic response of cortisol secretion to toxic stress (see above). The first time point may have captured the initial, cortisol-heightening phase in infants, whereas the second, cortisol-downregulating phase may have been captured at later ages.

In children and adolescents, conduct problems were almost invariably predicted by low cortisol at the first (predictor) time point. There were two exceptions only. In one, participants showed mixed externalizing and internalizing behaviors. As in this study, the former was roughly equivalent with conduct disorder, whereas the latter with mixed symptoms of anxiety and depression, the study strengthens the assumption that anxiety can reverse the cortisol–aggression relationship. In the second, patients were comorbid with depression, the symptoms of which led to discrepant associations with cortisol. This suggests that comorbid depression may also affect the cortisol–aggression relationship.

Overall, these findings suggest that in infancy, the subsequent development of aggression problems is predicted by increased cortisol secretion. The opposite appears to be true for later stages of life, when aggression problems appear to be predicted by low cortisol production. This age-dependent shift in the prediction power of cortisol may be related to the biphasic effect of toxic stressors on cortisol secretion.

6.3.4 Overview and Hypotheses

Many studies on the cortisol–aggression relationship started with an introductory sentence of the type "both high and low cortisol levels were associated with aggression..." and the experiments that followed strived at resolving the dispute. Other studies addressed the issue from a meta-analytic-like point of view, indirectly assuming that there is a "true" association and the major task was to find it. Such analyses, however, ended up with very low effect sizes (mostly in the "low cortisol" direction) or failed to find a significant association. However, the findings presented

Table 6.7 Cortisol as a predictor of aggression problems

Cortisol measurements in infancy					
Gender	*Studied at age (years)*		*Time span (years)*	*Prediction by cortisol*	
	Cortisol	*Aggression*		*Predicted*	*Predictor*
M, F [230]	0.5–1.25	7	6	CU	↑MB1[a]
M, F [231]	1–1.5	3	1.5–2	INT	↑
M, F [232]	1.25	6	5	CP-CU	↑
M, F [233]	1.4	5	3.5	INT + EXT	↑
M, F [231]	1–1.5	3	1.5–2	EXT	→
M, F [230]	0.5–1.25	7	6	CP	↓MB2[b]
M, F [234]	1.1	3	2	Anger	↓
Predictive for aggression problems - % share of studies				High cortisol	57
				No prediction	14
				Low cortisol	29
Cortisol measurements in childhood					
Gender	*Studied at age (years)*		*Time span (years)*	*Prediction by cortisol*	
	Cortisol	*Aggression*		*Predicted*	*Predictor*
M, F [235]	10	12	2	INT + EXT	↑
M [16]	2–4	4–6	2	DB	↓
[236]M, F	4–5	8	3	ADHD	↓
M, F [18]	5	7	2	AGG	↓CU
M, F [237]	6	9	3	AGG	↓
M, F [238]	6	12	5	EXT	↓PB3y
M, F [238]	6	12	5	INT	↓PB3y
M, F [239]	6–10	9–13	3	EXT	↓
M, F [239]	6–10	9–13	3	INT	↓
M, F [240]	7–8	8–9	1	DB	↓[c]
M [241]	10–12	15–17	5	AGG	↓
M, F [242]	10–12	12–14	2	DB	↓
Predictive for aggression problems - % share of studies				High cortisol	8
				No prediction	0
				Low cortisol	92
Cortisol measurements in adolescence					
Gender	Studied at age (years)		Time span (years)	Prediction by cortisol	
	Cortisol	Aggression		Predicted	Predictor
M, F [243]	6–16	8–18	2	EXT	↓
M, F [119]	15	17	2	AGG	↓
M, F [244]	15	17	2	AGG	↓
M, F [245]	15	18	3	AGG	↓ High DEP
M, F [245]	15	18	3	AGG	↑ Low DEP
Predictive for conduct problems - % share of studies				High cortisol	20
				No prediction	0
				Low cortisol	80

(continued)

Table 6.7 (continued)

Note: Except two (marked), all studies employed methodologies indicative of constitutive cortisol secretion. *Predictions*: ↑, high cortisol predicts aggression problems; ↑MB1, predictive if maternal behavior was characterized by harsh intrusion; ↑ low DEP, predictive in subject showing low depression; →, no prediction; ↓, low cortisol predicts conduct problems; ↓ CU, predictive in interaction with CU traits; ↓ PB3y, predictive in interaction with problem behaviors at age 3; ↓MB2, predictive if maternal behavior was characterized by high sensitivity;↓ DEP, predictive if associated with high depression; [a] stress response; [b] point measurement; [c] uniquely, this study showed the reverse relationship, i.e., psychopathologies at time point 1 predicted cortisol levels at time point 2. *Gender*: *M* male, *F* female, F̶ association not valid for females. *Behaviors predicted*: *ADHD* attention-deficit/hyperactivity disorder, *AGG* aggressiveness, *anger* prediction refers to this feeling, aggression not studied, *CD* conduct disorder, *CP* conduct problems, *CU* callous–unemotional traits, *DB* disruptive behavior, *EXT* externalizing behavior, *INT* internalizing behavior

above clearly demonstrate that the issue cannot be addressed in such simplistic ways.

Aggressiveness is not a stand-alone feature in psychiatric disorders but is embedded in a wide array of dysfunctions, which are disorder-specific and have a crucial impact on the cortisol–aggression relationship. It occurs that both the "high cortisol" and the "low cortisol" hypothesis were true but for different psychopathologies. This assumption is to certain extent thwarted by findings obtained in the same psychopathologies. As shown above, there is a "majority finding" for each disorder, but the share of "minority findings" is non-negligible for most disorders. Controversies may be attributed to experimental error, but a careful inspection of the studies does not support the assumption that good quality studies concentrate on either side, with the exception of point measurements, because these failed to find associations between cortisol and aggression at an unusually high rate. The share of indecisive studies based on point measurements was 81% for ADHD, 58% for various conduct problems displayed by children and adolescents, and 72% for ASPD. In the same disorders, the share of non-association studies was considerably lower when constitutive cortisol secretion patterns were evaluated more reliably or stress responses were studied (their share was around 20% in both). Considering these two measures together lowers the share of non-association studies even further because in many instances, unchanged constitutive cortisol secretion was "counteracted" by a change in stress responses.

To account for between-disorder and within-disorder discrepancies, we summarize the findings as follows.

Essentially, there are two major types of cortisol–aggression relationships in psychopathologies. Certain mental disorders preferentially associate with low cortisol secretion whereas others with high cortisol secretion. Importantly, psychopathologies are not aligned accidentally along this dichotomy. Downregulated cortisol secretion was primarily observed in psychopathologies where rule breaking, law infringements, and violence are among the major symptoms such as conduct problems in children and adolescents (externalizing and disruptive behavior and oppositional defiant and conduct disorders) and ASPD in adults. ADHD belongs to this class if comorbid with one of the conduct problems listed above. Upregulated cortisol secretion on its turn is regularly observed in patients with unstable mood, e.g., in ADHD not comorbid with aggression-related conduct problems, as well as in borderline personality disorder, and depression with manic or manic-like episodes ("micromania") that lead to aggressive outbursts. PTSD may also belong to this group although findings are mixed.

In summary, the "low cortisol hypothesis" appears valid for disorders where rule breaking is a core feature, whereas the "high cortisol hypothesis" appears valid for disorders that involve unstable mood. Findings incompatible with this dichotomy, i.e., those reported by a non-negligible minority of studies, might be explained by the differential genetic background of those experiencing adverse life events, differences in superimposed stressors, and comorbidities such as anxiety. It is also worth emphasizing that patients diagnosed with the same disorder might be quite different at phenotypic level, mostly because diagnoses require the presence of a subgroup of symptoms only. An illustrative example of this is PTSD, the symptoms of which are grouped into five clusters. The diagnosis requires the presence of one symptom from each of clusters A–C and two symptoms from clusters D to E (seven symptoms in total). The total number of symptoms being 24, diagnoses may be assigned to patients who are quite different. This might be one of the leading reasons for the high variability of cortisol associations in this disorder. The situation is not much better with other disorders. For instance, in ASPD, where three symptoms need to be present from the seven listed in cluster A, patients might fail to conform to social norms, might by irritable and aggressive, and might lack remorse (symptoms A1, A4, and A7 in DSM-5). Other patients, however, might be just deceitful, impulsive, and irresponsible (symptoms A2, A3, and A6, respectively).

Together, these considerations suggest that there are many reasons for which patients presenting with the same disorder can have divergent cortisol backgrounds. One can assume that differences in cortisol are associated with different types of aggression within the same psychopathology and, indeed, gain-oriented proactive aggression is associated with downregulated, whereas emotion-driven reactive aggression is associated with upregulated cortisol secretion, irrespective of psychopathologic background [35, 131, 246–252]. Noteworthy, a similar dichotomy was found in animal models [253]. This may explain why criminal violence is uniquely associated with low cortisol, because gain-oriented, proactive aggression is more likely apprehended than occasional outbursts of anger. Consequently, those with low cortisol profiles may be overrepresented in criminal populations.

Finally, the unique predictive power of low cortisol profiles may be due to the time required by this condition to induce those structural brain alterations which appear to mediate their behavioral effects in animals and which are commonly observed in humans as shown in the next section. The time required for changes in brain structure and consequently behavior may endow low cortisol secretion with a predictive power. On their turn, heightened cortisol stress responses might have an immediate effect on the brain circuitry of aggression as shown in animals and seen in humans. Due to this, endocrine and behavioral changes may occur concomitantly, which annuls the predictive power of cortisol upregulation.

The graphic summary of the main findings was presented in Fig. 6.2 through the lens of these hypotheses, which will be evaluated in the next section.

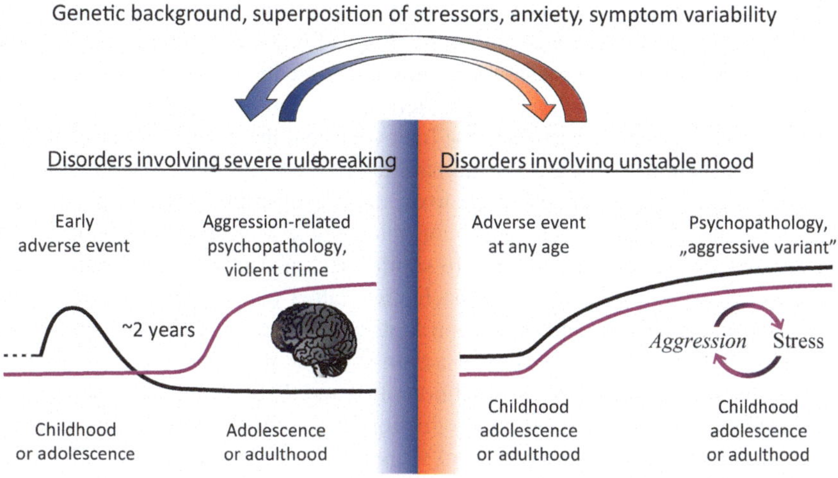

Fig. 6.2 The cortisol–aggression relationship in psychopathologies and crime. The two observed types of association between cortisol- (black) and psychopathology-driven aggression (magenta). Constitutive changes in secretion and cortisol stress responses were not differentiated for clarity. Note that in many cases, changes were similar in these two variables, and when constitutive changes were not apparent, stress responses showed the change typical to the disorder class. The graph was complemented with hypotheses on the mechanisms that make possible a switch from one type of association to the other (upper part of the schematic) and those that may mediate the impact of cortisol on aggression (shown below the "aggression curve"). The former explains why findings are not entirely congruent within disorders, whereas the latter may explain the unique predictive power of low cortisol backgrounds. For more explanations see text

6.4 General Overview and Interpretation

6.4.1 Epiphenomenon or Controlling Mechanism?

Ample evidence demonstrates that glucocorticoid production serves as a controlling mechanism in animals (see previous chapter). Acutely, the inhibition of glucocorticoid synthesis decreases, whereas the replacement of the glucocorticoid stress response by injections restores aggression. When the stress response was counteracted by glucocorticoid receptor blockade in the juvenile period, the behavioral effects of toxic stress did not develop in adulthood; moreover, glucocorticoid administration in critical periods mimicked the long-term effects of stressors. The behavioral effects of adrenalectomy and low glucocorticoid replacement were similarly inhibited by repeated glucocorticoid injections that mimicked stress responses in animals with non-reactive stress systems.

Similar experiments are extremely difficult if not impossible to perform in humans; therefore, most studies report simply associations, which as evidences for causal relationships are circumstantial only. Nevertheless, the associations seen in humans are highly similar to those seen in animals. Acutely, aggression associates with increased cortisol production in both animals and humans. The cortisol–aggression relationship observed in depression and bipolar disorder resembles the one observed in chronically restrained animals exposed to social challenge, i.e., to a heterotypic stressor. Finally, the long-term down- and upregulation of cortisol production in response to early adverse life events and the delayed development of abnormal (psychopathologic or criminal) aggression resemble the phenomena observed in animals submitted to early toxic stress. Not surprisingly, the schematics illustrating the glucocorticoid–aggression relationship were highly similar in this and the previous chapter. In addition to similarities, disparate human findings also suggest that cortisol is a controlling mechanism rather than an epiphenomenon. As shown above, cortisol administration and acute stressors promote human aggression acutely (see Sect. 6.2.2 above). The administration of a glucocorticoid agonist (hydrocortisone) ameliorated the condition of those PTSD patients who were characterized by downregulated cortisol production [254]. Finally, depression and bipolar disorder respond well to the cortisol secretion inhibitor metyrapone [255, 256] including the amelioration of "agitation," which often results in aggression. Although disparate, such findings still indicate that the role of glucocorticoids is similar in animals and humans: The totality of findings suggests cortisol serves as a controlling mechanism of aggression in humans.

6.4.2 The Mediators of Cortisol Effects

As with animals, findings on the brain mechanisms activated by cortisol will only be mentioned, because such mechanisms will be presented in detail in the following chapters. Here we refer to a few findings obtained with various paradigms, showing that they induce alterations in those brain areas that control aggression and are sensitive to cortisol actions.

As it regards acute effects, the amygdala showed increased activation in the Taylor Aggression Paradigm under high provocation [257], and acute glucocorticoid administrations also activated the amygdala [258]. These findings suggest that cortisol enhances the activity of a brain area which plays a role in aggressive responses in this paradigm. Downregulation of serotonin enhanced aggressive responses in the point subtraction paradigm [259], whereas cortisol downregulated serotonin neurotransmission acutely [260]. Similar examples are abundant in the literature, and all point to the assumption that acute cortisol responses elicited by aggression activate neural mechanisms associated with aggression.

Regarding long-term effects, we already mentioned that early adverse life events induce epigenetic modifications, which are mediated by cortisol [52]. Such changes may link cortisol stress responses to alterations that persist long after the triggering stressor vanished, an essential requirement of the so-called toxic stress.

Epigenetic changes generated by toxic stressors appear to have a dual target in humans. They may induce long-term alterations in the genes that control cortisol secretion and the responsiveness of neurons to cortisol, but they also affect brain development and structure [261, 262]. For instance, vulnerability to borderline personality disorder was associated with epigenetic changes in brain areas that are involved in the stress response [263]; moreover, the severity of the disorder was also associated with epigenetic events [264]. Associations between early adverse life events, epigenetics, and structural alterations in the brain were shown for all the disorders addressed above, e.g., ASPD [265], posttraumatic stress disorder [266], disruptive behavior in children [267], etc. Although these associations were recorded concomitantly in most cases, i.e., without the possibility of establishing the time course of events, recent studies address the development of aggressive traits from a neurodevelopmental perspective and suggest that changes in cortisol secretion are important mechanisms in this process. The predictive value of cortisol secretion patterns appears to be an important argument in favor of this hypothesis.

6.4.3 The U-Shaped Curve of the Cortisol–Aggression Relationship

As mentioned in the previous chapter, the cortisol–aggression relationship was recently visualized by a U-shaped curve suggesting that both low and high glucocorticoid secretion induces severe and abnormal forms of aggression in animals [268]. In the previous chapter, we used this "U-template" to describe the cortisol–aggression relationship not only from a quantitative point of view but also to characterize the type of aggression expressed by animals exposed to toxic stress in critical periods of life. In addition, we intercalated an inverted U-shaped curve between the arms of the "U" to account for acute cortisol–aggression relationships in animals undergoing normal development. The same template will be used here to illustrate the essence of human findings (see Fig. 6.3).

The inverted U-shaped "dose-response curve" for acute cortisol–aggression relationships was not demonstrated in humans, but the available findings do show that under conditions of social challenge, the cortisol stress response promotes aggression in psychologically healthy, non-criminal people. This assumption was based on laboratory models of experimental psychology where aggression was weak, often symbolic only, and participants did not violate the rules established by the experimenter. They only exploited the alternatives of responding, which were integral to the test. One can hypothesize that in real life situations, healthy subjects also use legally or morally acceptable forms of aggression to solve conflicts assertively, without damaging their social status or endangering their future.

The downregulated cortisol secretion arm of the U – the toxic stress eliciting this endocrine condition – is associated with mental disorders where rule breaking and aggression are among the main symptoms and which are associated primarily with proactive aggression. Based on the findings obtained so far, violent crime shows an exclusive association with downregulated cortisol secretion.

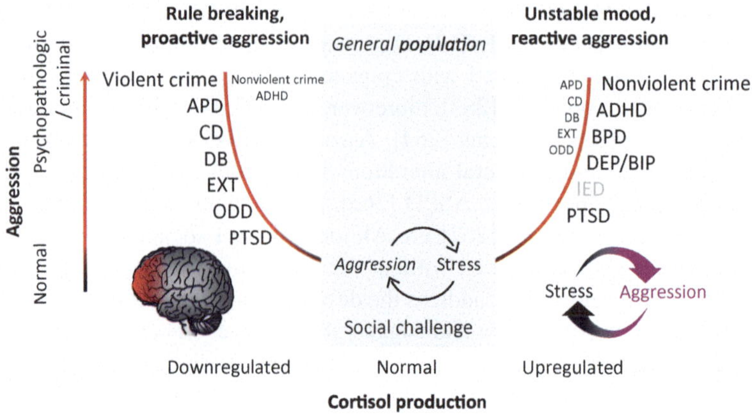

Fig. 6.3 The cortisol–aggression relationship in humans: an overview. Font size indicates the likelihood of a condition to belong to one of the two main cortisol backgrounds. The schematics placed below disorder acronyms symbolize the assumed mechanism: *brain drawing*, structural alterations in the central nervous system; *positive feedback loop*, enhanced acute activation of the aggression circuitry by enhanced cortisol. *ADHD*, attention-deficit/hyperactivity disorder; *APD*, antisocial personality disorder; *BPD*, borderline personality disorder; *CD*, conduct disorder; *DB*, disruptive behavior; *DEP/BIP*, depression and/or bipolar disorder; *EXT*, externalizing behavior; *IED*, intermittent explosive disorder (grey font because cortisol background is only assumed); *nV* crime, non-violent crime; *ODD*, oppositional defiant disorder; *PTSD*, posttraumatic stress disorder

We find disorders characterized by unstable mood on the right-hand arm of the U; these are most likely characterized by reactive aggression. The very same disorders may be found on both sides but with different likelihoods. Disorders associated with rule breaking may sometimes associate with upregulated cortisol secretion, especially when comorbid with anxiety and/or depression, i.e., when their condition involves periods of unstable mood. On the other hand, ADHD may be associated with downregulated cortisol secretion if comorbid with aggression problems; the same may apply to non-violent criminals who are occasionally violent.

Although some disorders may be placed on both sides of the U, each has a preferential association either with downregulated or with upregulated cortisol secretion. The only exception is PTSD, which is associated with the two endocrine backgrounds with equal chances. This may be explained by the high changeability of their symptomatology.

The main message conveyed by Fig. 6.3 is that while both downregulated and upregulated cortisol secretion may be associated with psychopathologic and criminal violence, the types of violence associated with the two cortisol conditions are *different*.

References

1. Dollard, J., Doob, L., Miller, N., Mowrer, O., & Sears, R. (1939). *Frustration and aggression*. Yale University Press.
2. Miller, N. E. (1941). The frustration-aggression hypothesis. *Psychological Review, 48*, 337–342.
3. Berkowitz, L. (1989). Frustration-aggression hypothesis: Examination and reformulation. *Psychological Bulletin, 106*, 59–73.
4. Henry, J. P. (1992). Biological basis of the stress response. *Integrative Physiological and Behavioral Science, 27*, 66–83.
5. Adam, E. K. (2006). Transactions among adolescent trait and state emotion and diurnal and momentary cortisol activity in naturalistic settings. *Psychoneuroendocrinology, 31*, 664–679.
6. Lopez-Duran, N. L., Olson, S. L., Hajal, N. J., Felt, B. T., & Vazquez, D. M. (2009). Hypothalamic pituitary adrenal axis functioning in reactive and proactive aggression in children. *Journal of Abnormal Child Psychology, 37*, 169–182.
7. Gallucci, A., Riva, P., Romero Lauro, L. J., & Bushman, B. J. (2019). Stimulating the ventrolateral prefrontal cortex (VLPFC) modulates frustration-induced aggression: A tDCS experiment. *Brain Stimulat*. https://doi.org/10.1016/j.brs.2019.10.015.
8. Virkkunen, M. (1985). Urinary free cortisol secretion in habitually violent offenders. *Acta Psychiatrica Scandinavica, 72*, 40–44.
9. Posner, I., & Conway, K. M. (1981). Arousal of sexual and aggressive contact by exposure to stressors in albino rats. *The Journal of General Psychology, 104*, 145–151.
10. Health promotion: Control of stress and violent behavior. Public Health Reports. Suppl, 167–176 (1983).
11. Mason, A., & Blankenship, V. (1987). Power and affiliation motivation, stress, and abuse in intimate relationships. *Journal of Personality and Social Psychology, 52*, 203–210.
12. Susman, E. J., Nottelmann, E. D., Dorn, L. D., Inoff-Germain, G., & Chrousos, G. P. (1988). Physiological and behavioral aspects of stress in adolescence. *Advances in Experimental Medicine and Biology., 245*, 341–352.
13. Zuckerman, M. (1989). Personality in the third dimension: A psychobiological approach. *Personality and Individual Differences, 10*, 391–418.
14. Vanyukov, M. M., et al. (1993). Antisocial symptoms in preadolescent boys and in their parents: Associations with cortisol. *Psychiatry Research, 46*, 9–17.
15. Haller, J., van de Schraaf, J., & Kruk, M. R. (2001). Deviant forms of aggression in glucocorticoid hyporeactive rats: A model for 'pathological' aggression? *Journal of Neuroendocrinology, 13*, 102–107.
16. McBurnett, K., Lahey, B. B., Rathouz, P. J., & Loeber, R. (2000). Low salivary cortisol and persistent aggression in boys referred for disruptive behavior. *Archives of General Psychiatry, 57*, 38–43.
17. Haller, J. (2018). The role of the lateral hypothalamus in violent intraspecific aggression-the glucocorticoid deficit hypothesis. *Frontiers in Systems Neuroscience, 12*, 26.
18. Wright, N., Hill, J., Pickles, A., & Sharp, H. (2019). Callous-unemotional traits, low cortisol reactivity and physical aggression in children: Findings from the Wirral child health and development study. *Translational Psychiatry, 9*, 79.
19. Strüber, N., Strüber, D., & Roth, G. (2014). Impact of early adversity on glucocorticoid regulation and later mental disorders. *Neuroscience and Biobehavioral Reviews, 38*, 17–37.
20. Brewer-Smyth, K., & Burgess, A. W. (2019). Neurobiology of female homicide perpetrators. *Journal of Interpersonal Violence*, 886260519860078. https://doi.org/10.1177/0886260519860078.
21. Taylor, S. P. (1967). Aggressive behavior and physiological arousal as a function of provocation and the tendency to inhibit aggression. *Journal of Personality, 35*, 297–310.
22. Cherek, D. R. (1992). *Point subtraction aggression paradigm (PSAP)*. University of Texas.

23. Güth, W., Schmittberger, R., & Schwarze, B. (1982). An experimental analysis of ultimatum bargaining. *Journal of Economic Behavior and Organization, 3*, 367–388.
24. Rapoport, A., & Chammah, A. M. (1966). The game of chicken. *The American Behavioral Scientist, 10*, 10–28.
25. Reijntjes, A., Dekovic, M., & Telch, M. J. (2007). Support for the predictive validity of the SASC-R: Linkages with reactions to an in vivo peer evaluation manipulation. *Journal of Anxiety Disorders, 21*, 903–917.
26. Eckhardt, C. I., Barbour, K. A., & Davison, G. C. (1998). Articulated thoughts of maritally violent and nonviolent men during anger arousal. *Journal of Consulting and Clinical Psychology, 66*, 259–269.
27. Rosenzweig, S. (1950). Revised norms for the adult form of the Rosenzweig picture-frustration study. *Journal of Personality, 18*, 344–346.
28. Salminen, M., & Ravaja, N. (2008). Increased oscillatory theta activation evoked by violent digital game events. *Neuroscience Letters, 435*, 69–72.
29. Harry, B. (1983). Obsessive video-game users. *JAMA, 249*, 473.
30. Böhnke, R., Bertsch, K., Kruk, M. R., & Naumann, E. (2010). The relationship between basal and acute HPA axis activity and aggressive behavior in adults. *Journal of Neural Transmission, 1996*(117), 629–637.
31. Goulter, N., Kimonis, E. R., Denson, T. F., & Begg, D. P. (2019). Female primary and secondary psychopathic variants show distinct endocrine and psychophysiological profiles. *Psychoneuroendocrinology, 104*, 7–17.
32. Gerra, G., et al. (2004). Aggressive responding in abstinent heroin addicts: Neuroendocrine and personality correlates. *Progress in Neuro-Psychopharmacology & Biological Psychiatry, 28*, 129–139.
33. Gerra, G., et al. (2001). Experimentally induced aggressive behavior in subjects with 3,4-methylenedioxy-methamphetamine ('ecstasy') use history: Psychobiological correlates. *Journal of Substance Abuse, 13*, 471–491.
34. Gerra, G., et al. (2001). Aggressive responding of male heroin addicts under methadone treatment: Psychometric and neuroendocrine correlates. *Drug and Alcohol Dependence, 65*, 85–95.
35. Geniole, S. N., Carré, J. M., & McCormick, C. M. (2011). State, not trait, neuroendocrine function predicts costly reactive aggression in men after social exclusion and inclusion. *Biological Psychology, 87*, 137–145.
36. Gerra, G., et al. (1997). Neurotransmitter-neuroendocrine responses to experimentally induced aggression in humans: Influence of personality variable. *Psychiatry Research, 66*, 33–43.
37. Gerra, G., et al. (2007). Experimentally induced aggressiveness in heroin-dependent patients treated with buprenorphine: Comparison of patients receiving methadone and healthy subjects. *Psychiatry Research, 149*, 201–213.
38. De Sousa Fernandes Perna, E. B., Theunissen, E. L., Kuypers, K. P. C., Toennes, S. W., & Ramaekers, J. G. (2016). Subjective aggression during alcohol and cannabis intoxication before and after aggression exposure. *Psychopharmacology, 233*, 3331–3340.
39. Probst, F., Golle, J., Lory, V., & Lobmaier, J. S. (2018). Reactive aggression tracks within-participant changes in women's salivary testosterone. *Aggressive Behavior, 44*, 362–371.
40. Gentile, D. A., Bender, P. K., & Anderson, C. A. (2017). Violent video game effects on salivary cortisol, arousal, and aggressive thoughts in children. *Computers in Human Behavior, 70*, 39–43.
41. Aliyari, H., et al. (2018). The beneficial or harmful effects of computer game stress on cognitive functions of players. *Basic and Clinical Neuroscience, 9*, 177–186.
42. Gunnar, M. R., Kryzer, E., Van Ryzin, M. J., & Phillips, D. A. (2010). The rise in cortisol in family day care: Associations with aspects of care quality, child behavior, and child sex. *Child Development, 81*, 851–869.
43. Murray-Close, D., Han, G., Cicchetti, D., Crick, N. R., & Rogosch, F. A. (2008). Neuroendocrine regulation and physical and relational aggression: The moderating roles of child maltreatment and gender. *Developmental Psychology, 44*, 1160–1176.

44. Blair, C., Granger, D., & Peters Razza, R. (2005). Cortisol reactivity is positively related to executive function in preschool children attending head start. *Child Development, 76*, 554–567.
45. Tout, K., de Haan, M., Campbell, E. K., & Gunnar, M. R. (1998). Social behavior correlates of cortisol activity in child care: Gender differences and time-of-day effects. *Child Development, 69*, 1247–1262.
46. Marsman, R., et al. (2008). HPA-axis activity and externalizing behavior problems in early adolescents from the general population: The role of comorbidity and gender the TRAILS study. *Psychoneuroendocrinology, 33*, 789–798.
47. Oberle, E., et al. (2017). Afternoon cortisol provides a link between self-regulated anger and peer-reported aggression in typically developing children in the school context. *Developmental Psychobiology, 59*, 688–695.
48. Böhnke, R., Bertsch, K., Kruk, M. R., Richter, S., & Naumann, E. (2010). Exogenous cortisol enhances aggressive behavior in females, but not in males. *Psychoneuroendocrinology, 35*, 1034–1044.
49. Verona, E., & Kilmer, A. (2007). Stress exposure and affective modulation of aggressive behavior in men and women. *Journal of Abnormal Psychology, 116*, 410–421.
50. Verona, E., & Curtin, J. J. (2006). Gender differences in the negative affective priming of aggressive behavior. *Emot. Wash. DC, 6*, 115–124.
51. Van Houdenhove, B., Van Den Eede, F., & Luyten, P. (2009). Does hypothalamic-pituitary-adrenal axis hypofunction in chronic fatigue syndrome reflect a 'crash' in the stress system? *Medical Hypotheses, 72*, 701–705.
52. Jiang, S., Postovit, L., Cattaneo, A., Binder, E. B., & Aitchison, K. J. (2019). Epigenetic modifications in stress response genes associated with childhood trauma. *Frontiers in Psychiatry, 10*, 808.
53. Kapoor, A., Petropoulos, S., & Matthews, S. G. (2008). Fetal programming of hypothalamic-pituitary-adrenal (HPA) axis function and behavior by synthetic glucocorticoids. *Brain Research Reviews, 57*, 586–595.
54. Buckingham-Howes, S., Mazza, D., Wang, Y., Granger, D. A., & Black, M. M. (2016). Prenatal drug exposure and adolescent cortisol reactivity: Association with Behavioral concerns. *Journal of Developmental & Behavioral Pediatrics, 37*, 565–572.
55. Zhang, C., et al. (2014). Prenatal xenobiotic exposure and intrauterine hypothalamus-pituitary-adrenal axis programming alteration. *Toxicology, 325*, 74–84.
56. Martin, C. G., Kim, H. K., Bruce, J., & Fisher, P. A. (2014). Child diurnal cortisol rhythms, parenting quality, and externalizing behaviors in preadolescence. *Psychoneuroendocrinology, 40*, 170–180.
57. McLaughlin, K. A., et al. (2015). Causal effects of the early caregiving environment on development of stress response systems in children. *Proceedings of the National Academy of Sciences of the United States of America, 112*, 5637–5642.
58. Koss, K. J., Hostinar, C. E., Donzella, B., & Gunnar, M. R. (2014). Social deprivation and the HPA axis in early development. *Psychoneuroendocrinology, 50*, 1–13.
59. van der Vegt, E. J. M., van der Ende, J., Kirschbaum, C., Verhulst, F. C., & Tiemeier, H. (2009). Early neglect and abuse predict diurnal cortisol patterns in adults a study of international adoptees. *Psychoneuroendocrinology, 34*, 660–669.
60. Elzinga, B. M., et al. (2008). Diminished cortisol responses to psychosocial stress associated with lifetime adverse events a study among healthy young subjects. *Psychoneuroendocrinology, 33*, 227–237.
61. Carpenter, L. L., et al. (2009). Effect of childhood emotional abuse and age on cortisol responsivity in adulthood. *Biological Psychiatry, 66*, 69–75.
62. Lovallo, W. R., Farag, N. H., Sorocco, K. H., Cohoon, A. J., & Vincent, A. S. (2012). Lifetime adversity leads to blunted stress axis reactivity: Studies from the Oklahoma family health patterns project. *Biological Psychiatry, 71*, 344–349.

63. Ouellet-Morin, I., et al. (2011). Blunted cortisol responses to stress signal social and behavioral problems among maltreated/bullied 12-year-old children. *Biological Psychiatry, 70*, 1016–1023.
64. Janusek, L. W., Tell, D., Gaylord-Harden, N., & Mathews, H. L. (2017). Relationship of childhood adversity and neighborhood violence to a proinflammatory phenotype in emerging adult African American men: An epigenetic link. *Brain, Behavior, and Immunity, 60*, 126–135.
65. Busso, D. S., McLaughlin, K. A., & Sheridan, M. A. (2017). Dimensions of adversity, physiological reactivity, and externalizing psychopathology in adolescence: Deprivation and threat. *Psychosomatic Medicine, 79*, 162–171.
66. Dayan, J., Rauchs, G., & Guillery-Girard, B. (2016). Rhythms dysregulation: A new perspective for understanding PTSD? *Journal of Physiology, Paris, 110*, 453–460.
67. Yehuda, R., et al. (1990). Low urinary cortisol excretion in patients with posttraumatic stress disorder. *The Journal of Nervous and Mental Disease, 178*, 366–369.
68. Pinto, R. J., Correia-Santos, P., Costa-Leite, J., Levendosky, A. A., & Jongenelen, I. (2016). Cortisol awakening response among women exposed to intimate partner violence. *Psychoneuroendocrinology, 74*, 57–64.
69. Buydens-Branchey, L., Branchey, M., Fergeson, P., Hudson, J., & McKernin, C. (1997). The meta-chlorophenylpiperazine challenge test in cocaine addicts: Hormonal and psychological responses. *Biological Psychiatry, 41*, 1071–1086.
70. Nijhof, S. L., et al. (2014). The role of hypocortisolism in chronic fatigue syndrome. *Psychoneuroendocrinology, 42*, 199–206.
71. Pruessner, M., Cullen, A. E., Aas, M., & Walker, E. F. (2017). The neural diathesis-stress model of schizophrenia revisited: An update on recent findings considering illness stage and neurobiological and methodological complexities. *Neuroscience and Biobehavioral Reviews, 73*, 191–218.
72. Kuhlman, K. R., Chiang, J. J., Horn, S., & Bower, J. E. (2017). Developmental psychoneuroendocrine and psychoneuroimmune pathways from childhood adversity to disease. *Neuroscience and Biobehavioral Reviews, 80*, 166–184.
73. Raymond, C., Marin, M.-F., Majeur, D., & Lupien, S. (2018). Early child adversity and psychopathology in adulthood: HPA axis and cognitive dysregulations as potential mechanisms. *Progress in Neuro-Psychopharmacology & Biological Psychiatry, 85*, 152–160.
74. Gunnar, M. R., & Vazquez, D. M. (2001). Low cortisol and a flattening of expected daytime rhythm: Potential indices of risk in human development. *Development and Psychopathology, 13*, 515–538.
75. Haller, J., Harold, G., Sandi, C., & Neumann, I. D. (2014). Effects of adverse early-life events on aggression and anti-social behaviours in animals and humans. *Journal of Neuroendocrinology, 26*, 724–738.
76. Miczek, K. A., de Boer, S. F., & Haller, J. (2013). Excessive aggression as model of violence: A critical evaluation of current preclinical methods. *Psychopharmacology, 226*, 445–458.
77. Fries, E., Hesse, J., Hellhammer, J., & Hellhammer, D. H. (2005). A new view on hypocortisolism. *Psychoneuroendocrinology, 30*, 1010–1016.
78. Doom, J. R., Cicchetti, D., & Rogosch, F. A. (2014). Longitudinal patterns of cortisol regulation differ in maltreated and nonmaltreated children. *Journal of the American Academy of Child and Adolescent Psychiatry, 53*, 1206–1215.
79. Bosch, N. M., et al. (2012). Timing matters: Long term effects of adversities from prenatal period up to adolescence on adolescents' cortisol stress response. The TRAILS study. *Psychoneuroendocrinology, 37*, 1439–1447.
80. Daskalakis, N. P., Bagot, R. C., Parker, K. J., Vinkers, C. H., & de Kloet, E. R. (2013). The three-hit concept of vulnerability and resilience: Toward understanding adaptation to early-life adversity outcome. *Psychoneuroendocrinology, 38*, 1858–1873.
81. Joos, C. M., McDonald, A., & Wadsworth, M. E. (2019). Extending the toxic stress model into adolescence: Profiles of cortisol reactivity. *Psychoneuroendocrinology, 107*, 46–58.

82. Peckins, M. K., Susman, E. J., Negriff, S., Noll, J., & Trickett, P. K. (2015). Cortisol profiles: A test for adaptive calibration of the stress response system in maltreated and nonmaltreated youth. *Development and Psychopathology, 27*, 1461–1470.
83. Haller, J. (2014). The glucocorticoid/aggression relationship in animals and humans: An analysis sensitive to behavioral characteristics, glucocorticoid secretion patterns, and neural mechanisms. *Current Topics in Behavioral Neurosciences, 17*, 73–109.
84. Khoury, J. E., et al. (2015). Summary cortisol reactivity indicators: Interrelations and meaning. *Neurobiol. Stress, 2*, 34–43.
85. Engert, V., et al. (2013). Differentiating anticipatory from reactive cortisol responses to psychosocial stress. *Psychoneuroendocrinology, 38*, 1328–1337.
86. Burke, H., Fernald, L., Gertler, P., & Adler, N. (2005). Depressive symptoms are associated with blunted cortisol stress responses in very low-income women. *Psychosomatic Medicine, 67*, 211–216.
87. *American Psychiatric Association: Diagnostic and Statistical Manual of Mental Disorders, Fifth Edition*. American Psychiatric Association, 2013.
88. *The ICD-10 Classification of Mental and Behavioral Disorders*. World Health Organization, 1999.
89. Mohr-Jensen, C., & Steinhausen, H.-C. (2016). A meta-analysis and systematic review of the risks associated with childhood attention-deficit hyperactivity disorder on long-term outcome of arrests, convictions, and incarcerations. *Clinical Psychology Review, 48*, 32–42.
90. Kaneko, M., Hoshino, Y., Hashimoto, S., Okano, T., & Kumashiro, H. (1993). Hypothalamic-pituitary-adrenal axis function in children with attention-deficit hyperactivity disorder. *Journal of Autism and Developmental Disorders, 23*, 59–65.
91. van West, D., Claes, S., & Deboutte, D. (2009). Differences in hypothalamic-pituitary-adrenal axis functioning among children with ADHD predominantly inattentive and combined types. *European Child & Adolescent Psychiatry, 18*, 543–553.
92. Palma, S. M. M., Fernandes, D. R. M., Muszkat, M., & Calil, H. M. (2012). The response to stress in Brazilian children and adolescents with attention deficit hyperactivity disorder. *Psychiatry Research, 198*, 477–481.
93. Lackschewitz, H., Hüther, G., & Kröner-Herwig, B. (2008). Physiological and psychological stress responses in adults with attention-deficit/hyperactivity disorder (ADHD). *Psychoneuroendocrinology, 33*, 612–624.
94. Palma, S. M. M., Natale, A. C. M. P., & Calil, H. M. (2015). A four-year follow-up controlled study of stress response and symptom persistence in Brazilian children and adolescents with attention deficit disorder and hyperactivity (ADHD). *Psychiatry Research, 230*, 227–232.
95. Maldonado, E. F., Trianes, M. V., Cortés, A., Moreno, E., & Escobar, M. (2009). Salivary cortisol response to a psychosocial stressor on children diagnosed with attention-deficit/hyperactivity disorder: Differences between diagnostic subtypes. *The Spanish Journal of Psychology, 12*, 707–714.
96. Schulz, K. P., Halperin, J. M., Newcorn, J. H., Sharma, V., & Gabriel, S. (1997). Plasma cortisol and aggression in boys with ADHD. *Journal of the American Academy of Child and Adolescent Psychiatry, 36*, 605–609.
97. Kariyawasam, S. H., Zaw, F., & Handley, S. L. (2002). Reduced salivary cortisol in children with comorbid attention deficit hyperactivity disorder and oppositional defiant disorder. *Neuro Endocrinology Letters, 23*, 45–48.
98. Işık, Ü., Bilgiç, A., Toker, A., & Kılınç, I. (2018). Serum levels of cortisol, dehydroepiandrosterone, and oxytocin in children with attention-deficit/hyperactivity disorder combined presentation with and without comorbid conduct disorder. *Psychiatry Research, 261*, 212–219.
99. Northover, C., Thapar, A., Langley, K., Fairchild, G., & van Goozen, S. H. M. (2016). Cortisol levels at baseline and under stress in adolescent males with attention-deficit hyperactivity disorder, with or without comorbid conduct disorder. *Psychiatry Research, 242*, 130–136.

100. Yang, S.-J., Shin, D. W., Noh, K. S., & Stein, M. A. (2007). Cortisol is inversely correlated with aggression for those boys with attention deficit hyperactivity disorder who retain their reactivity to stress. *Psychiatry Research, 153*, 55–60.
101. Stadler, C., et al. (2011). Cortisol reactivity in boys with attention-deficit/hyperactivity disorder and disruptive behavior problems: The impact of callous unemotional traits. *Psychiatry Research, 187*, 204–209.
102. Pesonen, A.-K., et al. (2011). Symptoms of attention deficit hyperactivity disorder in children are associated with cortisol responses to psychosocial stress but not with daily cortisol levels. *Journal of Psychiatric Research, 45*, 1471–1476.
103. Hastings, P. D., Fortier, I., Utendale, W. T., Simard, L. R., & Robaey, P. (2009). Adrenocortical functioning in boys with attention-deficit/hyperactivity disorder: Examining subtypes of ADHD and associated comorbid conditions. *Journal of Abnormal Child Psychology, 37*, 565–578.
104. King, J. A., Barkley, R. A., & Barrett, S. (1998). Attention-deficit hyperactivity disorder and the stress response. *Biological Psychiatry, 44*, 72–74.
105. Cicchetti, D., & Rogosch, F. A. (2001). The impact of child maltreatment and psychopathology on neuroendocrine functioning. *Development and Psychopathology, 13*, 783–804.
106. Klimes-Dougan, B., Hastings, P. D., Granger, D. A., Usher, B. A., & Zahn-Waxler, C. (2001). Adrenocortical activity in at-risk and normally developing adolescents: Individual differences in salivary cortisol basal levels, diurnal variation, and responses to social challenges. *Development and Psychopathology, 13*, 695–719.
107. Azar, R., et al. (2004). Cortisol levels and conduct disorder in adolescent mothers. *Journal of the American Academy of Child and Adolescent Psychiatry, 43*, 461–468; discussion 469-472.
108. Fairchild, G., et al. (2008). Cortisol diurnal rhythm and stress reactivity in male adolescents with early-onset or adolescence-onset conduct disorder. *Biological Psychiatry, 64*, 599–606.
109. Sondeijker, F. E. P. L., et al. (2007). Disruptive behaviors and HPA-axis activity in young adolescent boys and girls from the general population. *Journal of Psychiatric Research, 41*, 570–578.
110. Oosterlaan, J., Geurts, H. M., Knol, D. L., & Sergeant, J. A. (2005). Low basal salivary cortisol is associated with teacher-reported symptoms of conduct disorder. *Psychiatry Research, 134*, 1–10.
111. Puetz, V. B., et al. (2017). Altered brain network integrity after childhood maltreatment: A structural connectomic DTI-study. *Human Brain Mapping, 38*, 855–868.
112. Puetz, V. B., et al. (2016). Multidimensional assessment of neuroendocrine and psychopathological profiles in maltreated youth. *Journal of Neural Transmission, 1996*(123), 1095–1106.
113. van de Wiel, N. M. H., van Goozen, S. H. M., Matthys, W., Snoek, H., & van Engeland, H. (2004). Cortisol and treatment effect in children with disruptive behavior disorders: A preliminary study. *Journal of the American Academy of Child and Adolescent Psychiatry, 43*, 1011–1018.
114. van Bokhoven, I., et al. (2005). Salivary cortisol and aggression in a population-based longitudinal study of adolescent males. *Journal of Neural Transmission, 1996*(112), 1083–1096.
115. Stoppelbein, L., Greening, L., Luebbe, A., Fite, P., & Becker, S. P. (2014). The role of cortisol and psychopathic traits in aggression among at-risk girls: Tests of mediating hypotheses. *Aggressive Behavior, 40*, 263–272.
116. Kohrt, B. A., et al. (2015). Child abuse, disruptive behavior disorders, depression, and salivary cortisol levels among institutionalized and community-residing boys in Mongolia. *Asia-Pacific Psychiatry, 7*, 7–19.
117. Popma, A., et al. (2007). The diurnal cortisol cycle in delinquent male adolescents and normal controls. *Neuropsychopharmacol, 32*, 1622–1628.
118. Loney, B. R., Butler, M. A., Lima, E. N., Counts, C. A., & Eckel, L. A. (2006). The relation between salivary cortisol, callous-unemotional traits, and conduct problems in an adolescent non-referred sample. *Journal of Child Psychology and Psychiatry, 47*, 30–36.

119. Platje, E., et al. (2013). Longitudinal associations in adolescence between cortisol and persistent aggressive or rule-breaking behavior. *Biological Psychology, 93*, 132–137.
120. Pajer, K., Gardner, W., Rubin, R. T., Perel, J., & Neal, S. (2001). Decreased cortisol levels in adolescent girls with conduct disorder. *Archives of General Psychiatry, 58*, 297–302.
121. Pajer, K., et al. (2006). Adrenal androgen and gonadal hormone levels in adolescent girls with conduct disorder. *Psychoneuroendocrinology, 31*, 1245–1256.
122. Grotzinger, A. D., et al. (2018). Hair and salivary testosterone, hair cortisol, and externalizing Behaviors in adolescents. *Psychological Science, 29*, 688–699.
123. von Polier, G. G., et al. (2013). Reduced cortisol in boys with early-onset conduct disorder and callous-unemotional traits. *BioMed Research International, 2013*(349530).
124. Poustka, L., et al. (2010). Negative association between plasma cortisol levels and aggression in a high-risk community sample of adolescents. *Journal of Neural Transmission, 1996*(117), 621–627.
125. van Goozen, S. H., Matthys, W., Cohen-Kettenis, P. T., Buitelaar, J. K., & van Engeland, H. (2000). Hypothalamic-pituitary-adrenal axis and autonomic nervous system activity in disruptive children and matched controls. *Journal of the American Academy of Child and Adolescent Psychiatry, 39*, 1438–1445.
126. Kobak, R., Zajac, K., & Levine, S. (2009). Cortisol and antisocial behavior in early adolescence: The role of gender in an economically disadvantaged sample. *Development and Psychopathology, 21*, 579–591.
127. van Goozen, S. H., et al. (1998). Salivary cortisol and cardiovascular activity during stress in oppositional-defiant disorder boys and normal controls. *Biological Psychiatry, 43*, 531–539.
128. Feilhauer, J., Cima, M., Korebrits, A., & Nicolson, N. A. (2013). Salivary cortisol and psychopathy dimensions in detained antisocial adolescents. *Psychoneuroendocrinology, 38*, 1586–1595.
129. Scerbo, A. S., & Kolko, D. J. (1994). Salivary testosterone and cortisol in disruptive children: Relationship to aggressive, hyperactive, and internalizing behaviors. *Journal of the American Academy of Child and Adolescent Psychiatry, 33*, 1174–1184.
130. Susman, E. J., et al. (2010). Cortisol and alpha amylase reactivity and timing of puberty: Vulnerabilities for antisocial behaviour in young adolescents. *Psychoneuroendocrinology, 35*, 557–569.
131. McBurnett, K., et al. (2005). Mood and hormone responses to psychological challenge in adolescent males with conduct problems. *Biological Psychiatry, 57*, 1109–1116.
132. Schaefer, J. M., et al. (2013). Corticotropin (ACTH)-reactive immunoglobulins in adolescents in relation to antisocial behavior and stress-induced cortisol response. The TRAILS study. *Psychoneuroendocrinology, 38*, 3039–3047.
133. Schoorl, J., van Rijn, S., de Wied, M., van Goozen, S., & Swaab, H. (2016). The role of anxiety in cortisol stress response and cortisol recovery in boys with oppositional defiant disorder/conduct disorder. *Psychoneuroendocrinology, 73*, 217–223.
134. Moss, H. B., Vanyukov, M. M., & Martin, C. S. (1995). Salivary cortisol responses and the risk for substance abuse in prepubertal boys. *Biological Psychiatry, 38*, 547–555.
135. Snoek, H., et al. (2002). Serotonergic functioning in children with oppositional defiant disorder: A sumatriptan challenge study. *Biological Psychiatry, 51*, 319–325.
136. Popma, A., et al. (2006). Hypothalamus pituitary adrenal axis and autonomic activity during stress in delinquent male adolescents and controls. *Psychoneuroendocrinology, 31*, 948–957.
137. Portnoy, J., et al. (2015). Digit ratio (2D:4D) moderates the relationship between cortisol reactivity and self-reported externalizing behavior in young adolescent males. *Biological Psychology, 112*, 94–106.
138. Fazel, S., & Danesh, J. (2002). Serious mental disorder in 23000 prisoners: A systematic review of 62 surveys. *Lancet, 359*, 545–550.
139. Sansone, R. A., & Sansone, L. A. (2009). Borderline personality and criminality. *Psychiatry Edgmont Pa Townsh., 6*, 16–20.

140. Alegria, A. A., et al. (2013). Sex differences in antisocial personality disorder: Results from the National Epidemiological Survey on alcohol and related conditions. *Personality Disorders, 4*, 214–222.
141. Sansone, R. A., & Sansone, L. A. (2011). Gender patterns in borderline personality disorder. *Innovations in Clinical Neuroscience, 8*, 16–20.
142. Moran, P. (1999). The epidemiology of antisocial personality disorder. *Social Psychiatry and Psychiatric Epidemiology, 34*, 231–242.
143. Hare, R. D. (2003). *Hare psychopathy checklist-revised* (2nd ed.). Ann Arbor.
144. Welker, K. M., Lozoya, E., Campbell, J. A., Neumann, C. S., & Carré, J. M. (2014). Testosterone, cortisol, and psychopathic traits in men and women. *Physiology & Behavior, 129*, 230–236.
145. Vaillancourt, T., & Sunderani, S. (2011). Psychopathy and indirect aggression: The roles of cortisol, sex, and type of psychopathy. *Brain and Cognition, 77*, 170–175.
146. O'Leary, M. M., Taylor, J., & Eckel, L. (2010). Psychopathic personality traits and cortisol response to stress: The role of sex, type of stressor, and menstrual phase. *Hormones and Behavior, 58*, 250–256.
147. Glenn, A. L., Raine, A., Schug, R. A., Gao, Y., & Granger, D. A. (2011). Increased testosterone-to-cortisol ratio in psychopathy. *Journal of Abnormal Psychology, 120*, 389–399.
148. Loomans, M. M., Tulen, J. H. M., de Rijke, Y. B., & van Marle, H. J. C. (2016). A hormonal approach to anti-social behaviour. *Criminal Behaviour and Mental Health, 26*, 380–394.
149. Sorocco, K. H., Lovallo, W. R., Vincent, A. S., & Collins, F. L. (2006). Blunted hypothalamic-pituitary-adrenocortical axis responsivity to stress in persons with a family history of alcoholism. *International Journal of Psychophysiology, 59*, 210–217.
150. Fishbein, D. H., Dax, E., Lozovsky, D. B., & Jaffe, J. H. (1992). Neuroendocrine responses to a glucose challenge in substance users with high and low levels of aggression, impulsivity, and antisocial personality. *Neuropsychobiology, 25*, 106–114.
151. Holi, M., Auvinen-Lintunen, L., Lindberg, N., Tani, P., & Virkkunen, M. (2006). Inverse correlation between severity of psychopathic traits and serum cortisol levels in young adult violent male offenders. *Psychopathology, 39*, 102–104.
152. Lindman, R. E., Aromäki, A. S., & Eriksson, C. J. (1997). Sober-state cortisol as a predictor of drunken violence. *Alcohol Alcohol. Oxf. Oxfs., 32*, 621–626.
153. Bergman, B., & Brismar, B. (1994). Hormone levels and personality traits in abusive and suicidal male alcoholics. *Alcoholism, Clinical and Experimental Research, 18*, 311–316.
154. Roy, A. R. K., Cook, T., Carré, J. M., & Welker, K. M. (2019). Dual-hormone regulation of psychopathy: Evidence from mass spectrometry. *Psychoneuroendocrinology, 99*, 243–250.
155. Glenn, A. L., et al. (2015). Alpha-amylase reactivity in relation to psychopathic traits in adults. *Psychoneuroendocrinology, 54*, 14–23.
156. Johnson, M. M., Mikolajewski, A., Shirtcliff, E. A., Eckel, L. A., & Taylor, J. (2015). The association between affective psychopathic traits, time incarcerated, and cortisol response to psychosocial stress. *Hormones and Behavior, 72*, 20–27.
157. O'Leary, M. M., Loney, B. R., & Eckel, L. A. (2007). Gender differences in the association between psychopathic personality traits and cortisol response to induced stress. *Psychoneuroendocrinology, 32*, 183–191.
158. Almeida, M., Lee, R., & Coccaro, E. F. (2010). Cortisol responses to ipsapirone challenge correlate with aggression, while basal cortisol levels correlate with impulsivity, in personality disorder and healthy volunteer subjects. *Journal of Psychiatric Research, 44*, 874–880.
159. Buydens-Branchey, L., & Branchey, M. (2004). Cocaine addicts with conduct disorder are typified by decreased cortisol responsivity and high plasma levels of DHEA-S. *Neuropsychobiology, 50*, 161–166.
160. Rausch, J., et al. (2015). Increased testosterone levels and cortisol awakening responses in patients with borderline personality disorder: Gender and trait aggressiveness matter. *Psychoneuroendocrinology, 55*, 116–127.

161. Wingenfeld, K., Driessen, M., Adam, B., & Hill, A. (2007). Overnight urinary cortisol release in women with borderline personality disorder depends on comorbid PTSD and depressive psychopathology. *European Psychiatry, 22*, 309–312.
162. Jogems-Kosterman, B. J. M., de Knijff, D. W. W., Kusters, R., & van Hoof, J. J. M. (2007). Basal cortisol and DHEA levels in women with borderline personality disorder. *Journal of Psychiatric Research, 41*, 1019–1026.
163. van Heeringen, K., Audenaert, K., Van de Wiele, L., & Verstraete, A. (2000). Cortisol in violent suicidal behaviour: Association with personality and monoaminergic activity. *Journal of Affective Disorders, 60*, 181–189.
164. Simeon, D., Knutelska, M., Smith, L., Baker, B. R., & Hollander, E. (2007). A preliminary study of cortisol and norepinephrine reactivity to psychosocial stress in borderline personality disorder with high and low dissociation. *Psychiatry Research, 149*, 177–184.
165. Nater, U. M., et al. (2010). Increased psychological and attenuated cortisol and alpha-amylase responses to acute psychosocial stress in female patients with borderline personality disorder. *Psychoneuroendocrinology, 35*, 1565–1572.
166. Carvalho Fernando, S., et al. (2012). Associations of childhood trauma with hypothalamic-pituitary-adrenal function in borderline personality disorder and major depression. *Psychoneuroendocrinology, 37*, 1659–1668.
167. Sinai, C., et al. (2014). Hypothalamic pituitary thyroid axis and exposure to interpersonal violence in childhood among women with borderline personality disorder. *European Journal of Psychotraumatology, 5*.
168. Minzenberg, M. J., et al. (2006). Blunted hormone responses to Ipsapirone are associated with trait impulsivity in personality disorder patients. *Neuropsychopharmacology, 31*, 197–203.
169. Schweitzer, I., Tuckwell, V., Maguire, K., & Tiller, J. (2001). Personality pathology, depression and HPA axis functioning. *Human Psychopharmacology, 16*, 303–308.
170. Wingenfeld, K., Hill, A., Adam, B., & Driessen, M. (2007). Dexamethasone suppression test in borderline personality disorder: Impact of PTSD symptoms. *Psychiatry and Clinical Neurosciences, 61*, 681–683.
171. Rinne, T., et al. (2002). Hyperresponsiveness of hypothalamic-pituitary-adrenal axis to combined dexamethasone/corticotropin-releasing hormone challenge in female borderline personality disorder subjects with a history of sustained childhood abuse. *Biological Psychiatry, 52*, 1102–1112.
172. Engström, G., Alling, C., Gustavsson, P., Oreland, L., & Träskman-Bendz, L. (1997). Clinical characteristics and biological parameters in temperamental clusters of suicide attempters. *Journal of Affective Disorders, 44*, 45–55.
173. Banki, C. M., & Arató, M. (1983). Amine metabolites and neuroendocrine responses related to depression and suicide. *Journal of Affective Disorders, 5*, 223–232.
174. Ehrenthal, J. C., Levy, K. N., Scott, L. N., & Granger, D. A. (2018). Attachment-related regulatory processes moderate the impact of adverse childhood experiences on stress reaction in borderline personality disorder. *Journal of Personality Disorders, 32*, 93–114.
175. Van den Bergh, B. R. H., Van Calster, B., Pinna Puissant, S., & Van Huffel, S. (2008). Self-reported symptoms of depressed mood, trait anxiety and aggressive behavior in post-pubertal adolescents: Associations with diurnal cortisol profiles. *Hormones and Behavior, 54*, 253–257.
176. Dedovic, K., & Ngiam, J. (2015). The cortisol awakening response and major depression: Examining the evidence. *Neuropsychiatric Disease and Treatment, 11*, 1181–1189.
177. Sher, L., et al. (2005). Higher cortisol levels in spring and fall in patients with major depression. *Progress in Neuro-Psychopharmacology & Biological Psychiatry, 29*, 529–534.
178. Dietrich, A., et al. (2013). Cortisol in the morning and dimensions of anxiety, depression, and aggression in children from a general population and clinic-referred cohort: An integrated analysis. The TRAILS study. *Psychoneuroendocrinology, 38*, 1281–1298.
179. Soderstrom, H., et al. (2004). A controlled study of tryptophan and cortisol in violent offenders. *Journal of Neural Transmission, 1996*(111), 1605–1610.

180. Van Praag, H. M. (2001). Anxiety/aggression—Driven depression. A paradigm of functionalization and verticalization of psychiatric diagnosis. *Progress in Neuro-Psychopharmacology & Biological Psychiatry, 25*, 893–924.
181. van Praag, H. M. (1998). Anxiety and increased aggression as pacemakers of depression. *Acta Psychiatrica Scandinavica. Supplementum, 393*, 81–88.
182. López-Ibor, J. J., Saiz-Ruiz, J., & Pérez de los Cobos, J. C. (1985). Biological correlations of suicide and aggressivity in major depressions (with melancholia): 5-hydroxyindoleacetic acid and cortisol in cerebral spinal fluid, dexamethasone suppression test and therapeutic response to 5-hydroxytryptophan. *Neuropsychobiology, 14*, 67–74.
183. Jokinen, J., & Nordström, P. (2009). HPA axis hyperactivity and attempted suicide in young adult mood disorder inpatients. *Journal of Affective Disorders, 116*, 117–120.
184. Johnson, D. M., Delahanty, D. L., & Pinna, K. (2008). The cortisol awakening response as a function of PTSD severity and abuse chronicity in sheltered battered women. *Journal of Anxiety Disorders, 22*, 793–800.
185. Lindauer, R. J. L., Olff, M., van Meijel, E. P. M., Carlier, I. V. E., & Gersons, B. P. R. (2006). Cortisol, learning, memory, and attention in relation to smaller hippocampal volume in police officers with posttraumatic stress disorder. *Biological Psychiatry, 59*, 171–177.
186. Austin-Ketch, T. L., et al. (2012). Addictions and the criminal justice system, what happens on the other side? Post-traumatic stress symptoms and cortisol measures in a police cohort. *Journal of Addictions Nursing, 23*, 22–29.
187. Pico-Alfonso, M. A., Garcia-Linares, M. I., Celda-Navarro, N., Herbert, J., & Martinez, M. (2004). Changes in cortisol and dehydroepiandrosterone in women victims of physical and psychological intimate partner violence. *Biological Psychiatry, 56*, 233–240.
188. Shaheen, M., et al. (2018). Victims of war-Psychoendocrine evidence for the impact of traumatic stress on psychological Well-being of adolescents growing up during the Israeli-Palestinian conflict. *Psychophysiology*, e13271. https://doi.org/10.1111/psyp.13271.
189. Young, E. A., & Breslau, N. (2004). Saliva cortisol in posttraumatic stress disorder: A community epidemiologic study. *Biological Psychiatry, 56*, 205–209.
190. Boeckel, M. G., Viola, T. W., Daruy-Filho, L., Martinez, M., & Grassi-Oliveira, R. (2017). Intimate partner violence is associated with increased maternal hair cortisol in mother-child dyads. *Comprehensive Psychiatry, 72*, 18–24.
191. Pinna, K. L. M., Johnson, D. M., & Delahanty, D. L. (2014). PTSD, comorbid depression, and the cortisol waking response in victims of intimate partner violence: Preliminary evidence. *Anxiety, Stress, and Coping, 27*, 253–269.
192. Nicolson, N. A., & Ponnamperuma, T. (2019). Gender moderates diurnal cortisol in relation to trauma and PTSD symptoms: A study in Sri Lankan adolescents. *Psychoneuroendocrinology, 104*, 122–131.
193. Schindler, L., et al. (2019). Victims of war: Dehydroepiandrosterone concentrations in hair and their associations with trauma Sequelae in Palestinian adolescents living in the West Bank. *Brain Sciences, 9*.
194. Spivak, B., Maayan, R., Mester, R., & Weizman, A. (2003). Plasma testosterone levels in patients with combat-related posttraumatic stress disorder. *Neuropsychobiology, 47*, 57–60.
195. van der Hal-Van Raalte, E. A. M., Bakermans-Kranenburg, M. J., & van Ijzendoorn, M. H. (2008). Diurnal cortisol patterns and stress reactivity in child holocaust survivors reaching old age. *Aging & Mental Health, 12*, 630–638.
196. Young, E. A., Tolman, R., Witkowski, K., & Kaplan, G. (2004). Salivary cortisol and posttraumatic stress disorder in a low-income community sample of women. *Biological Psychiatry, 55*, 621–626.
197. Cordero, M. I., et al. (2017). Effects of interpersonal violence-related post-traumatic stress disorder (PTSD) on mother and child diurnal cortisol rhythm and cortisol reactivity to a laboratory stressor involving separation. *Hormones and Behavior, 90*, 15–24.

198. Suglia, S. F., Staudenmayer, J., Cohen, S., & Wright, R. J. (2010). Posttraumatic stress symptoms related to community violence and children's diurnal cortisol response in an urban community-dwelling sample. *International Journal of Behavioral Medicine, 17*, 43–50.
199. Bierer, L. M., et al. (2006). Clinical correlates of 24-h cortisol and norepinephrine excretion among subjects seeking treatment following the world trade center attacks on 9/11. *Annals of the New York Academy of Sciences, 1071*, 514–520.
200. Yehuda, R., Golier, J. A., & Kaufman, S. (2005). Circadian rhythm of salivary cortisol in holocaust survivors with and without PTSD. *The American Journal of Psychiatry, 162*, 998–1000.
201. Basu, A., Levendosky, A. A., & Lonstein, J. S. (2013). Trauma sequelae and cortisol levels in women exposed to intimate partner violence. *Psychodynamic Psychiatry, 41*, 247–275.
202. Yehuda, R., et al. (1995). Low urinary cortisol excretion in holocaust survivors with posttraumatic stress disorder. *The American Journal of Psychiatry, 152*, 982–986.
203. Wessa, M., Rohleder, N., Kirschbaum, C., & Flor, H. (2006). Altered cortisol awakening response in posttraumatic stress disorder. *Psychoneuroendocrinology, 31*, 209–215.
204. Witteveen, A. B., et al. (2010). Associations of cortisol with posttraumatic stress symptoms and negative life events: A study of police officers and firefighters. *Psychoneuroendocrinology, 35*, 1113–1118.
205. Fazel, S., et al. (2015). Depression and violence: A Swedish population study. *Lancet Psychiatry, 2*, 224–232.
206. Kofler, M. J., et al. (2011). Depression and delinquency covariation in an accelerated longitudinal sample of adolescents. *Journal of Consulting and Clinical Psychology, 79*, 458–469.
207. Látalová, K. (2009). Bipolar disorder and aggression. *International Journal of Clinical Practice, 63*, 889–899.
208. Volavka, J. (2013). Violence in schizophrenia and bipolar disorder. *Psychiatria Danubina, 25*, 24–33.
209. Corry, N. H., Kulka, R., & Fairbank, J. A. (2016). Forty years after the war: How are Vietnam veterans doing today? *PTSD Res. Q., 27*, 1050–1835.
210. Kessler, R. C., et al. (2017). Trauma and PTSD in the WHO world mental health surveys. *European Journal of Psychotraumatology, 8*, 1353383.
211. MacManus, D., et al. (2015). Aggressive and violent behavior among military personnel deployed to Iraq and Afghanistan: Prevalence and link with deployment and combat exposure. *Epidemiologic Reviews, 37*, 196–212.
212. Javidi, H., & Yadollahie, M. (2012). Post-traumatic stress disorder. *International Journal of Occupational and Environmental Medicine, 3*, 2–9.
213. Fairchild, G. (2012). Hypothalamic-pituitary-adrenocortical axis function in attention-deficit hyperactivity disorder. *Current Topics in Behavioral Neurosciences, 9*, 93–111.
214. Coccaro, E. F. (2019). Psychiatric comorbidity in intermittent explosive disorder. *Journal of Psychiatric Research, 118*, 38–43.
215. McElroy, S. L., Soutullo, C. A., Beckman, D. A., Taylor, P., & Keck, P. E. (1998). DSM-IV intermittent explosive disorder: A report of 27 cases. *The Journal of Clinical Psychiatry, 59*, 203–210; quiz 211.
216. McElroy, S. L. (1999). Recognition and treatment of DSM-IV intermittent explosive disorder. *The Journal of Clinical Psychiatry, 60*(Suppl 15), 12–16.
217. Coccaro, E. F. (2012). Intermittent explosive disorder as a disorder of impulsive aggression for DSM-5. *The American Journal of Psychiatry, 169*, 577–588.
218. Taft, C. T., et al. (2007). Posttraumatic stress disorder symptoms, physiological reactivity, alcohol problems, and aggression among military veterans. *Journal of Abnormal Psychology, 116*, 498–507.
219. Murakami, S., Rappaport, N., & Penn, J. V. (2006). An overview of juveniles and school violence. *The Psychiatric Clinics of North America, 29*, 725–741.
220. Couture, S., et al. (2008). Hypothalamic-pituitary-adrenal axis response to stress in male DUI recidivists. *Accident; Analysis and Prevention, 40*, 246–253.

221. Gowin, J. L., et al. (2013). The role of cortisol and psychopathy in the cycle of violence. *Psychopharmacology, 227*, 661–672.
222. Cima, M., Smeets, T., & Jelicic, M. (2008). Self-reported trauma, cortisol levels, and aggression in psychopathic and non-psychopathic prison inmates. *Biological Psychology, 78*, 75–86.
223. Brewer-Smyth, K., Burgess, A. W., & Shults, J. (2004). Physical and sexual abuse, salivary cortisol, and neurologic correlates of violent criminal behavior in female prison inmates. *Biological Psychiatry, 55*, 21–31.
224. Dabbs, J. M., Jurkovic, G. J., & Frady, R. L. (1991). Salivary testosterone and cortisol among late adolescent male offenders. *Journal of Abnormal Child Psychology, 19*, 469–478.
225. van der Meij, L., et al. (2015). Football fan aggression: The importance of low basal cortisol and a fair referee. *PLoS One, 10*, e0120103.
226. Gostisha, A. J., et al. (2014). Beyond physiological hypoarousal: The role of life stress and callous-unemotional traits in incarcerated adolescent males. *Hormones and Behavior, 65*, 469–479.
227. Halpern, C. T., Campbell, B., Agnew, C. R., Thompson, V., & Udry, J. R. (2002). Associations between stress reactivity and sexual and nonsexual risk taking in young adult human males. *Hormones and Behavior, 42*, 387–398.
228. Couture, S., et al. (2018). Blunted cortisol reactivity and risky driving in young offenders - a pilot study. *International Journal of Adolescent Medicine and Health*. https://doi.org/10.1515/ijamh-2017-0123.
229. Horn, M., et al. (2014). Male inmate profiles and their biological correlates. *The Canadian Journal of Psychiatry, 59*, 441–449.
230. Wagner, N. J., Mills-Koonce, W. R., Willoughby, M. T., Cox, M. J., & Family Life Project Key Investigators. (2019). Parenting and cortisol in infancy interactively predict conduct problems and callous-unemotional behaviors in childhood. *Child Development, 90*, 279–297.
231. Saridjan, N. S., et al. (2014). The longitudinal association of the diurnal cortisol rhythm with internalizing and externalizing problems in pre-schoolers. The Generation R Study. *Psychoneuroendocrinology, 50*, 118–129.
232. Mills-Koonce, W. R., et al. (2015). Greater fear reactivity and psychophysiological hyperactivity among infants with later conduct problems and callous-unemotional traits. *Journal of Child Psychology and Psychiatry, 56*, 147–154.
233. Nofech-Mozes, J., Pereira, J., Gonzalez, A., & Atkinson, L. (2019). Cortisol secretion moderates the association between mother-infant attachment at 17 months and child behavior at age 5 years. *Developmental Psychobiology, 61*, 239–253.
234. Frost, A., Jelinek, C., Bernard, K., Lind, T., & Dozier, M. (2018). Longitudinal associations between low morning cortisol in infancy and anger dysregulation in early childhood in a CPS-referred sample. *Developmental Science, 21*, e12573.
235. Shirtcliff, E. A., & Essex, M. J. (2008). Concurrent and longitudinal associations of basal and diurnal cortisol with mental health symptoms in early adolescence. *Developmental Psychobiology, 50*, 690–703.
236. Pauli-Pott, U., Schloß, S., Skoluda, N., Nater, U. M., & Becker, K. (2019). Low hair cortisol concentration predicts the development of attention deficit hyperactivity disorder. *Psychoneuroendocrinology, 110*, 104442.
237. Salis, K. L., Bernard, K., Black, S. R., Dougherty, L. R., & Klein, D. (2016). Examining the concurrent and longitudinal relationship between diurnal cortisol rhythms and conduct problems during childhood. *Psychoneuroendocrinology, 71*, 147–154.
238. Frost, A., et al. (2019). Homotypic and heterotypic continuity of internalizing and externalizing symptoms from ages 3 to 12: The moderating role of diurnal cortisol. *Development and Psychopathology, 31*, 789–798.
239. Ruttle, P. L., et al. (2011). Disentangling psychobiological mechanisms underlying internalizing and externalizing behaviors in youth: Longitudinal and concurrent associations with cortisol. *Hormones and Behavior, 59*, 123–132.

240. Alink, L. R. A., Cicchetti, D., Kim, J., & Rogosch, F. A. (2012). Longitudinal associations among child maltreatment, social functioning, and cortisol regulation. *Developmental Psychology, 48*, 224–236.
241. Shoal, G. D., Giancola, P. R., & Kirillova, G. P. (2003). Salivary cortisol, personality, and aggressive behavior in adolescent boys: A 5-year longitudinal study. *Journal of the American Academy of Child and Adolescent Psychiatry, 42*, 1101–1107.
242. Sondeijker, F. E. P. L., et al. (2008). HPA-axis activity as a predictor of future disruptive behaviors in young adolescents. *Psychophysiology, 45*, 398–404.
243. Shirtcliff, E. A., Granger, D. A., Booth, A., & Johnson, D. (2005). Low salivary cortisol levels and externalizing behavior problems in youth. *Development and Psychopathology, 17*, 167–184.
244. Platje, E., et al. (2013). A longitudinal biosocial study of cortisol and peer influence on the development of adolescent antisocial behavior. *Psychoneuroendocrinology, 38*, 2770–2779.
245. Yu, R., Branje, S., Meeus, W., Cowen, P., & Fazel, S. (2019). Depression, violence and cortisol awakening response: A 3-year longitudinal study in adolescents. *Psychological Medicine, 49*, 997–1004.
246. Kempes, M., Matthys, W., de Vries, H., & van Engeland, H. (2005). Reactive and proactive aggression in children--a review of theory, findings and the relevance for child and adolescent psychiatry. *European Child & Adolescent Psychiatry, 14*, 11–19.
247. Lopez-Duran, N. L., Olson, S. L., Hajal, N. J., Felt, B. T., & Vazquez, D. M. (2009). Hypothalamic pituitary adrenal axis functioning in reactive and proactive aggression in children. *Journal of Abnormal Child Psychology, 37*, 169–182.
248. McBurnett, K., King, J., & Scarpa, A. (2003). The HPA and the development of aggressive, antisocial, and substance abuse disorders. In D. Cicchetti & E. Walker (Eds.), *Neurodevelopmental mechanisms in psychopathology* (pp. 324–344). Cambridge University Press, Cambridge.
249. O'Neal, C. R., et al. (2010). Understanding relations among early family environment, cortisol response, and child aggression via a prevention experiment. *Child Development, 81*, 290–305.
250. Poustka, L., et al. (2010). Negative association between plasma cortisol levels and aggression in a high-risk community sample of adolescents. *Journal of Neural Transmission, 1996*(117), 621–627.
251. van Bokhoven, I., et al. (2005). Salivary cortisol and aggression in a population-based longitudinal study of adolescent males. *Journal of Neural Transmission, 112*, 1083–1096.
252. van Honk, J., Harmon-Jones, E., Morgan, B. E., & Schutter, D. J. L. G. (2010). Socially explosive minds: The triple imbalance hypothesis of reactive aggression. *Journal of Personality, 78*, 67–94.
253. Haller, J. (2018). Preclinical models of conduct disorder - principles and pharmacologic perspectives. *Neuroscience and Biobehavioral Reviews, 91*, 112–120.
254. Yehuda, R., et al. (2015). Cortisol augmentation of a psychological treatment for warfighters with posttraumatic stress disorder: Randomized trial showing improved treatment retention and outcome. *Psychoneuroendocrinology, 51*, 589–597.
255. Kling, M. A., Coleman, V. H., & Schulkin, J. (2009). Glucocorticoid inhibition in the treatment of depression: Can we think outside the endocrine hypothalamus? *Depression and Anxiety, 26*, 641–649.
256. Sigalas, P. D., Garg, H., Watson, S., McAllister-Williams, R. H., & Ferrier, I. N. (2012). Metyrapone in treatment-resistant depression. *Therapeutic Advances in Psychopharmacology, 2*, 139–149.
257. Repple, J., et al. (2018). Sex differences in the neural correlates of aggression. *Brain Structure & Function, 223*, 4115–4124.
258. Buades-Rotger, M., Serfling, G., Harbeck, B., Brabant, G., & Krämer, U. M. (2016). Prednisolone increases neural reactivity to negative socio-emotional stimuli in healthy young men. *European Neuropsychopharmacology, 26*, 1176–1189.

259. Moeller, F. G., et al. (1996). Tryptophan depletion and aggressive responding in healthy males. *Psychopharmacology, 126*, 97–103.
260. Tafet, G. E., Toister-Achituv, M., & Shinitzky, M. (2001). Enhancement of serotonin uptake by cortisol: A possible link between stress and depression. *Cognitive, Affective, & Behavioral Neuroscience, 1*, 96–104.
261. Waltes, R., Chiocchetti, A. G., & Freitag, C. M. (2016). The neurobiological basis of human aggression: A review on genetic and epigenetic mechanisms. *American Journal of Medical Genetics Part B, 171*, 650–675.
262. Lupien, S. J., McEwen, B. S., Gunnar, M. R., & Heim, C. (2009). Effects of stress throughout the lifespan on the brain, behaviour and cognition. *Nature Reviews. Neuroscience, 10*, 434–445.
263. Cattane, N., Rossi, R., Lanfredi, M., & Cattaneo, A. (2017). Borderline personality disorder and childhood trauma: Exploring the affected biological systems and mechanisms. *BMC Psychiatry, 17*, 221.
264. Martín-Blanco, A., et al. (2014). Association between methylation of the glucocorticoid receptor gene, childhood maltreatment, and clinical severity in borderline personality disorder. *Journal of Psychiatric Research, 57*, 34–40.
265. Raine, A. (2018). Antisocial personality as a neurodevelopmental disorder. *Annual Review of Clinical Psychology, 14*, 259–289.
266. Labonté, B., Azoulay, N., Yerko, V., Turecki, G., & Brunet, A. (2014). Epigenetic modulation of glucocorticoid receptors in posttraumatic stress disorder. *Translational Psychiatry, 4*, e368.
267. Wang, D., et al. (2012). Peripheral SLC6A4 DNA methylation is associated with in vivo measures of human brain serotonin synthesis and childhood physical aggression. *PLoS One, 7*, e39501.
268. Walker, S. E., Papilloud, A., Huzard, D., & Sandi, C. (2018). The link between aberrant hypothalamic-pituitary-adrenal axis activity during development and the emergence of aggression-animal studies. *Neuroscience and Biobehavioral Reviews, 91*, 138–152.

Chapter 7
The Aggression Circuitry in Animals

Introduction

The brain control of aggression has been studied for nearly a hundred years with a number of technologies that have become increasingly sophisticated. During this long period, there were several phases when the issue seemed to have been solved: aggression control appeared to have been revealed; however, novel research methodologies have refuted this feeling time and time again. Today, we are witnessing an advance in research technologies that we would have thought unimaginable only a decade ago. As usual, these new technologies put a question mark on what was thought true and reliable earlier; however, there also is a consistency in knowledge. New discoveries did not entirely invalidate previous ones but added new details, explored unknown mechanisms, and incorporated the approaches from other fields.

The purpose of this chapter is to integrate old and new discoveries into a single concept that accounts for, on the one hand, the complexity of neurons and network architectures and, on the other, the complexity of aggressive behavior. The created template will be used in subsequent chapters to understand what goes wrong with neural control in models of abnormal aggression and how normal and abnormal human aggression is controlled.

7.1 A Brief History

The history of research into the neurobiology of aggression can be divided into four epochs. The first began in 1928 when the Swiss Nobel laureate Walter Rudolf Hess studied the role of the diencephalon in the control of internal organs and observed that the electric stimulation of particular hypothalamic regions elicited excitement

J. Haller, *Neurobiopsychosocial Perspectives on Aggression and Violence*,
Advances in Preventing and Treating Violence and Aggression,
https://doi.org/10.1007/978-3-030-46331-1_7

and a series of behaviors reminiscent of attack and escape [1]. Subsequent research identified a hypothalamic subregion – the "hypothalamic attack area" – which is tightly involved in the control of biting attacks. Hess's discovery developed later into a research field that ultimately outlined the neural circuitry underlying aggressive behaviors in animals, mostly cats and rats. Notable scientists of this field include John P. Flynn, who together with various coauthors discovered the role of the amygdala in the circuitry [2] and described the sensory control of hypothalamic attack sites [3]; David B. Adams [4] and Richard J. Bandler Jr. [5] who recognized the role of the periaqueductal gray; Menno R. Kruk, who mapped and differentiated hypothalamic areas involved in the control of various behaviors [6] and described the hormonal (e.g., androgenic [7]) and pharmacologic (e.g., serotonergic [8]) control of the hypothalamic attack area; and many other eminent scientists the work of whom is difficult to disentangle after such a long time. One of the pinnacles of this research was the work by Alan Siegel, whose systematic research spanned more than four decades [9, 10] and decisively contributed to our understanding of the brain circuitry of aggressive behavior. The basic methodologies employed included electric stimulation, brain lesion, pathway mapping, and the local administration of various chemicals, including neurotransmitters and hormones. The end product of this research line was a map of the aggression circuitry, with indications on the neurochemical processes involved. This map is highly influential even today for both animal and human research. From a human perspective, important by-products were techniques that aimed at controlling pathological forms of human aggression. This issue will be addressed in the next section.

The "brain stimulation epoch" was followed by the "neurochemistry/pharmacology epoch" which was initiated in the 1960s by important discoveries concerning the roles of dopamine [11], norepinephrine [12], serotonin [13], and other neurotransmitters later on. Studies of this kind did not strive at anatomical precision although the application of the microinjection technique in behavioral studies one decade later [14] and the development of the punch sampling technique almost two decades later [15] did allow for such investigations. Basically, researchers measured neurotransmitter levels and neurotransmitter turnover rates (in simple terms the ratio of the neurotransmitter and its key metabolites) and corroborated their level with the level of aggressive behaviors or administered pharmacological agents to alter neurotransmission and to investigate behavioral consequences. The end products of this research line were treatments employed clinically. The agents developed include the D2 dopamine receptor antagonist haloperidol and the mixed D2/5-HT2A serotonin antagonist olanzapine which are considered the best choices for acute outbursts of aggression, even today [16], and serotonin reuptake inhibitors and antagonists of the 5-HT1B serotonin and β norepinephrine receptors for more chronic aggression problems [17]. Later, research into the pharmacology of aggression was extended towards other neurotransmitter systems, e.g., vasopressin [18–20], oxytocin [20–22], γ-aminobutyric acid (GABA) [23, 24], endocannabinoid signaling [25], etc. Research into these neurotransmitter systems also provided leads to the development of anti-aggression treatments [26–28].

The next epoch was allowed by the study of immediate early genes, first by bacteriologists and [29] then by neuroscientists [30]. This class of genes includes about 40 members, which are activated rapidly and transiently, and the protein products of which are transcription factors. The best known member of the family, the c-Fos, was studied in aggression research from the mid-1990s onwards [31, 32]. Essentially, animals were exposed to the resident–intruder test; their brain was sampled, sliced, and stained for the c-Fos protein. As the protein specifically concentrates in the nuclei of those neurons, which were intensely active during conflict, the technique allowed for the mapping of the neuron populations which played roles in the behavioral response, e.g., aggression. The technique significantly contributed to the mapping of the aggression circuitry, especially as it was combined with neurochemical markers to uncover both the location and the neurochemical identity of the neurons activated by aggression. The end products of the technology were also maps as with brain stimulations, which, however, were more comprehensive and detailed.

Finally, current aggression research, the "fourth epoch," heavily relies on several modern technologies, including optogenetics, the Designer Receptors Exclusively Activated by Designer Drugs (DREADD) technology, and epigenetics. Optogenetics can be traced back to the 1970s when light-sensitive ion-trafficking proteins were discovered in the cellular membranes of microorganisms [33]. The insertion of the genes of such proteins into neurons made these neurons light-sensitive, offering a unique way to stimulate and inhibit or "silence" neurons by channelrhodopsin-2 [34] and halorhodopsin [35], respectively. In aggression research, the technique was first employed in 2011 [36], 4 years after its introduction into behavioral science [37]. The combination of optogenetics with other advanced gene engineering techniques makes the technology one of the most powerful tools of neuroscientific research developed so far. The core of the DREADD technology is the engineering of G protein-coupled receptors such to respond exclusively to synthetic ligands, e.g., clozapine N-oxide. The systemic injection of the ligand activates the neurons that were made to express the engineered receptors, by this allowing their selective study. The combination of this with other advanced gene technologies can make stimulation exquisitely selective.

DREADD is technically simpler than optogenetics and almost does not disturb the animal, yet its time resolution is considerably poorer. Optogenetics allows the free choice of stimulation frequencies, and the start and end of the stimulation can also be controlled as desired. In contrast, the effect of the DREADD ligand develops gradually over 30 min, and the time course of the effect cannot be changed; the stimulation lasts about an hour. The technology was first used in aggression research in 2016 [38], but only three studies were published with this technology so far.

In its turn, epigenetics – the remodeling of the chromatin after birth – has a long history in virology and cancerology [39, 40] but was introduced into aggression research in 2008 only [41]. Since then, it became very popular and was used considerably more frequently than the two technologies briefly described above. In fact, epigenetics offers molecular genetic mechanisms for neural plasticity, which was studied earlier to explain long-term alterations in aggression [42]. The short history of optogenetics, DREADD, and epigenetic research does not allow estimates on their end products. So far, findings are like pieces of a mosaic where the picture is not discernable yet, but they allow the understanding of aggression control with unprecedented detail.

Naturally, there is no clear demarcation line between the four epochs; the various technologies were used in parallel, often in combination. In addition, there are a series of other technologies – e.g., immunohistochemistry – which were continuously used over time. Nevertheless, each epoch had its leading technology and unique contributions for understanding the neural control of aggression.

7.2 Theoretical Considerations

7.2.1 Simple Networks for Complex Neurons?

According to the biological approach, aggression is triggered by the perception of a competitive situation and consists in a series of muscle contractions that are organized into behaviors that ensure benefit – the exclusion of competitors from the enjoyment of resources. The task of neural mechanisms is to link perceptions to muscle contractions, interpret the former, compare them with memory traces and the actual physiological state of the organism, elaborate decisions, and implement them as muscle contractions in accordance with opponent behavior and environmental events. The neural mechanisms also evaluate the outcome of the conflict to generate subsequent actions. The basics of this up- and downward information flow were summarized in Fig. 7.1.

According to the classical view, the neural mechanisms of aggression are organized hierarchically at both neuronal and brain levels. Neuron A – for instance, a sensory neuron – sends an impulse to neuron B, which transmits it to neuron C and so forth till neuron N elicits muscle contraction. Along the way, information is processed by local microcircuits and the accumulation of information that arrives from different sources. This implies that there is a bottom-up stream of information that informs the prefrontal cortex – the highest decision-making area of the brain – and a top-down flux of "commands" that transmits the decision to executory neural elements and finally to the muscles. This approach was adopted early on and constitutes the backbone of the present view on the circuits that control aggression (Fig. 7.2, left-hand panel).

Although it is not necessarily false, the structure of neurons (Fig. 7.2, right-hand panel) suggests that the classical approach to the mechanisms of aggression is rather simplistic. For instance, information is not transmitted linearly along pathways. Instead of being part of the "A → B → C → […] → N" type of information chain, each neuron forms itself an immensely complex network by receiving thousands of synaptic inputs from and sending out thousands of synaptic efferents to other neurons [44, 45]. Although about half of the contacts are established with neighboring neurons, the other half links neurons that are located far away in diverse areas of the brain, and instead of having a clear direction (e.g., bottom-up or top-down),

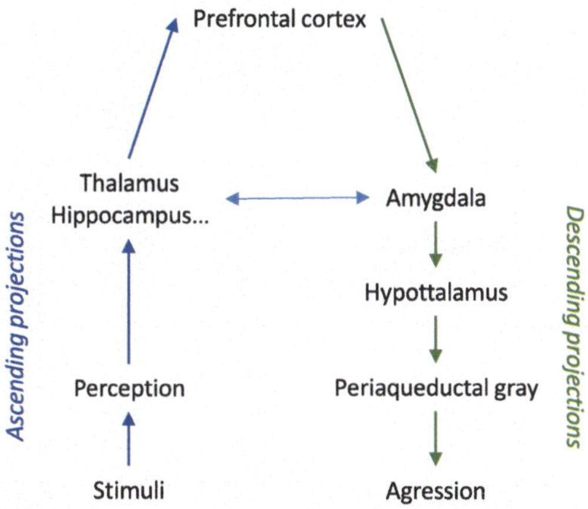

Fig. 7.1 The general organization of aggression control. It is generally believed that the mechanisms controlling behavior are organized into ascending pathways that process information coming from internal and external organs and terminate in the prefrontal cortex, which makes decisions that are transmitted to executory organs via descending pathways as commands. Commands are on their turn also processed along their way to executory organs and may or may not lead to action depending on the circumstances. The schematic shows the main centers of the pathways, which are specific to aggression only on the right-hand (downstream) side. The thalamus and hippocampus process all information before they reach the prefrontal cortex and can at the same time activate memories, attribute value to possible actions, etc. irrespective to the behavior to be controlled. Therefore, we will focus on the downstream pathways in the following

projections may go either or both ways. Without going into technical detail, it is also worth to note that the location of the synapse has a large impact on the consequences of information transfer. For example, an inhibitory input blocks a subgroup of other inputs, if it is located on the apical segment of a dendritic branch, but it may block all efferents if located at the apical segment of the axon. In addition to this complex synaptic organization, neurons are also influenced non-synaptically via neurotransmitter receptors located outside the synapse [46]. This non-synaptic communication, renamed later "volume transmission," [47] is common with serotonergic and noradrenergic neurotransmission [48] but was observed in several other systems, including opiate neurotransmission in various brain areas [47] and GABAergic communication in the neocortex [49]. In addition to complications derived from the complex synaptic network of neurons, and distant and concomitant influences received non-synaptically, the whole brain is subject to a complex array of hormonal effects, including glucocorticoids which were described in detail above.

Each neuron is a nonlinear computing machine, rather than a link in a chain. Consequently, it is highly unlikely that the aggression circuitry is organized hierarchically into ascending and descending pathways, as will be shown below, primarily for the hypothalamic attack area. Each node of the circuitry is influenced by and influences a myriad of other neurons located upstream, downstream, or horizontally. Aggression results from a multidirectional and multidimensional neural communication network, and the complexities of which are just emerging.

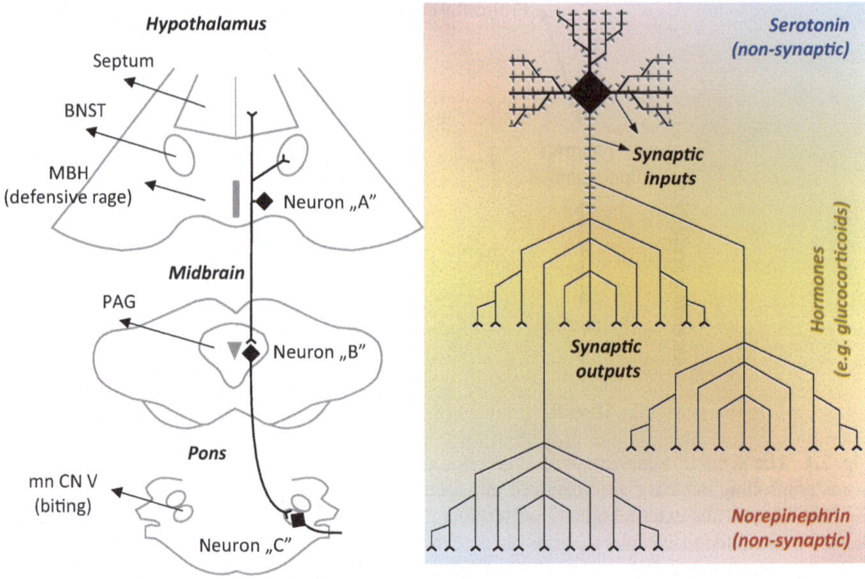

Fig. 7.2 The hierarchical control concept vis-a-vis neuron structure. *Left-hand panel.* Fragment of the circuit that controls aggression (compiled based on Siegel and Kruk [43]). It shows how hypothalamic stimulation leads to biting in cats by a microcircuit encompassing the mediobasal hypothalamus (MBH), periaqueductal gray (PAG), and the motor nucleus of the fifth cranial nerve (mn CN V). The stimulus also reaches the bed nucleus of stria terminalis (BNST) and septum. *Right-hand panel.* A schematic representation of a typical neuron, which receives thousands of synaptic inputs (only 137 shown in the figure) and establishes thousands of synapses with other neurons (only 32 shown in the figure). Inputs were not shown on axonal branches for clarity. The neuron is surrounded by a "bath" of neurotransmitters that affect its functions non-synaptically and hormones that affect its function and molecular microstructure non-genomically and genomically, respectively

7.2.2 The Organization of the Circuitry: A Hypothesis

Aggression research failed so far to incorporate ideas as complex as those presented above. This is not surprising as the intricacies of neural network building are a hot area of neuroscience that has much to discover before being able to penetrate behavioral science. In view of this complexity and on findings obtained so far, however, one can hypothesize that the circuitry of aggression has four domains.

1. A "core circuitry" that processes environmental and internal information, elaborates decisions, and controls aggressive responses. Within this circuitry, information transfer may not be unidirectional, and pathways may branch out, but without this circuitry, aggressive behavior cannot be performed.
2. An "accessory system" consisting of synaptic inputs that affect the function of the core circuitry. Instead of controlling behavior, they control those neurons that

control behavior. One can assume that the elements of this system do not form a unitary network as the core circuitry does. It is more likely that it is composed of independent local circuits and distant influence areas as those proposed below for the prefrontal cortex and the hypothalamic attack area, respectively. This system is highly specific as its effects are exerted on specific neurons and specific neuron parts. Nevertheless, aggression can be performed and can be more easily performed without these accessory areas, as shown by lesion experiments.

3. An "attuning system" consisting mainly of the monoaminergic systems, primarily those parts of these that communicate non-synaptically. They affect extended brain areas concomitantly which excludes specific behavioral effects; consequently, their effects cover most if not all aspects of cognition, emotion, and behavior. Instead of controlling behaviors directly, this system attunes neural circuits to momentary external influences and internal states.
4. An "organizing system," which includes hormones that reach the brain via the circulation. Glucocorticoids were presented in detail above. Testosterone is another important organizing hormone that affects aggressive behavior from birth to elderly and programs brain development on the long run and brain function on the medium term. This system is differentiated from the previous one by its complex structural and functional organizing role that extends well beyond momentary events. Another difference relates to tie-ins by which neural "commands" elaborated under hormonal influences are supported by their own somatic effects.

7.3 Core Networks

7.3.1 *Behaviors Controlled by the Core Networks*

The core networks presented below refer to three forms of aggression: male rivalry aggression; predatory aggression, which is displayed by both genders but is mostly studied in males; and maternal aggression displayed by females when protecting pups from potentially infanticidal males.

Rivalry aggression is prototypically biological as it is tightly connected to resource competition. The neural background of this aggression type was studied by electric stimulation, mostly in cats and rats, and by means of the resident–intruder test in various rodent species. Although aggression elicited by electric stimulation is not competitive – i.e., it is not induced by a social challenge – and does not lead to benefit, it is also highly similar to rivalry aggression in terms of the attack behaviors displayed [50, 51], hormonal backgrounds [7, 52, 53], pharmacologic responsiveness [43, 54], and brain mechanisms [55]. As such, the neural background of natural rivalry aggression and of attacks induced by electric stimulation will be discussed together.

Predatory aggression – although a form of feeding – falls within the scope of this chapter because its neural mechanisms are operational under certain conditions in real competitive situations, i.e., when the members of the same species fight for resources. In addition, similarities in the neural mechanisms of predation are seen in abnormal rivalry aggression as shown in the next section. This behavior was studied mostly by stimulation techniques, but many studies investigated more naturalistic behaviors, e.g., spontaneous mouse or frog killing by rats and cricket killing by rats and mice.

Maternal aggression serves inclusive fitness, i.e., the transmission of genes to the next generation, and, as such, it fulfils the requirements of the biological approach. It consists in violent attacks on unfamiliar male intruders, which are likely to kill pups to increase the mother's inclusive fitness. Dams do not attack virgin female intruders; virgin females are not infanticidal and hence not a threat to the inclusive fitness of the dam. Therefore, in experiments, virgin females were often used as comparisons.

The three behaviors can be divided into two major groups, with rivalry aggression on one side and predatory and maternal aggressions on the other. The grouping factors are the nature of attack and its glucocorticoid background. In contrast to rivalry aggression, predatory and maternal attacks are poorly signaled by social threats, are potentially life-threatening, and are performed on the background of low glucocorticoid stress responses [56, 57].

7.3.2 Overview

It is widely accepted that the core circuitry of aggression includes the following five levels and functions (in blunt terms): (1) the prefrontal cortex where decisions are made; (2) the amygdala, which transmits the decision by adding an emotional component; (3) the hypothalamus, which elicits complete movement patterns that consist in biting attacks (the essence of aggression in the species studied); (4) the periaqueductal gray, which integrates autonomic and behavioral responses; and (5) executory neural centers including those involved in autonomic control (e.g., spinal ganglions), biting (motor nucleus of the trigeminal nerve, cranial nerve V), and movements (spinal cord).

The core circuits of rivalry (intraspecific) and predatory (interspecific) aggression are different but are located in close vicinity (Fig. 7.3). The connectivity was deduced from co-stimulation and lesion studies (see below) and based on structural equation modeling of brain activation patterns [58]. Notably, the neural mechanisms underlying maternal aggression incorporate both circuits as shown below.

Both arms of the schematic were described already by the Siegel group over several decades of systematic research (see Siegel and Kruk [43] for a review). In addition to showing that the stimulation of the mediobasal hypothalamus and dorsal periaqueductal gray elicits a behavior called "defensive rage" (emotional aggression), the stimulation of lateral hypothalamus and ventral periaqueductal gray elic-

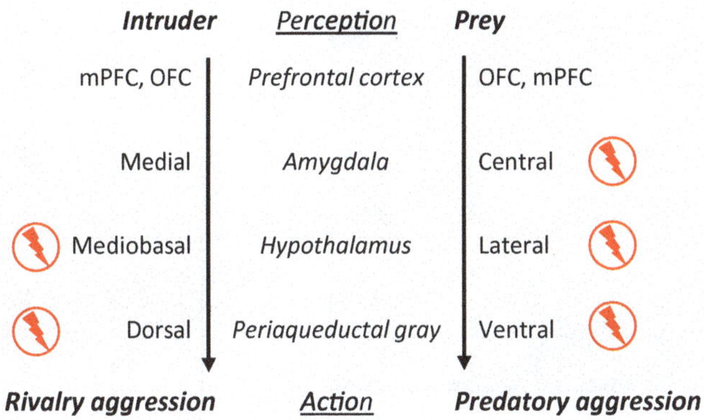

Fig. 7.3 Core circuits of rivalry and predatory aggressions. The composite figure summarizes findings obtained in a variety of species by several neuroscientific methods. *Arrow* assumed flow of information, *encircled lightning symbol* structures from where the respective form of attack can be elicited by electric stimulation, *mPFC, OFC* medial prefrontal cortex, orbitofrontal cortex. Note that attack type-specific prefrontal regions were not differentiated so far

its mouse killing (predatory aggression). Siegel's group also traced the anatomical connections and the major neurotransmitters operating within this circuit. This group, however, discovered a reciprocal inhibitory mechanism of the two pathways at the level of the hypothalamus [59]. This mechanism seems to be absent in rodents as shown by the coactivation of the two pathways in maternal aggression and the glucocorticoid deficit model of abnormal aggression [60]. This group did not directly include the prefrontal cortex in this pathway. They assumed that this brain area affects aggression by a multi-synaptic pathway encompassing the medial prefrontal cortex, mediodorsal thalamus, nucleus reuniens of the thalamus, and hypothalamic attack centers [61].

Subsequent developments incorporated the prefrontal cortex into the circuitry by showing that it projects directly to both the medial and central amygdala [62], and to the mediobasal and lateral hypothalamus, and controls both the rivalry and predatory pathways [63]. The predatory pathway described in cats is also operational in rats [64]. Electric stimulation of the central amygdala elicits the whole behavioral sequence of predatory aggression in mice, the key behavioral element being a rapid bite on the head that kills the prey [65]. Finally, brain activation patterns associated with maternal aggression [66–68] revealed that the neural control of this behavior is similar to that observed in predatory aggression, as it involves the activation of the central amygdala and lateral hypothalamus rather than the medial amygdala and mediobasal hypothalamus [69]. For a 3D representation of the system, see Fig. 7.4.

Optogenetic techniques have contributed considerably to the elucidation of the core pathways in the control of aggression. These new developments together with further details on the core networks will be presented in the subsequent sections which analyze in detail the role of the main components of the core networks.

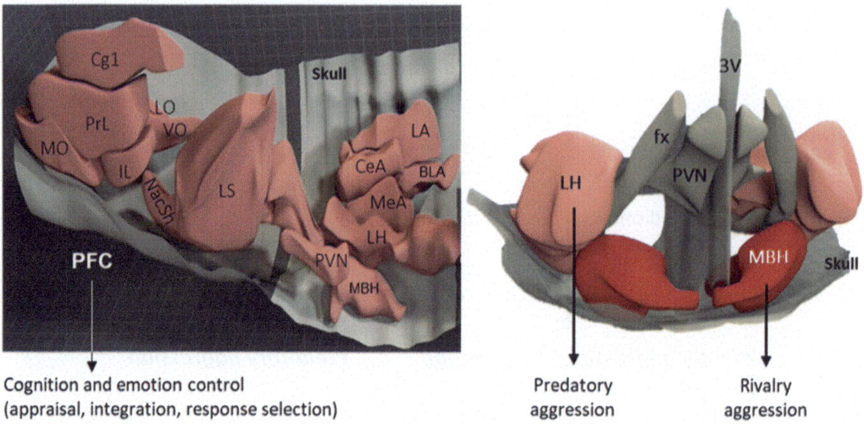

Fig. 7.4 A 3D view on the core circuitry and some accessory systems in the rat. The figure is not comprehensive; it was compiled to give a feeling of the size and spatial location of some of the main elements of the aggression circuitry. All these regions are activated while the animals fight, together with other areas as shown below. *Left-hand panel.* A general view of the system from the prefrontal cortex to the hypothalamus. Only one side of the brain was shown. The remote and long periaqueductal gray was not included to maintain the distinctness of more frontal regions. *Right-hand panel.* A closer look at the circuitry at the hypothalamic level. 3V third ventricle, BLA basolateral amygdala, CeA central amygdala, Cg1 anterior cingulate, fx fornix, IL infralimbic cortex, LA lateral amygdala, LH lateral hypothalamus, LO lateral orbitofrontal cortex, LS lateral septum, MBH mediobasal hypothalamus, MeA medial amygdala, MO medial orbitofrontal cortex, NacSh nucleus accumbens shell, PFC prefrontal cortex, PrL prelimbic cortex, PVN paraventricular nucleus of the hypothalamus, VO ventral orbitofrontal cortex. The authors thanks Áron Tulogdi for compiling this 3D figure based on the atlas of Paxinos and Watson [70]. Versions of this figure were published earlier [71]

7.3.3 The Prefrontal Cortex

The prefrontal cortex (PFC) is the main locus of control for higher cognitive and emotional processes and goal directed behaviors [72, 73]. It is widely accepted that, except for reflexive behavioral responses, the monitoring of ongoing environmental events, the assessment and anticipation of the value of different behavioral options, and behavioral response selection are performed at this level [74–76].

The involvement of the prefrontal cortex in aggression is usually indicated by the phrases "inhibitory control" or "prefrontal deficit theory" involving that this brain area has the role of inhibiting those brain mechanisms that control aggression, primarily the amygdala. The main arguments supporting this assumption are twofold: (1) the stimulation of prefrontal areas in cats inhibited the execution of aggression that was elicited by the stimulation of the hypothalamus [77], and (2) prefrontal lesions increased aggression in various species (e.g., rats [78–80] and monkeys [81, 82]). All these studies assigned a role for the ventral (orbitofrontal) prefrontal cortex; the medial prefrontal cortex did not seem to affect aggression.

If the inhibitory control theory was true, the prefrontal cortex was better placed among the brain areas that belong to the accessory system of the aggression circuitry, as aggression could have been performed without its contribution; moreover, aggression was more intense if the orbitofrontal cortex was eliminated from the circuitry. The negative modulation of aggression by the prefrontal cortex suggests that this brain area is the highest order accessory area of those mechanisms that actually control aggression.

There is, however, recurrent evidence that demonstrates that the prefrontal cortex is activated when animals fight, as shown in rats [71, 83–85] and mice [86–89]. The prefrontal cortex was also activated by hypothalamic stimulation [55], maternal aggression [90], and predation, e.g., mouse killing [64] and insect hunting [91]. In contrast with lesion studies, where the critical area was the orbitofrontal cortex, increased activations were reported also in the medial prefrontal cortex (anterior cingulate, prelimbic, and infralimbic cortices). Note that many of the cited studies focused on abnormal aggression, but here we refer to findings obtained in control animals.

These findings demonstrate that the prefrontal cortex is activated by aggressive encounters, which is at variance with the prefrontal deficit hypothesis of aggression. In theory, one may still assume that this brain area was activated to limit aggression, as aggression has to be stopped once it achieved its goal, e.g., the rival male submitted, the potentially infanticidal male was chased away, or the prey was killed. As such, one can hypothesize that prefrontal activation had the role of limiting aggression when this had to be stopped rather than controlling the fight when it unfolded. Yet, the prefrontal cortex was activated in animals that had no opportunity to fight because they were separated from the opponent by a partition [83, 89] or their head was immobilized to allow for brain imaging [92]. In these cases, there was no aggression to be limited, yet the prefrontal cortex was activated. This evidence suggests that the prefrontal cortex may regulate aggression beyond the mechanism called inhibitory control.

More direct evidence was provided for this assumption by a study employing pathway analysis and axonal optogenetic stimulation techniques in rats [63]. It was established that the mediobasal and lateral hypothalamus, locations associated with rivalry and predatory aggressions, respectively, are innervated by intermingled but predominantly distinct neuron populations of the medial prefrontal cortex, which constitute about 20% of all neurons. In the next step, the stimulatory opsin channelrhodopsin-2 was expressed in neurons of the prelimbic and infralimbic cortices, and their axons were optically stimulated in the mediobasal and lateral hypothalamus. This procedure allowed for the specific upregulation of the prefrontal cortex–mediobasal hypothalamus and the prefrontal cortex–lateral hypothalamus pathways, respectively, without affecting other circuits in the brain. The stimulation of axons in the mediobasal hypothalamus dramatically increased bite counts, whereas axonal stimulation in the lateral hypothalamus specifically increased violent bites on vulnerable body parts of opponents that were poorly signaled socially – i.e., bites reminiscent of predatory attacks. These findings suggest that rats possess distinct prefrontal mechanisms that can stimulate either rivalry or predatory-like attacks by projections that target hypothalamic brain structures specialized for the control of these behaviors. The stimulatory role of distinct prefrontal neural populations is at variance with the prefrontal deficit theory of aggression but does not necessarily disprove it. It is more likely that the prefrontal cortex can do both: it can stimulate aggression by specific subgroups of neurons and can also inhibit it by other neuron subgroups. This possibility was indirectly supported by the anti-aggressive effect of indiscriminate prefrontal stimulations [93]. In this study, optogenetic stimulation targeted the prefrontal cortex, which activated all output regions of the area, as opposed to the previous study, which focused on specific pathways by stimulating remote axon terminals.

The dual ability of stimulating and inhibiting aggression removes the prefrontal cortex from the "accessory system" and establishes it as a true mechanism of control. The findings also explain why no aggression-specific subareas were evidenced earlier in the prefrontal cortex because the specific neurons are intermingled and offer some hints on how decisions are taken. Tentatively, the decision on fighting and its strategy may be limited to selecting the appropriate neuron populations. If the incoming information and its processing by the local cortical networks activate those prefrontal populations that inhibit aggression, then the animals will refrain from fighting; if neurons projecting to the mediobasal or lateral hypothalamus were activated, animals will fight more intensely or more viciously. According to this scenario, the decision is in the hands of local circuits, which ultimately elicit the activation of ruling local neuron populations which generate commands to lower brain areas.

7.3.4 The Amygdala

Following confusing early studies performed in cats, it was gradually recognized that the internal organization of the amygdala has an impact on its role in aggression; however, the roles of various amygdala subregions are different [94]. Rivalry aggression is supported by the cortical, basolateral, and medial part of the cat amygdala, as defensive rage (rivalry-like aggression), which was elicited electrically from the mediobasal hypothalamus and was facilitated when these amygdala regions were co-stimulated [95]. In line with this finding, the destruction of the basolateral or medial amygdala reduced rivalry aggression [96–99], whereas the stimulation of the cortical and medial amygdala facilitated rivalry aggression [100]. In contrast, quiet biting and mouse killing were facilitated by the co-stimulation of the central amygdala and lateral hypothalamus in cats [101] and rats [102], and the destruction of the central amygdala abolished naturally occurring predatory aggression in rodents [103], whereas the stimulation of the central amygdala alone induced predatory attacks in mice [65]. Notably, this is the only amygdala region from where any form of attack can be elicited by electric stimulation. The medial and central amygdala reciprocally inhibit each other's impact on aggression [95, 104], but this seems to be secondary to mutual inhibitions observed at the level of their downstream hypothalamic projections [40].

These results argue for the roles of the two amygdala subregions outlined in Fig. 7.3 and are fully supported by brain activation studies utilizing immediate early gene immunohistochemistry. Rivalry aggression preferentially activates the medial amygdala in all the species studied so far including hamsters [105, 106], mice [88], rats [107, 108], and voles [109, 110]. Notably, aggression and sexual behaviors recruited distinct neuron populations within the medial amygdala [36, 108], and the level of aggression correlated positively with the level of medial amygdala activation [88, 107, 111], suggesting that the association of the medial amygdala with rivalry aggression was specific and not secondary to overall effects on arousal. The basolateral and cortical nuclei were also activated by the resident–intruder test in the very same studies. Predatory aggression was less well studied, but two studies show that mouse killing [64] and insect hunting [91] activate the central amygdala. Notably, the attack type-unspecific amygdala region (e.g., the central amygdala in the case of rivalry and the medial amygdala for predatory aggression) was either not activated or showed a much weaker activation than the attack type-specific amygdala region. Finally, maternal aggression appears to show similarities with the predatory pattern. In contrast to non-lactating females, dams protecting their pups showed a robust activation in the central amygdala [66–68]. Notably, the medial amygdala was also activated, showing that maternal aggression recruits both pathways concurrently.

The amygdala regions involved in the control of aggression – in addition to processing and transmitting commands from the prefrontal cortex to the hypothalamus – appear to integrate social memory to adjust aggressive behavior to memory traces [98] and also appear to integrate the entire spectrum of social behaviors as the decrease in aggression that followed amygdala lesions was associated with an increase in affiliative behaviors [112]. In a somewhat similar vein, lesions placed in the medial amygdala of golden hamsters suggested that this brain region not only reduces pre- and post-copulatory aggression in females but also promotes sexual behaviors [113]. Taken together, these findings suggest that the amygdala augments the command received from the prefrontal cortex by integrating aggressive behavior with other behavioral domains. This is likely achieved by those amygdala inputs that influence the function of the amygdala and which may be parts of the accessory system of the aggression circuitry.

7.3.5 The Hypothalamus

Being the first brain areas connected to the execution of aggression, hypothalamic attack centers remain the focus of research attention, albeit that subsequent research showed that attacks can be elicited by the stimulation of other brain areas such as the central amygdala and the periaqueductal gray (see below). Nevertheless, the hypothalamus remains the major attack-eliciting brain area, due to the reliability of findings and its ubiquitous involvement in aggression [51].

There are two regions of interest: one is situated ventromedially to the fornix and induces affective aggression and another that is located laterally to the fornix and elicits emotionally neutral predatory attacks in a variety of species. The former was named the "hypothalamic attack area" in the rat but identified by the name of the anatomical region in other species (e.g., mediobasal hypothalamus), whereas the latter is usually called simply the lateral hypothalamus. We prefer the anatomy-linked names over behaviorally descriptive appellations.

The electrical stimulation of the mediobasal hypothalamus elicited biting attacks in all the species studied so far, including cats [1], chicken [114], cichlid fish [115], guinea pig [116], lizards [117], marmoset monkeys [118], mice [36], opossum [119], and rats [120]. In rats, for example, the behavioral response starts with a brief orienting response by which the stimulated rat locates the opponent, approaches it, and delivers the biting attack, occasionally by overcoming resistance. The first bite is delivered after about 3–5 seconds, and bites are repeated at intervals of about the same length, although brief episodes of serial biting may also occur. Once stimulation is stopped, animals cease to attack so abruptly that even initiated movements are suspended. The rat never loses contact with the environment – no empty biting occurs, the opponent is followed, its actions are observed, etc. – yet the abrupt ending of attack behavior shows its tight dependence on stimulation. If no opponent was present, the rat remained motionless after a brief orienting response.

The studied vertebrates belong to very different taxa; therefore, the exact anatomical matching of attack sites is difficult; however, it is obvious that small differences in the size and shape of attack-eliciting hypothalamic sites occur even in closely related species. In the rat, these include the posterior part of the anterior hypothalamus, the tuber cinereum, and the ventrolateral aspects of the ventromedial hypothalamus [54], whereas in mice they are restricted to a narrow strip in the ventrolateral part of the ventromedial hypothalamus [36]. Nevertheless, all these and other species have hypothalamic sites from where biting attacks can be elicited by electric stimulation. It remains to be seen whether there are similar hypothalamic regions in species which attack differently, e.g., by butting, but as far as bites are concerned, the mediobasal hypothalamic control appears universal. The lateral hypothalamus was studied less often, but predatory aggression was elicited from lateral hypothalamic sites in at least two species – the cat [43] and the rat [102, 121–123].

In the rat, where the issue was systematically studied, the two "attack areas" are embedded in a hypothalamic region from where a variety of other behaviors can be elicited, including escape jumps [124], feeding [125], food hoarding [126], self-grooming [127], social grooming [6], teeth-chattering [6], and rivalry-like and predatory attacks. Each behavior has its own area within the hypothalamus, although adjacent areas may overlap to a certain extent. Note that rivalry-like, and predatory attack sites are not only distinct but are separated by a strip of neural tissue from where neither behaviors can be elicited. Even when areas do overlap, the behavioral outcome of stimulation can be separated by the intensity of the current that elicits responses. For instance, teeth chattering is elicited by lower current intensities, whereas aggression is elicited by higher current intensities where their control regions overlap. The same applies to overlaps between escape and aggression sites, the former being elicited by approximately five times higher current intensities than attacks. Thus, behaviorally relevant hypothalamic sites are distinct primarily by their specific anatomical location but also by their sensitivity to stimulation.

The universal nature and spatial specificity of hypothalamic attack sites alone suggest that the effects of electric stimulations are not artifacts as suggested for a while. These arguments are strengthened by several other findings, for instance, that attacks can be elicited neurochemically from hypothalamic attack sites in freely moving animals, i.e., without electric currents. In the mediobasal hypothalamus, rivalry aggression can be enhanced by disabling local inhibitory (GABAergic) networks [128, 129] and by stimulating of local stimulatory (glutamatergic) networks [130]. In the lateral hypothalamus, cholinergic agents induced mouse killing in freely moving rats that would not ordinarily kill mice [122]. These findings demonstrate that hypothalamic mechanisms of attack do exist as they can be activated under rather natural circumstances by influencing neural communication. Attacks can also be evoked by optogenetics [36], a technique which eliminates many deficiencies of electric stimulations (e.g., they do not affect nearby, passing fibers). Finally, immediate early gene expression studies show that hypothalamic attack sites are dramatically activated by aggressive encounters. This was true for the activation of the mediobasal hypothalamus by rivalry aggression in cats [131], chicken [132], fish [133], rats [107], golden hamsters [134], Mongolian gerbils [135], Syrian hamsters [105], etc. and for the activation of the lateral hypothalamus by mouse killing [64] and insect hunting in rats [91] and mice [136]. Interestingly, the role of the lateral hypothalamus appears to be overtaken, at least partly, by the medial preoptic area in mice that hunt for insects [137]. In maternal aggression, both the mediobasal and lateral hypothalamus are activated [66], strengthening the view that this type of aggression recruits the rivalry and the predatory circuitry concurrently.

While there remains little doubt regarding the control of attacks by the hypothalamic attack centers, it is entirely unclear how the behavioral response is elicited at this level. The rat has to perform a complex sequence of movements and to adjust its behavior to circumstances and to the behavior of the opponent. For instance, in rats, clinch fights involve bending over the opponent from one side, snatching its flank with teeth on the opposite side, pulling the victim in the air with teeth, and kicking with hind paws to throw the opponent away, all this being performed while the opponent implements countermeasures. This precise sequence of behaviors is inherited because it occurs in animals reared in isolation, i.e., which did not witness it.

Such fixed action patterns (FAPs) require a dedicated neural network that is permanently informed about the location and actions of the opponent. Yet, the whole movement sequence can be evoked by stimulating only a few hundred neurons unilaterally anywhere in the mediobasal hypothalamus [6]. This means that either the dedicated network is present in the hypothalamus in several copies to allow for evoking aggression from anywhere and also to ensure that each copy receives the same input or, alternatively, the FAP is elicited from elsewhere and the hypothalamus serves only as a triggering mechanism. As the former assumption is highly unlikely, one must conclude that biting attacks are triggered rather than regulated by the hypothalamus. If so, what does the mediobasal hypothalamus do?

It was hypothesized early on that hypothalamic centers involved in the control of goal-directed behavior, e.g., aggression, in fact increase the motivation for a particular behavior rather than controlling it directly [138]. This assumption seems to be supported by recent optogenetic evidence. For instance, the stimulation of the hypothalamic attack site made male mice to self-initiate stimulation to gain brief and repeated access to a weaker male that they could attack [139]. A motivational aspect controlled by the ventromedial hypothalamus seems to be present here. Another study from the same group showed that a subpopulation of ventromedial hypothalamic neurons become activated by the mere sensing of the opponent, i.e., before the attack started. Moreover, this apparently premature activation was predictive of the intensity of subsequent aggressive responses, again suggesting a role in motivation [140]. Finally, another optogenetic study revealed that the role of the ventromedial nucleus is exerted in conjunction with impulsiveness, i.e., a motivational aspect [141]. These findings suggest that hypothalamic attack sites control motivation. In its turn, however, the motivational hypothesis cannot explain all the effects of hypothalamic stimulations because the interruption of stimulation instantaneously stops behavior and such abrupt changes are not typical to motivational systems. The second counterargument is that, at least in the rat, bites are not associated with piloerection or other typical displays of emotion. Teeth chattering may occur, but this behavior has its own hypothalamic site and co-occurs with bites only when an overlapping area is stimulated.

Taken together, the "where?" question was answered, but the "how?" question was not or at least not convincingly. The explanation may lay in hypothalamic connectivity. The mediobasal hypothalamus receives inputs from dozens of brain areas both up- and downstream and sends projections to a similarly large number and similarly scattered brain areas [142, 143]. On one hand, this shows that attack sites integrate rather than transmit information, whereas, on the other, these connections may provide hints on how the hypothalamus works. This issue will be addressed below.

7.3.6 The Periaqueductal Gray

The periaqueductal gray surrounds the aqueduct that connects the third and fourth ventricles and is organized into four rostro-caudal columns. Behaviors controlled by it also have a columnar arrangement, with an overlaying rostro-caudal organization.

In the cat, affective and predatory aggressions can be evoked by the stimulation of the dorsolateral and ventrolateral columns, respectively [43]. These columns are under the influence of the mediobasal and lateral hypothalamus, respectively, and their stimulation results in behaviors similar to those elicited at hypothalamic level. Note that the behavioral effects of electric and neurochemical stimulations are similar [144], showing that the putative artifacts of electrical stimulations do not play important roles.

Stimulation and lesion techniques were less frequently used to study the role of the periaqueductal gray in rat aggression, and the two available studies focused on affective aggression only [145, 146]. Stimulations did evoke affective bites, but only 10% of the electrode placements were effective. Offensive threats were more commonly observed. Subsequent publications by the same authors used these findings to refute the idea that bites can be evoked from the periaqueductal gray in rats due to the low effectiveness of stimulations. In our view, however, they actually proved it.

The periaqueductal gray is a very complex structure which is at the crossroads of many behavioral and physiological control mechanisms that can easily cancel out each other when the area is stimulated electrically. As it regards behavior, the periaqueductal gray in fact balances opposite responses to challenges, as it controls all three passive defense (freezing), active defense (flight), and aggression, by circuitries that overlap spatially to a great extent. For instance, an optogenetic study showed that a pathway that connects the ventromedial nucleus of the hypothalamus to the dorsal nucleus of the periaqueductal gray, which in principle is along the aggression pathway, elicited freezing, i.e., a defensive response [147]. Those ventromedial neurons that target the periaqueductal gray and elicit freezing appear to be located in the anterior part of the hypothalamic ventromedial nucleus [148], whereas those that control aggression are located in the ventrolateral aspect. Such intricacies are difficult to disentangle with methodologies as indiscriminative as electric stimulation, because the pathways that control opposite responses appear intermingled. This may explain the low share of locations that resulted in attacks. On the other hand, the fact that some electrodes did evoke aggression, despite circuit intermingling, shows that the periaqueductal gray does contain neuron populations that can elicit attacks in conjunction with commands received from the hypothalamus.

The first added value of the periaqueductal gray in the control of aggression is the association of bites with affective behaviors, which was not seen at hypothalamic level in rodents. In addition, the periaqueductal gray appears to be a link to mechanisms that control glucose metabolism [149] and emotion-related autonomic responses [150, 151] that fuel aggressive behavior by increasing energy metabolism. Finally, the periaqueductal gray has links to facial and somatic motor neurons that can elicit the muscle contractions typical to aggressive behavior [151]. One is tempted to believe that the dedicated network that serves the execution of FAPs, and which is unlikely to be located in hypothalamic attack sites, is hosted by the periaqueductal gray, which as a consequence appears to be a multifaceted execution-bound section of the aggression circuitry.

Unfortunately, those who employ modern neuroscientific methodologies, e.g., optogenetics, paid far less attention to the role of the periaqueductal gray in aggressive behavior than to its role in defense, anxiety, and depression. Therefore, the role of this brain area in aggression and the precise connectivity that controls it remain poorly known, although its involvement appears ensured. Again, the questions "where?" and "what?" appear answered, but the question "how exactly?" was not.

7.4 Accessory, Attuning, and Organizing Systems

7.4.1 Overview

The networks underlying aggression cannot be discovered without lesion, brain stimulation, and local inhibition experiments, but for technical reasons, such studies cannot address the role of more than one or very few brain areas at a time. In addition, it is sensible to preselect the areas of interest based on current knowledge, quite often on the early "electrophysiological maps" of the aggression circuitry, which introduces a certain degree of bias.

Although in many respects inferior, immediate early gene expression studies eliminate these deficiencies. They allow the identification of all the neuron populations activated by fights in one single experiment (in theory at least), and studies are guided by the brain activation patterns observed rather than by earlier discoveries. Although still incomplete, such studies were used here to outline those brain areas that may constitute the pool of accessory and attuning systems (see Table 7.1).

The table clearly shows that the number of brain areas implicated in or at least activated by aggression is very large. Note that the list is incomplete. First, empty cells in the table are most often due to missing data rather than to the lack of activation. Second, there are a series of brain areas, e.g., the habenula, which were not in the focus of immediate early gene expression studies yet which still play important roles in aggression [154]. This table, however, was not compiled to list all the brain areas that may play roles in aggression but to allow a first glance on the complexity of the circuitry. What is the role of this wide array of brain regions?

Based on early electrophysiological work and subsequent studies, we outlined in the previous section the "core circuitry," i.e., the one that bridges decision and execution. To account for the roles of other areas, e.g., of the areas listed above, we hypothesized that they control the functioning of the core circuitry either directly by targeted synapses (accessory system), indirectly by non-targeted volume transmission (attuning system), or by their neural organizing roles (hormones).

A comprehensive account of the systems associated with core circuitries is difficult for two reasons. First, information on many accessory/attuning/organizing systems is incomplete. Second, such a broad approach would stretch the boundaries of this book. Therefore, we chose three areas as examples to illustrate the complexity of aggression control and to reveal the nature of the gaps that exist in present knowledge. In addition to being illustrative, we believe that these examples are also important for understanding aggression control.

7.4.2 The Hypothalamus and Its Accessory Systems

As shown above, the stimulation of the hypothalamus elicits an inborn FAP – the attack – which consists of a succession of complex movements that are continuously adapted to environmental events and the actions of the opponents. How is this

Table 7.1 The c-Fos map of the aggression circuitry in three closely related species

Brain area	Rats [71, 83, 107]	Hamsters [105, 134, 152]	Mice [36, 88, 153]
Agranular insular cortex	X		
Anterior cingulate	X		X
Anterior hypothalamic area	X	X	X
Arcuate nucleus of the hypothalamus	X		X
Basolateral amygdala	X		X
Bed nucleus of stria terminalis	X	X	X
CA1-4 region of the hippocampus	X		X
Central nucleus of the amygdala	X		
Cingulate cortex	X	X	X
Cortical nucleus of the amygdala	X	X	
Dentate gyrus of the hippocampus	X		X
Dorsolateral periaqueductal grey	X	X	X
Dorsomedial hypothalamic nucleus	X		X
Dorsomedial periaqueductal grey	X		
Facial somatosensory cortex			X
Infralimbic cortex	X	X	X
Lateral hypothalamic area	X		
Lateral nucleus of the amygdala	X		
Lateral orbitofrontal cortex	X		
Lateral periaqueductal grey	X		X
Lateral preoptic area	X		
Lateral septum	X	X	X
Locus coeruleus	X		
Medial nucleus of the amygdala	X	X	X
Medial orbitofrontal cortex	X		
Medial preoptic area	X	X	X
Medial septum	X		
Median preoptic nucleus	X		
Mediobasal hypothalamus	X		
Nucleus accumbens shell	X	X	
Paraventricular nucleus of the hypothalamus	X	X	X
Parvocellular subparafascicular nucleus			X
Piriform cortex	X		
Prelimbic cortex	X	X	X
Premammillary nucleus of the hypothalamus		X	
Sensory cortices (visual and auditory)			X
Retrosplenial cortex			X
Suprachiasmatic nucleus	X		
Supraoptic nucleus	X		

(continued)

Table 7.1 (continued)

Brain area	Rats [71, 83, 107]	Hamsters [105, 134, 152]	Mice [36, 88, 153]
Ventral orbitofrontal cortex	X		
Ventral tegmental area	X	X	
Ventrolateral periaqueductal grey	X		X
Ventrolateral hypothalamic nucleus	X	X	

Areas were ordered alphabetically because this table does not aim at conveying mechanistic information. The magnitude of activation was not indicated for the same reason. *X* – activated by aggression

role achieved? As suggested above, the explanation may lie in the complex connectivity of the hypothalamus (see Table 7.2).

The mediobasal hypothalamus, the "center" for rivalry attacks, establishes contacts with nearly 100 brain areas, one-third of these contacts being two-sided. Contacts cover the whole brain from the olfactory bulb to the pons; moreover, mediobasal hypothalamic projections may reach the medulla. These are not shown in the table because of inconsistent labelling. All connections are synaptic; as such, the listed brain areas can be considered as accessory systems of the aggression circuitry.

One can discover a directionality of information transfer, primarily in the case of cortical regions, which send dense projections to the mediobasal hypothalamus but receive none from it, and the periaqueductal gray which is densely innervated from the mediobasal hypothalamus but "sends back" very few projections. In these two cases, the expected top-down information transfer appears evident. A hypothalamus → thalamus directionality is also obvious, although this goes bottom-up. The amygdala in contrast establishes bidirectional connections with the mediobasal hypothalamus, which are typically very strong both ways. Other connections of the mediobasal hypothalamus may go both up- and downstream, without any evident directionality.

Taken together, these findings show that the mediobasal hypothalamus is surprisingly strongly connected to other brain regions. Some major pathways are directed as expected (top-down), but unexpected bottom-up pathways are too frequent to be considered exceptions. Particularly remarkable is the amygdala, which appears to be in a dialog with the mediobasal hypothalamus instead of controlling it. Note that the directionality of contacts was deduced from the intensity ratio of input and output connections.

Importantly, about half of the areas connected to the mediobasal hypothalamus are activated in fighting animals. This share is likely higher because many of the projection areas are outside the usual focus of aggression research and consequently were not investigated when activation patterns were studied. Remarkably, the mirror relationship is almost exclusive: nearly all brain areas activated by fighting are in contact with the mediobasal hypothalamus suggesting that the connections are indeed relevant for aggression control. Thus, the hypothalamus appears to play that kind of crucial role that was assumed by early brain stimulation studies.

Table 7.2 Input and output areas of the hypothalamus

Brain area	Mediobasal hypothalamic projections	
	Inputs[143]	Outputs[142]
Cortex		
Agranular insular cortex	±	
Bed nucleus accessory olfactory tract	++	
Dorsal endopiriform cortex	±	
Dorsal peduncular cortex	++	
Dorsal tenia tecta	+	
Ectorhinal cortex	±	
Infralimbic cortex	+++	
Medial orbitofrontal cortex	++	
Olfactory bulb	±	
Olfactory-limbic transitional zone	+	
Perirhinal cortex	±	
Piriform cortex	±	
Prelimbic cortex	++	
Septofimbrial nucleus	+	
Subfornical organ	±	
Basal ganglia		
Periaccumbens area	++	
Substantia innominate	±	XX
Septum		
Lateral septum, dorsal part	±	XX
Lateral septum, intermediate part	+++	XXX
Lateral septum, ventral part	+++	XX
Medial nucleus of the septum		XXX
Hippocampus		
CA1 area of the hippocampus		XXX
Subiculum	++++	
Amygdala		
Amygdalo-hippocampal transitional area	++++	XXX
Amygdalo-piriform transitional area	+	
Anterior amygdala		X
Basolateral nucleus of the amygdala, posterior part	+	XX
Bed nucleus of the stria terminalis, intraamygdalar	±	XXX
Bed nucleus of the stria terminalis, lateral	±	XXX
Bed nucleus of the stria terminalis, medial	++++	XXX
Central nucleus of the amygdala,		XX
Cortical nucleus of the amygdala, anterior part	++	
Cortical nucleus of the amygdala, posterior part	±	

Table 7.2 (continued)

Diencephalon		
Habenular nucleus	±	xx
Peripeduncular area	±	
Posterior intralaminar thalamic nucleus	±	
Precomissural nucleus	±	xxx
Subparafascicular area	+	
Thalamus, central nucleus		xx
Thalamus, mediodorsal nucleus		xxx
Thalamus, nucleus reuniens		xxx
Thalamus, parataenial nucleus		xxx
Thalamus, paraventricular nucleus	+	xxx
Thalamus, rhomboid nucleus		x
Thalamus, stria medullaris		x
Zona incerta		xx
Hypothalamus		
Anterior nucleus of the hypothalamus	++	xx
Anteroventral periventricular nucleus	++	
Arcuate nucleus	++	xx
Dorsal tuberomammillary nucleus	+	
Dorsomedial nucleus of the hypothalamus	++	xx
Lateral hypothalamic area	±	xx
Lateral preoptic area	±	xxx
Medial preoptic area	++++	xxx
Medial preoptic nucleus of the hypothalamus	++++	
Median eminence		x
Median preoptic nucleus of the hypothalamus	+	
Paraventricular nucleus, magnocellular part	+	
Paraventricular nucleus, parvocellular part	++	
Periventricular nucleus of the hypothalamus	++	
Posterior nucleus of the hypothalamus	++	
Premammillary nucleus, dorsal		xxx
Premammillary nucleus, ventral	++	xx
Retrochiasmatic area	±	
Striohypothalamic nucleus	+++	
Suprachiasmatic nucleus	±	
Supramamillary nucleus	±	
Supraoptic nucleus	+	
Ventromedial nucleus of the hypothalamus	+++	xxx

Table 7.2 (continued)

Midbrain		
Cuneiform nucleus	+	xxx
Deep mesencephalic nucleus	±	
Periaqueductal gray, dorsolateral	±	xx
Periaqueductal gray, dorsomedial	±	x
Periaqueductal gray, lateral	±	xxx
Periaqueductal gray, ventral	±	xx
Dorsal raphe	±	xx
Raphe magnus		xx
Median raphe		xx
Pons		
Barrington's nucleus		x
Köllike-Fuse nucleus	++	
Locus coeruleus	±	xx
Noradrenergic A5 area		xx
Parabrachial nuclus, lateral	+++	xx
Parabrachial nuclus, medial		xx
Paralemniscal nucleus	+	
Pedunculopontine tegmental nucleus	+	xx
Tegmental nuclei (4th ventricle)	±	xxx
Ventrolateral tegmental area		xx

The strength of contacts. Retrograde labeling was ± sparse; +, weak; ++, significant; +++, dense, ++++, very dense. Innervation was x, sparse; *xx*, moderate; *xxx*, dense. Note that the scales slightly differ in the in- and output columns. *Outlines*. activated by aggression (see Table 7.1); reciprocal innervation.

Studies on the in- and output areas of the mediobasal hypothalamus shed light on the organization of biting attacks in two ways. (1) The mediobasal hypothalamus is part of a circuit that controls adaptive navigation which explains how attack behavior remains in permanent contact with environment when elicited from the hypothalamus. This assumption was based on studies showing that flexible and adaptive behavioral responses are controlled by a circuit composed of the hypothalamus, thalamus, and the prefrontal cortex, with ramifications to the hippocampus, septum, and amygdala [155]. The connectivity map outlined in Table 7.2 suggests the existence of a mediobasal hypothalamus → thalamus → prefrontal cortex → mediobasal hypothalamus triangle which is similar to the one that plays important roles in cue discrimination, cue-reward processing, and cue-responses [156]. The hypothalamus is able to integrate all the key elements of the circuitry, i.e., the thalamus, hippocampus, amygdala, and via the thalamus the prefrontal cortex. (2) Retrograde and anterograde tracing studies may also explain why is the same behavior elicited by the stimulation of various small parts of the mediobasal hypothalamus. As suggested above, the hypothalamus cannot be the site which hosts the neural circuitries of behaviors as complex as biting attacks. A close inspection of connectivity studies, however, revealed that the in- and output projections of the mediobasal hypothalamus are rather uniformly distributed within the area. This is indicated by the similarity of connections labelled by different injection sites. Injection site differences result from the technical impossibility of injecting tracers exactly into the same place. In tracing studies, tracers were always injected within the boundaries of the mediobasal hypothalamus but into different parts of it. Yet, in- and output areas showed only minor individual variation, suggesting that neurons are not compartmentalized within the area and the connectivity of each mediobasal hypothalamic subregion is roughly the same. This may explain why different electrode placements elicit the same behavioral response provided that they are within the boundaries of the area.

Classical approaches were inappropriate to sort out interactions as complex as those that are suggested by the intricate in- and output connections of the mediobasal hypothalamus. This may explain why the "where?" question was answered but the "how?" question was not: there was a mismatch between the complexity of the system and the resolution capacities of earlier methodologies. The few optogenetic studies performed so far, however, suggest that intricacies can be untangled by more sophisticated approaches. This takes time, but one can see the light at the end of the tunnel.

7.4.3 Associated and Attuning Pathways in the Raphe Nuclei

The role of serotonergic system in aggression control was indicated by early studies published in the 1970s. These revealed that lesions placed within the main serotonergic nuclei, i.e., the median and dorsal raphe, increased rivalry aggression [157], whereas the depletion of serotonin by para-chlorophenylalanine induced predatory attacks [158]. Subsequent research confirmed these findings and established that the serotonin is among the main determinants of aggression control [159]. Some even suggested that other neurotransmitters affect aggression only by affecting serotonergic neurotransmission [160], i.e., indirectly. This research line concluded that all novel anti-aggression drugs should target the serotonergic system [161].

The field, however, was not devoid of contradictory findings. For instance, the pharmacological reduction of serotonin availability in some instances decreased aggression whereas in others increased it [162].

As an example of such contradictory findings, it was reported that agonists of the 5-HT_{1B} serotonin receptor decreased aggression when injected into the infralimbic region of the prefrontal cortex but also when the agent was injected into the dorsal raphe [163]. Ostensibly, the two findings reported in the same study are consistent, but in fact they highlight the contradiction mentioned above. This is due to the differential consequences of post- and presynaptic receptors and to the differential expression of these receptors in the prefrontal cortex and dorsal raphe [164]. Postsynaptic 5-HT_{1B} receptors mediate serotonin effects, but the same receptor inhibits serotonin release when located presynaptically, because such receptors (often called autoreceptors) regulate neurotransmitter release by negative feedback.

Thus, post- and presynaptic receptors have diametrically opposed roles. The prefrontal cortex – one of the target areas of raphe nuclei – contains mainly postsynaptic 5-HT_{1B} receptors, whereas the raphe nuclei contain mainly presynaptic receptors. As such, agonists of the 5-HT_{1B} receptor elicit in the prefrontal cortex effects typical of serotonin, but they inhibit serotonin release when injected into raphe nuclei. Consequently, the anti-aggressive effect of prefrontal treatments suggests that serotonin decreases aggression, whereas the anti-aggressive effect of dorsal raphe injections suggests the opposite. The inhibition of serotonin release reduces aggression, although it should increase it if the classical view on the serotonin–aggression relationship was right.

Without entering further detail, one can clearly perceive hidden and often neglected discrepancies in the general view on the serotonin–aggression relationship. Such discrepancies are clinically relevant as several serotonin-enhancing agents, e.g., selective serotonin reuptake inhibitors are used as therapies for aggression-related psychopathologies, yet the very same agents induced outbursts of anger and moreover homicide in a few well-documented cases [165–168]. As such, understanding the role of serotonin in aggression control is not a purely academic endeavor.

Classical neuroscientific tools were sufficient to reveal basic mechanisms and even to detect hidden discrepancies, but the elucidation of the intricate neural circuits that stand behind the observed phenomena remains to more modern approaches. Below we present three recent studies that are illustrative in this respect.

The first study aimed at understanding how synaptic and non-synaptic serotonergic communication by the two serotonergic nuclei affect aggression [169]. Note that there are two distinct serotonergic systems in the brain, which differ in their topographic organization, electrophysiological characteristics, morphology, and sensitivity to psychoactive agents [170]. One system originates from the dorsal raphe and communicates mainly non-synaptically with extended brain regions, whereas the other originates from the median raphe and consists of projections that establish synapses at specific target structures. Based on these differences, it was hypothesized that the two nuclei play different roles in the control of aggressive behavior. The hypothesis was studied by optogenetic methods to reveal effects on both behavior and neurotransmission in the prefrontal cortex. The stimulation of the median raphe region decreased aggression in a phasic-like manner without affecting social behaviors. Aggression was inhibited within 1 min after the start of stimulations and vanished similarly rapidly when stimulations were stopped. In contrast, the stimulation of the dorsal raphe led to tonic effects that were behaviorally less specific: amiable social interactions were promoted, whereas agonistic social behaviors were inhibited. These effects persisted long after the stimulations were stopped; moreover, some effects were observable days later. As expected based on behavioral responses, serotonin release in the prefrontal cortex was transiently and lastingly increased by median and dorsal raphe stimulation, respectively. In addition, median but not dorsal raphe stimulations increased prefrontal glutamate release.

Together, these findings show that the median raphe belongs to the accessory system of the aggression core circuitry, as it specifically and phasically decreases aggression likely via synaptic communication, because this is the overwhelming mode of communication of this brain area. In contrast, the dorsal raphe appears to belong to the attuning system, as it induces lasting and aggression-nonspecific changes in social behavior via non-synaptic communication. Moreover, the dorsal raphe might even affect neuronal plasticity as shown by its persistent effects. One remarkable finding of the study was the increase of glutamate release in the prefrontal cortex by the median raphe stimulation, which might have been a secondary response, if the raphe nuclei were composed exclusively of serotonergic neurons. This, however, is not so.

In addition to serotonergic neurons, both the dorsal [171, 172] and median raphe [173, 174] contain neurons that communicate via the excitatory neurotransmitter glutamate, via the inhibitory neurotransmitter GABA, or via several other neurotransmitters. Serotonergic neurons are not only complemented by a few other neuron types but are outnumbered by these; some studies suggest that the share of serotonergic neurons in raphe nuclei is as low as 10% [175]. Moreover, serotonergic neurons often co-express other neurotransmitters suggesting that even serotonergic neurons release non-serotonergic neurotransmitters [175, 176]. This complicates the involvement of raphe neurons in aggression control and also the elucidation of the roles of serotonin.

The second study presented here [177] used the DREADD technique to study the role of the median raphe in genetically engineered mice. The authors used a Cre strain to allow the selective stimulation of glutamatergic neurons of the median raphe. The stimulation of this neuron subpopulation dramatically *increased* aggression. The glutamatergic neurons of the median raphe target the lateral habenula, ventral tegmental area, and hippocampus, which on their turn establish reciprocal connections with the mediobasal hypothalamus as accessory systems (see Table 7.2). In addition, the hippocampus [178] also projects to the prefrontal cortex. As such, medial amygdala glutamatergic neurons are the accessory system of the accessory systems of the aggression core circuitry. In contrast, the *serotonergic* neurons of the median raphe send efferents to the prefrontal cortex [179], basolateral amygdala [180], and anterior hypothalamus [181], all belonging to the core aggression circuitry in the rat.

The third study [182] employed complex intersectional genetic tools that allowed the silencing of serotonergic neurons depending on the co-expression of various genes. Silencing did not differentiate neurons based on their anatomical location, i.e., the neurons may have been in either or both the dorsal and median raphe. The study showed that a subpopulation of serotonergic neurons that expressed the genes of the D1 and D2 dopamine receptors (thus putatively being sensitive to dopamine influences) has a specific aggression-inhibiting effect, as their silencing increased aggression, whereas the silencing of other subpopulations did not affect aggressiveness in this study.

The three studies briefly reviewed above are seemingly conflicting as two were in favor of an aggression-inhibitory role of the raphe nuclei and of the serotonergic neurons they contain, whereas another lead to the opposite conclusion. There were, however, considerable differences between the three studies. The first separately studied the two serotonergic nuclei, but stimulation affected all neuron types within. The second studied glutamatergic neurons of the median raphe, whereas the third studied dopamine receptor-expressing serotonergic neurons irrespective to their anatomical location. Tentatively, the inhibition of aggression by all neurons and by a subpopulation of serotonergic neurons and the stimulation of aggression by a subgroup of neurons suggest that there are two subpopulations within the median raphe: one inhibits aggression, whereas the other stimulates it. As the stimulation of the entire nucleus decreased aggression, one can speculate that the aggression-inhibiting neurons of the median raphe – likely including the serotonergic ones – are "stronger" than the aggression-increasing glutamatergic cell population. Importantly, the differential projections of the median raphe serotonergic and glutamatergic neurons suggest that their effects are exerted at different brain levels and consequently are mediated by different mechanisms.

Findings obtained over several decades of research make the role of serotonin in aggression unquestionable; however, findings like those presented above reveal that this role is poorly understood at mechanistic level. One can even speculate that the upregulation of serotonin release (e.g., by selective serotonin reuptake inhibitors) inhibits aggression indirectly by silencing median raphe glutamatergic neurons either by local circuits or by serotonin receptors located on glutamatergic cells. As mentioned above, however, the role of serotonin in aggression and the precise mechanisms mediating it are not academic questions as many anti-aggressive drugs are serotonergic, and these sometimes elicit strange effects. One can assume that understanding the internal organization of raphe nuclei and the roles of various cell types may even lead to novel, better treatments. This work, however, is in the future.

7.4.4 Organizing the Circuitry: Testosterone

The organizing and mechanistic roles of glucocorticoids in aggression were addressed in two separate chapters; here we focus on another important hormone that was associated with aggression, in fact one that was studied before glucocorticoids. Arnold Berthold showed in 1847 that castration decreased while the re-implantation of testes restored aggression [183], and exactly 100 years later, Beeman [184] revealed that the role of testes is mediated by testosterone, the hormone secreted by them.

The main role of testosterone in the organism is to support the development of primary and secondary sexual characteristics and to promote sexual behavior. Its effects on aggression appear useful tie-ins, because males usually need to fight each other off to get access to females. The role of testosterone in aggression was supported by innumerable studies, but doubts regarding its role are recurrent, and these doubts are fueled mainly by studies showing that aggression is independent of testosterone production in several species or under particular conditions. For instance, the association is confusing and inconsistent in humans [185–187]. One can argue that humans are special, but they are still mammals. To confirm that the confusing association of testosterone with aggression is not a purely human characteristic, we refer to several mammalian and non-mammalian species that fight without being helped by testosterone. In the non-breading season, for instance, aggression is controlled by the adrenal steroid dehydroepiandrosterone in several bird and mammal species [188]. In several seasonally breeding hamster species, the main activator is the day length, which modifies melatonin secretion [189], which in its turn affects aggression by influencing the production of nitric oxide [190], a molecule produced by particular neurons to evoke the release of several neurotransmitters [191, 192]. Without entering into detail, there are ample examples where aggression was controlled independently of testosterone.

The controversy is regularly recalled by new studies that confirm and refute the role of testosterone in aggression again and again. We suggest, however, that controversies surrounding the association derive from a faulty understanding of the biological roles of aggression and from a failure of discriminating the organizing and mechanistic roles of hormones. Two lines of evidence support this view.

1. If aggression was very tightly linked to testosterone production, females would be unable to compete for resources; moreover, males would be less aggressive outside the breeding season when testosterone production is low. Neither prediction is true. Maternal aggression is probably the most violent form of aggression out of those that occur under natural conditions, whereas aggressiveness was not decreased by castration in a variety of species from lizards [193] to California mice [194] and mandarin voles [195] outside the breeding season and in species that breed across the year.

   If aggression was uniquely tied to testosterone, its biological definition would have to be changed. Instead of being a behavioral mechanism of resource competition, aggression would be a behavioral mechanism of competition for females. Such a restriction of the scope of the behavior is incompatible with the facts. Both genders are aggressive, and neither links this behavior exclusively to sexually relevant situations.
2. As opposed to glucocorticoids, the mechanistic roles of testosterone appear minimal. Glucocorticoids can affect the functioning of the aggression circuitry, while aggression unfolds by their non-genomic and early genomic effects. This results in the aggression → glucocorticoid production → aggression positive feedback loop mentioned above. Attempts were made to assign testosterone similar roles, but the supporting arguments were indirect and unconvincing in the case of aggression [196, 197], although testosterone might influence other behaviors non-genomically [198]. As testosterone appears to control aggression primarily by its long-term neural organizing roles, there is no need for an actual association between testosterone and aggression levels. One and the same testosterone level may be associated with both low and high levels of aggression depending on how the hormone prepared the brain in early stages of development or changed its function in response to life events.

The primary period for testosterone action is related to birth, when testosterone production transiently increases in males for a few hours, which has a long-term impact on adult aggressive behavior [199–201]. The blockade of testosterone production or testosterone receptors in this sensitive period decreased male aggression in adulthood, whereas testosterone treatments administered to female fetuses induced male-typical aggression in later stages of life (e.g., females engaged in hierarchy fights with males). The consequences of this early testosterone surge become apparent in adolescence when testosterone production increases more durably. From this age onwards, testosterone affects male-typical behaviors only if the brain was sensitized to its effects in the neonatal period. The second period when testosterone affects aggression is breeding [202]. This a is clearly distinguishable period in many species, which is associated with a series of neural changes that are supported by increased testosterone production [183], which prepares the field for increased male–male competition. The third period when aggression and testosterone become associated cannot be connected to a specific life stage except that it usually happens in adulthood. Particularly, testosterone increases after winning an aggressive encounter and decreases after this was lost, which influences subsequent aggressiveness [203–205].

In conclusion, negative findings demonstrate that testosterone is not among the universal mechanisms of aggression control in the way in which the core aggression circuitry or even glucocorticoids are. Yet, testosterone (i) constitutes an important mechanism of brain development that contributes to the emergence of male-typical behaviors in adulthood including aggression and (ii) is important for the activation of male-typical behaviors in the breeding season, and (iii) it is a tool by which male-typical behaviors are adapted to social conditions, e.g., to the experience of winning or losing. In this respect, corticosterone is also important as shown above; thus, current theories emphasize the role of the testosterone/cortisol ratio [206].

As such, the question should be reformulated: instead of asking how testosterone affects aggression, one should ask how testosterone affects brain structure and function to promote the development and maintenance of male-typical behaviors including competition for females. An adequate approach to the issue requires epigenetic studies, which, however, rarely if ever focused on aggression specifically.

The sexual differentiation of the brain in contrast has received some attention recently. A study published almost 50 years ago by Raisman and Field [207] showed that the sexual dimorphism of the brain is due to neonatal androgen production, i.e., to the aforementioned transient increase in testosterone production by males. Epigenetics was unknown by that time, but later research demonstrated that the testosterone-dependent rearrangement of chromatin plays a major role in the sexual differentiation of the brain [208]. Interestingly, some studies showed that epigenetic changes in the DNA are not detectable till adulthood, suggesting that the methylation of nucleobases and the acetylation of histones are produced with a considerable delay due to some unknown process. One cannot exclude that early epigenetic changes – the ones that triggered those occurring later – remained undetected or, alternatively, epigenetics was triggered by the emergence of testosterone production in adolescence in interaction with an unknown latent factor.

Epigenetic events contributing to the masculinization of the brain are not known in detail, primarily because male and female brains differ in many respects and only a few brain areas and processes have been studied in detail. Nevertheless, the available findings can be perceived as important preludes of an emerging field that on the long run may clarify the neonatal epigenetics of brain development. One study focused on the sex hormone-dependent organization of the arcuate nucleus and median eminence neurokinin B system, which are sexually dimorphic in adulthood [209]. The study was not directly relevant to aggression control but demonstrated that neuronal organization is responsive to alterations in testosterone production both perinatally and around puberty. The finding is important because the post-neonatal epigenetic roles of testosterone had not been investigated so far. This study suggests that the epigenetics of breeding season- and defeat-induced changes in testosterone production are worthwhile studying. Another study, albeit not focusing on aggression, showed that testosterone had a role in the sex-dependent development of the bed nucleus of stria terminalis, preoptic area, and striatum [210], which all are implicated in the control of aggression. The study investigated DNA-methylation genome-wide and found that methylation increased considerably (sometimes even 20-fold) in many genes under the influence of testosterone. Another study revealed that not only DNA methylation but also histone deacetylation plays important roles in the sexual differentiation of the bed nucleus of stria terminalis [211]. Finally, a recent study [212] investigated the balance between DNA methyltransferases and ten-eleven translocation methylcytosine dioxygenases in the sexual differentiation of the hypothalamus. The former enzyme places methyl marks on the DNA, whereas the latter removes them. As such, this study did not investigate the methylation of particular DNA segments but the enzymatic processes that control this and showed that early testosterone affects enzyme expression over the life course. The investigated brain areas were the preoptic area, the ventromedial nucleus of the hypothalamus, and the hippocampus, i.e., three areas important for aggression control.

7.5 Overview: A New Approach to the Circuity

Early studies outlined the core circuitry of aggression control, which was used subsequently as a template for guiding studies and understanding aggression control even by those who addressed human aggression. In blunt terms, reactive and proactive human aggressions were differentiated, and the former was attributed to the "rivalry aggression circuitry" whereas the latter to the "predatory aggression circuitry." Others suggested that the rivalry aggression circuitry is operational in normally aggressive humans, whereas pathological and criminal forms of aggression occur when the predatory circuitry is activated.

Such generalizations are not necessarily false, but the number of areas recognized for participating in aggression control has increased over time, and their connectivity has gradually become better understood. As such the classical view on the aggression circuitry became outdated. Below we provide an integrated view of old and new discoveries, as a trial to create a template more compatible with recent findings (see Figs. 7.5 and 7.6). Note that the concept does not deviate from the classical

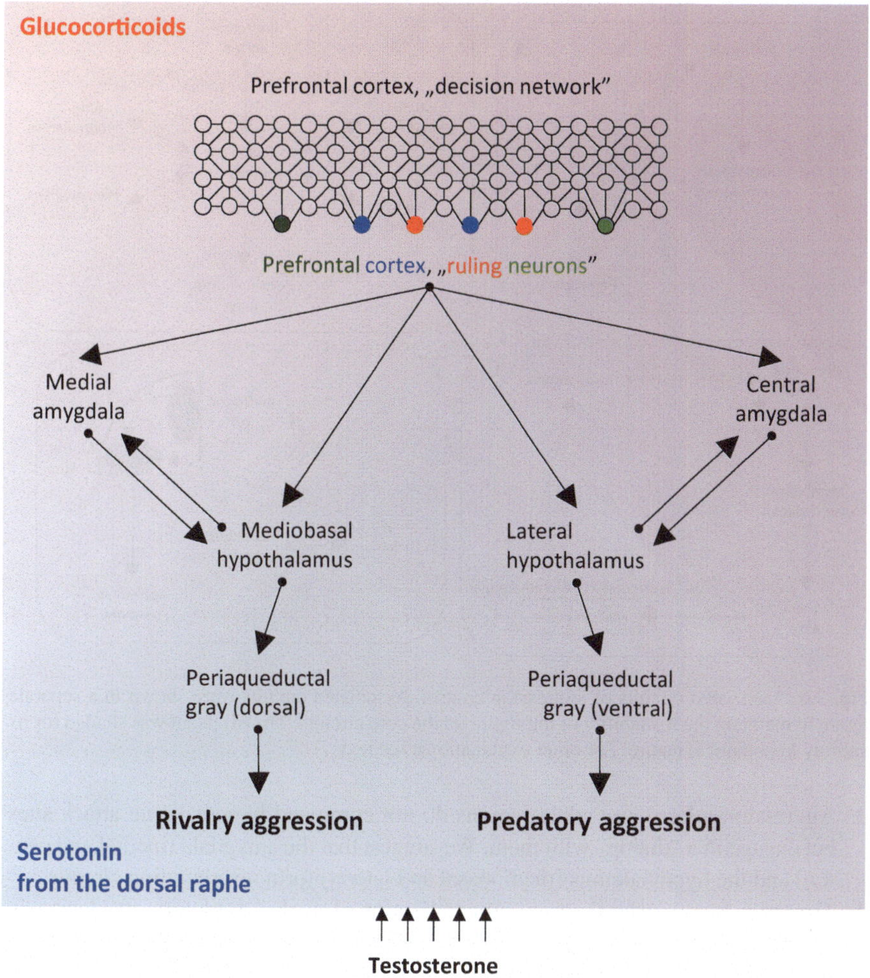

Fig. 7.5 The core circuitry re-mapped. The circuit contains several new elements, including the distinction of "decision networks" and "ruling neurons" in the prefrontal cortex and the direct projection of the latter to the hypothalamus. For other explanations, see text

view on the core circuitry but complements it with important details concerning their organization into a network. The differences from earlier versions of similar schematics are as follows:

1. The prefrontal cortex was not considered solely an inhibitory component of the network as it can both inhibit and stimulate aggression.
2. The prefrontal cortex was divided into "decision networks" that integrate information received from various brain areas and specific "ruling" neuron populations that project to downstream nuclei to control particular behaviors in a highly selective way. Decisions are taken by "decision networks" simply by activating those "ruling" neuron populations that are appropriate for the task at the moment.

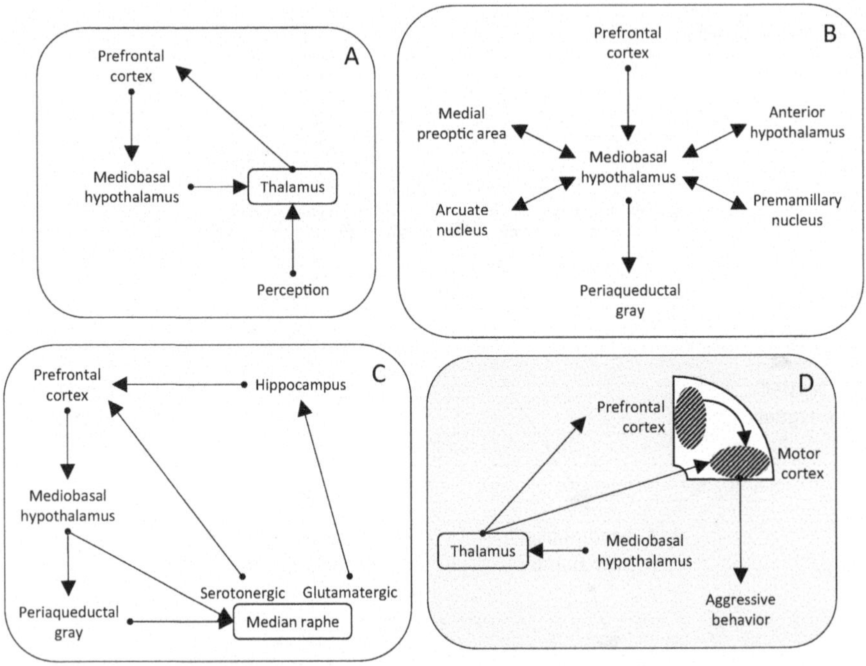

Fig. 7.6 Associated circuits of aggression control. Associated circuits were shown in a separate figure to maintain the readability of the figure on the core circuits. The (**d**) panel was shaded for its entirely hypothetical nature. For other explanations, see text

3. Aggression-related amygdala regions do not command hypothalamic attack sites but engage in a "dialog" with them. We suggest that the amygdala (medial and central) and the hypothalamus (mediobasal and lateral) form reverberating circuits.
4. The strict dorsal–ventral compartmentalization of rivalry–predatory attack sites in the periaqueductal gray was downscaled as aggression-induced activation patterns only partially support the narrow specialization of dorsoventrally columns.
5. Finally, the whole circuitry appears bathed in serotonin that is released from the non-synaptic terminals of the dorsal raphe. This mechanism exerts tonic influences on the circuit, which are behaviorally nonspecific. Such serotonergic effects appear conceptually similar to those exerted by hormones. Only glucocorticoids and testosterone were shown in the figure, but other hormones may play similar roles.

There are a series of microcircuits associated with the core circuitry; we outline four of these in Fig. 7.6. These were shown separately to ensure the readability of the figures, but in fact all of the circuits are parts of the same unitary circuit.

The first microcircuit (Fig. 7.6a) includes the triangle composed of a one-way connectivity that links the mediobasal hypothalamus, thalamic relay nuclei, and prefrontal cortex. The key component of this triangle appears to be the thalamus, which in addition to mediobasal hypothalamic inputs receives a series of sensory inputs from lower brain centers. As such, it is in a key position to integrate the functioning of the attack site with events occurring in the environment.

The second circuitry (Fig. 7.6b) includes those hypothalamic nuclei that establish bidirectional contacts with the mediobasal hypothalamus and at the same time are activated while the animals fight. Although attacks cannot be elicited from any of these, the local circuit likely plays a role in the excitability of the attack site.

The third circuitry (Fig. 7.6c) depicts the ambivalent role of the median raphe in aggression control. This brain area establishes synaptic contacts with target areas, and as such it belongs to the accessory system of the core circuitry, as opposed to the dorsal raphe, which appears to be an attuning system. Recent studies suggest that median raphe serotonergic nuclei decrease aggression by direct effects on the prefrontal cortex, amygdala, and hypothalamus, whereas its glutamatergic neurons increase aggression via influencing the functioning of the ventral tegmental area, habenula, and hippocampus. Note that connections were simplified to maintain the figure readable. In addition to these connections justified above, we also showed a pathway that connects the periaqueductal gray to the median raphe [213], because this may also be important for the functioning of the system.

Finally, we propose the almost heretic view that the muscle movements that constitute aggressive behavior are controlled from the motor cortex (Fig. 7.6d). This possibility never occurred in any concept on aggression control so far and is entirely hypothetical. To emphasize this, the background of this panel was shaded. We have only two arguments to support the involvement of the motor cortex: (i) this area is under the control of both the prefrontal cortex and the thalamus [214, 215], and (ii) the motor cortex is the most appropriate area of the brain to organize complex movements.

We acknowledge that the attempt to renew the concept of aggression circuitry is in many ways hypothetical and incomplete in the sense that it has not integrated all available new results. Yet, it has the advantage of illustrating the complexity of the network and provides a framework for integrating separate discoveries into a common scheme.

References

1. Hess, W. R. (1928). Stammganglien-Reizversuche. *Berichte über die gesamte Physiologie, 42*, 554–555.
2. Egger, M. D., & Flynn, J. P. (1962). Amygdaloid suppression of hypothalamically elicited attack behavior. *Science, 136*, 43–44.
3. MacDonnell, M., & Flynn, J. P. (1966). Sensory control of hypothalamic attack. *Animal Behaviour, 14*, 399–405.
4. Adams, D. B. (1968). Cells related to fighting behavior recorded from midbrain central gray neuropil of cat. *Science, 159*, 894–896.
5. Bandler, R. J., Chi, C. C., & Flynn, J. P. (1972). Biting attack elicited by stimulation of the ventral midbrain tegmentum of cats. *Science, 177*, 364–366.
6. Lammers, J. H., Kruk, M. R., Meelis, W., & van der Poel, A. M. (1988). Hypothalamic substrates for brain stimulation-induced attack, teeth-chattering and social grooming in the rat. *Brain Research, 449*, 311–327.

7. Bermond, B., Mos, J., Meelis, W., van der Poel, A. M., & Kruk, M. R. (1982). Aggression induced by stimulation of the hypothalamus: Effects of androgens. *Pharmacology, Biochemistry, and Behavior, 16*, 41–45.
8. van der Poel, A. M., et al. (1982). Anti-aggressive effect of a new phenylpiperazine compound (DU27716) on hypothalamically induced behavioural activities. *Pharmacology, Biochemistry, and Behavior, 17*, 147–153.
9. Siegel, A., & Flynn, J. P. (1968). Differential effects of electrical stimulation and lesions of the hippocampus and adjacent regions upon attack behavior in cats. *Brain Research, 7*, 252–267.
10. Siegel, A., & Douard, J. (2011). Who's flying the plane: Serotonin levels, aggression and free will. *International Journal of Law and Psychiatry, 34*, 20–29.
11. Lamprecht, F., Eichelman, B., Thoa, N. B., Williams, R. B., & Kopin, I. J. (1972). Rat fighting behavior: Serum dopamine--hydroxylase and hypothalamic tyrosine hydroxylase. *Science, 177*, 1214–1215.
12. Goldberg, M. E., & Salama, A. I. (1969). Norepinephrine turnover and brain monoamine levels in aggressive mouse-killing rats. *Biochemical Pharmacology, 18*, 532–534.
13. Welch, A. S., & Welch, B. L. (1968). Effect of stress and para-chlorophenylalanine upon brain serotonin, 5-hydroxyindoleacetic acid and catecholamines in grouped and isolated mice. *Biochemical Pharmacology, 17*, 699–708.
14. Inoue, N., Tsukada, Y., & Barbeau, A. (1975). Behavioral effects in rats following intrastriatal microinjection of manganese. *Brain Research, 95*, 103–124.
15. Palkovits, M. (1983). Punch sampling biopsy technique. *Methods in Enzymology, 103*, 368–376.
16. Bak, M., et al. (2019). The pharmacological management of agitated and aggressive behaviour: A systematic review and meta-analysis. *European Psychiatry: The Journal of the Association of European Psychiatrists, 57*, 78–100.
17. Goedhard, L. E., et al. (2006). Pharmacotherapy for the treatment of aggressive behavior in general adult psychiatry: A systematic review. *The Journal of Clinical Psychiatry, 67*, 1013–1024.
18. Ferris, C. F., Meenan, D. M., Axelson, J. F., & Albers, H. E. (1986). A vasopressin antagonist can reverse dominant/subordinate behavior in hamsters. *Physiology & Behavior, 38*, 135–138.
19. Ferris, C. F., & Delville, Y. (1994). Vasopressin and serotonin interactions in the control of agonistic behavior. *Psychoneuroendocrinology, 19*, 593–601.
20. Haller, J., et al. (1996). Compression of the pituitary stalk elicits chronic increases in CSF vasopressin, oxytocin as well as in social investigation and aggressiveness. *Journal of Neuroendocrinology, 8*, 361–365.
21. Winslow, J. T., & Insel, T. R. (1991). Social status in pairs of male squirrel monkeys determines the behavioral response to central oxytocin administration. *Journal of Neuroscience: The Official Journal of the Society for Neuroscience, 11*, 2032–2038.
22. Winslow, J. T., Shapiro, L., Carter, C. S., & Insel, T. R. (1993). Oxytocin and complex social behavior: Species comparisons. *Psychopharmacology Bulletin, 29*, 409–414.
23. Weerts, E. M., Tornatzky, W., & Miczek, K. A. (1993). 'Anxiolytic' and 'anxiogenic' benzodiazepines and beta-carbolines: Effects on aggressive and social behavior in rats and squirrel monkeys. *Psychopharmacology, 110*, 451–459.
24. Weerts, E. M., Miller, L. G., Hood, K. E., & Miczek, K. A. (1992). Increased GABAA-dependent chloride uptake in mice selectively bred for low aggressive behavior. *Psychopharmacology, 108*, 196–204.
25. Aliczki, M., Varga, Z. K., Balogh, Z., & Haller, J. (2015). Involvement of 2-arachidonoylglycerol signaling in social challenge responding of male CD1 mice. *Psychopharmacology, 232*, 2157–2167.
26. Miczek, K. A., DeBold, J. F., van Erp, A. M., & Tornatzky, W. (1997). Alcohol, GABAA-benzodiazepine receptor complex, and aggression. *Recent Developments in Alcoholism: An Official Publication of the American Medical Society on Alcoholism, the Research Society on Alcoholism, and the National Council on Alcoholisms, 13*, 139–171.

27. Griebel, G., Stemmelin, J., Gal, C. S.-L., & Soubrié, P. (2005). Non-peptide vasopressin V1b receptor antagonists as potential drugs for the treatment of stress-related disorders. *Current Pharmaceutical Design, 11*, 1549–1559.
28. Ji, N. Y., & Findling, R. L. (2016). Pharmacotherapy for mental health problems in people with intellectual disability. *Current Opinion in Psychiatry, 29*, 103–125.
29. Jayaraman, R. (1972). Transcription of bacteriophage T4 DNA by Escherichia coli RNA polymerase in vitro: Identification of some immediate-early and delayed-early genes. *Journal of Molecular Biology, 70*, 253–263.
30. Morgan, J. I., & Curran, T. (1988). Calcium as a modulator of the immediate-early gene cascade in neurons. *Cell Calcium, 9*, 303–311.
31. Joppa, M. A., Meisel, R. L., & Garber, M. A. (1995). Fos expression in female hamster brain following sexual and aggressive behaviors. *Neuroscience, 68*, 783–792.
32. Potegal, M., Ferris, C. F., Hebert, M., Meyerhoff, J., & Skaredoff, L. (1996). Attack priming in female Syrian golden hamsters is associated with a c-fos-coupled process within the corticomedial amygdala. *Neuroscience, 75*, 869–880.
33. Oesterhelt, D., & Stoeckenius, W. (1971). Rhodopsin-like protein from the purple membrane of Halobacterium halobium. *Nature: New Biology, 233*, 149–152.
34. Boyden, E. S., Zhang, F., Bamberg, E., Nagel, G., & Deisseroth, K. (2005). Millisecond-timescale, genetically targeted optical control of neural activity. *Nature Neuroscience, 8*, 1263–1268.
35. Schobert, B., & Lanyi, J. K. (1982). Halorhodopsin is a light-driven chloride pump. *The Journal of Biological Chemistry, 257*, 10306–10313.
36. Lin, D., et al. (2011). Functional identification of an aggression locus in the mouse hypothalamus. *Nature, 470*, 221–226.
37. Adamantidis, A. R., Zhang, F., Aravanis, A. M., Deisseroth, K., & de Lecea, L. (2007). Neural substrates of awakening probed with optogenetic control of hypocretin neurons. *Nature, 450*, 420–424.
38. Hattori, T., et al. (2016). Self-exposure to the male pheromone ESP1 enhances male aggressiveness in mice. *Current Biology: CB, 26*, 1229–1234.
39. Chu, E. H., Trosko, J. E., & Chang, C. C. (1977). Mutational approaches to the study of carcinogenesis. *Journal of Toxicology and Environmental Health, 2*, 1317–1334.
40. Rubinstein, L. J. (1976). Current concepts in neuro-oncology. *Advances in Neurology, 15*, 1–25.
41. Partecke, J., & Schwabl, H. (2008). Organizational effects of maternal testosterone on reproductive behavior of adult house sparrows. *Developmental Neurobiology, 68*, 1538–1548.
42. Ferris, C. F. (2000). Adolescent stress and neural plasticity in hamsters: A vasopressin-serotonin model of inappropriate aggressive behaviour. *Experimental Physiology, 85 Spec No*, 85S–90S.
43. Siegel, A., Roeling, T. A., Gregg, T. R., & Kruk, M. R. (1999). Neuropharmacology of brain-stimulation-evoked aggression. *Neuroscience and Biobehavioral Reviews, 23*, 359–389.
44. David, B., Idan, S., & Michael, L. (2019). Single cortical neurons as deep artificial neural networks. *bioRxiv*, 613141. https://doi.org/10.1101/613141.
45. Shadlen, M. N., & Newsome, W. T. (1998). The variable discharge of cortical neurons: Implications for connectivity, computation, and information coding. *Journal of Neuroscience: The Official Journal of the Society for Neuroscience, 18*, 3870–3896.
46. Vizi, E. S. (1982). Non-synaptic intercellular communication: Presynaptic inhibition. *Acta Biologica Academiae Scientiarum Hungaricae, 33*, 331–351.
47. Agnati, L. F., et al. (1986). A correlation analysis of the regional distribution of central enkephalin and beta-endorphin immunoreactive terminals and of opiate receptors in adult and old male rats. Evidence for the existence of two main types of communication in the central nervous system: The volume transmission and the wiring transmission. *Acta Physiologica Scandinavica, 128*, 201–207.
48. Vizi, E. S., & Kiss, J. P. (1998). Neurochemistry and pharmacology of the major hippocampal transmitter systems: Synaptic and nonsynaptic interactions. *Hippocampus, 8*, 566–607.

49. Oláh, S., et al. (2009). Regulation of cortical microcircuits by unitary GABA-mediated volume transmission. *Nature, 461*, 1278–1281.
50. Kruk, M. R., et al. (1984). Comparison of aggressive behaviour induced by electrical stimulation in the hypothalamus of male and female rats. *Progress in Brain Research, 61*, 303–314.
51. Kruk, M. R. (2014). Hypothalamic attack: A wonderful artifact or a useful perspective on escalation and pathology in aggression? A viewpoint. *Current Topics in Behavioral Neurosciences, 17*, 143–188.
52. Kruk, M. R., et al. (1998). The hypothalamus: Cross-roads of endocrine and behavioural regulation in grooming and aggression. *Neuroscience and Biobehavioral Reviews, 23*, 163–177.
53. Kruk, M. R., Halász, J., Meelis, W., & Haller, J. (2004). Fast positive feedback between the adrenocortical stress response and a brain mechanism involved in aggressive behavior. *Behavioral Neuroscience, 118*, 1062–1070.
54. Kruk, M. R. (1991). Ethology and pharmacology of hypothalamic aggression in the rat. *Neuroscience and Biobehavioral Reviews, 15*, 527–538.
55. Halász, J., Liposits, Z., Meelis, W., Kruk, M. R., & Haller, J. (2002). Hypothalamic attack area-mediated activation of the forebrain in aggression. *Neuroreport, 13*, 1267–1270.
56. Parmigiani, S., Brain, P. F., Mainardi, D., & Brunoni, V. (1988). Different patterns of biting attack employed by lactating female mice (Mus domesticus) in encounters with male and female conspecific intruders. *Journal of Comparative Psychology (Washington, D.C.: 1983), 1983*(102), 287–293.
57. Neumann, I. D. (2001). Alterations in behavioral and neuroendocrine stress coping strategies in pregnant, parturient and lactating rats. *Progress in Brain Research, 133*, 143–152.
58. Biro, L., et al. (2017). Structural and functional alterations in the prefrontal cortex after post-weaning social isolation: Relationship with species-typical and deviant aggression. *Brain Structure & Function, 222*, 1861–1875.
59. Cheu, J. W., & Siegel, A. (1998). GABA receptor mediated suppression of defensive rage behavior elicited from the medial hypothalamus of the cat: Role of the lateral hypothalamus. *Brain Research, 783*, 293–304.
60. Tulogdi, A., et al. (2010). Brain mechanisms involved in predatory aggression are activated in a laboratory model of violent intra-specific aggression. *The European Journal of Neuroscience, 32*, 1744–1753.
61. Brutus, M., et al. (1984). A [14C]2-deoxyglucose analysis of the functional neural pathways of the limbic forebrain in the rat. IV. A pathway from the prefrontal cortical-medial thalamic system to the hypothalamus. *Brain Research, 310*, 279–293.
62. LeDoux, J. (2007). The amygdala. *Current Biology: CB, 17*, R868–R874.
63. Biro, L., et al. (2018). Task division within the prefrontal cortex: Distinct neuron populations selectively control different aspects of aggressive behavior via the hypothalamus. *Journal of Neuroscience: The Official Journal of the Society for Neuroscience, 38*, 4065–4075.
64. Tulogdi, A., et al. (2015). Neural mechanisms of predatory aggression in rats-implications for abnormal intraspecific aggression. *Behavioural Brain Research, 283*, 108–115.
65. Han, W., et al. (2017). Integrated control of predatory hunting by the central nucleus of the amygdala. *Cell, 168*, 311–324.e18.
66. Hasen, N. S., & Gammie, S. C. (2006). Maternal aggression: New insights from Egr-1. *Brain Research, 1108*, 147–156.
67. Hasen, N. S., & Gammie, S. C. (2005). Differential fos activation in virgin and lactating mice in response to an intruder. *Physiology & Behavior, 84*, 681–695.
68. Gammie, S. C., & Nelson, R. J. (2001). cFOS and pCREB activation and maternal aggression in mice. *Brain Research, 898*, 232–241.
69. Haller, J. (2018). The role of central and medial amygdala in normal and abnormal aggression: A review of classical approaches. *Neuroscience and Biobehavioral Reviews, 85*, 34–43.
70. Paxinos, G., & Watson, C. (2013). *The rat brain in stereotaxic coordinates* (7th ed.). San Diego: Academic.

71. Toth, M., et al. (2012). The neural background of hyper-emotional aggression induced by post-weaning social isolation. *Behavioural Brain Research, 233*, 120–129.
72. Ray, R. D., & Zald, D. H. (2012). Anatomical insights into the interaction of emotion and cognition in the prefrontal cortex. *Neuroscience and Biobehavioral Reviews, 36*, 479–501.
73. Pessoa, L. (2015). Précis on the cognitive-emotional brain. *The Behavioral and Brain Sciences, 38*, e71.
74. Vertes, R. P. (2006). Interactions among the medial prefrontal cortex, hippocampus and midline thalamus in emotional and cognitive processing in the rat. *Neuroscience, 142*, 1–20.
75. Bonini, F., et al. (2014). Action monitoring and medial frontal cortex: Leading role of supplementary motor area. *Science, 343*, 888–891.
76. Saunders, B., Lin, H., Milyavskaya, M., & Inzlicht, M. (2017). The emotive nature of conflict monitoring in the medial prefrontal cortex. *International Journal of Psychophysiology: Official Journal of the International Organization of Psychophysiology, 119*, 31–40.
77. Siegel, A., Edinger, H., & Dotto, M. (1975). Effects of electrical stimulation of the lateral aspect of the prefrontal cortex upon attack behavior in cats. *Brain Research, 93*, 473–484.
78. de Bruin, J. P., van Oyen, H. G., & Van de Poll, N. (1983). Behavioural changes following lesions of the orbital prefrontal cortex in male rats. *Behavioural Brain Research, 10*, 209–232.
79. Kolb, B. (1974). Social behavior of rats with chronic prefrontal lesions. *Journal of Comparative and Physiological Psychology, 87*, 466–474.
80. Rudebeck, P. H., et al. (2007). Distinct contributions of frontal areas to emotion and social behaviour in the rat. *The European Journal of Neuroscience, 26*, 2315–2326.
81. Izquierdo, A., Suda, R. K., & Murray, E. A. (2005). Comparison of the effects of bilateral orbital prefrontal cortex lesions and amygdala lesions on emotional responses in rhesus monkeys. *Journal of Neuroscience: The Official Journal of the Society for Neuroscience, 25*, 8534–8542.
82. Machado, C. J., & Bachevalier, J. (2006). The impact of selective amygdala, orbital frontal cortex, or hippocampal formation lesions on established social relationships in rhesus monkeys (Macaca mulatta). *Behavioral Neuroscience, 120*, 761–786.
83. Halász, J., Tóth, M., Kalló, I., Liposits, Z., & Haller, J. (2006). The activation of prefrontal cortical neurons in aggression – A double labeling study. *Behavioural Brain Research, 175*, 166–175.
84. Beiderbeck, D. I., et al. (2012). High and abnormal forms of aggression in rats with extremes in trait anxiety – Involvement of the dopamine system in the nucleus accumbens. *Psychoneuroendocrinology, 37*, 1969–1980.
85. Clinton, S. M., et al. (2011). Pattern of forebrain activation in high novelty-seeking rats following aggressive encounter. *Brain Research, 1422*, 20–31.
86. Haller, J., Tóth, M., Halasz, J., & De Boer, S. F. (2006). Patterns of violent aggression-induced brain c-fos expression in male mice selected for aggressiveness. *Physiology & Behavior, 88*, 173–182.
87. Wall, V. L., Fischer, E. K., & Bland, S. T. (2012). Isolation rearing attenuates social interaction-induced expression of immediate early gene protein products in the medial prefrontal cortex of male and female rats. *Physiology & Behavior, 107*, 440–450.
88. Duncan, G. E., Inada, K., Farrington, J. S., Koller, B. H., & Moy, S. S. (2009). Neural activation deficits in a mouse genetic model of NMDA receptor hypofunction in tests of social aggression and swim stress. *Brain Research, 1265*, 186–195.
89. Ago, Y., et al. (2013). Role of social encounter-induced activation of prefrontal serotonergic systems in the abnormal behaviors of isolation-reared mice. *Neuropsychopharmacology: Official Publication of the American College of Neuropsychopharmacology, 38*, 1535–1547.
90. Caffrey, M. K., Nephew, B. C., & Febo, M. (2010). Central vasopressin V1a receptors modulate neural processing in mothers facing intruder threat to pups. *Neuropharmacology, 58*, 107–116.

91. Comoli, E., Ribeiro-Barbosa, E. R., Negrão, N., Goto, M., & Canteras, N. S. (2005). Functional mapping of the prosencephalic systems involved in organizing predatory behavior in rats. *Neuroscience, 130*, 1055–1067.
92. Ferris, C. F., et al. (2008). Imaging the neural circuitry and chemical control of aggressive motivation. *BMC Neuroscience, 9*, 111.
93. Takahashi, A., Nagayasu, K., Nishitani, N., Kaneko, S., & Koide, T. (2014). Control of intermale aggression by medial prefrontal cortex activation in the mouse. *PLoS One, 9*, e94657.
94. Egger, M. D., & Flynn, J. P. (1963). Effects of electrical stimulation of the amygdala on hypothalamically elicited attack behavior in Cats. *Journal of Neurophysiology, 26*, 705–720.
95. Shaikh, M. B., & Siegel, A. (1994). Neuroanatomical and neurochemical mechanisms underlying amygdaloid control of defensive rage behavior in the cat. *Brazilian Journal of Medical and Biological Research = Revista brasileira de pesquisas médicas e biológicas, 27*, 2759–2779.
96. McGregor, A., & Herbert, J. (1992). Differential effects of excitotoxic basolateral and corticomedial lesions of the amygdala on the behavioural and endocrine responses to either sexual or aggression-promoting stimuli in the male rat. *Brain Research, 574*, 9–20.
97. Noack, J., Murau, R., & Engelmann, M. (2015). Consequences of temporary inhibition of the medial amygdala on social recognition memory performance in mice. *Frontiers in Neuroscience, 9*, 152.
98. Vochteloo, J. D., & Koolhaas, J. M. (1987). Medial amygdala lesions in male rats reduce aggressive behavior: Interference with experience. *Physiology & Behavior, 41*, 99–102.
99. Wang, Y., He, Z., Zhao, C., & Li, L. (2013). Medial amygdala lesions modify aggressive behavior and immediate early gene expression in oxytocin and vasopressin neurons during intermale exposure. *Behavioural Brain Research, 245*, 42–49.
100. Potegal, M., Hebert, M., DeCoster, M., & Meyerhoff, J. L. (1996). Brief, high-frequency stimulation of the corticomedial amygdala induces a delayed and prolonged increase of aggressiveness in male Syrian golden hamsters. *Behavioral Neuroscience, 110*, 401–412.
101. Block, C. H., Siegel, A., & Edinger, H. (1980). Effects of amygdaloid stimulation upon trigeminal sensory fields of the lip that are established during hypothalamically-elicited quiet biting attack in the cat. *Brain Research, 197*, 39–55.
102. Vergnes, M., & Karli, P. (1969). Interspecific rat-mice aggression behavior: Effects of electric stimulation of the lateral hypothalamus, amygdala and hippocampus. *Journal of Physiology (Paris), 61*(Suppl 2), 425.
103. Karli, P. M., Vergnes, M., Eclancher, F., Schmitt, P., & Chawerand, I. P. (1972). Role of amygdala in the control of mouse-killing behavior in the rat. *Advances in Behavioral Biology, 2*, 533–580.
104. Han, Y., Shaikh, M. B., & Siegel, A. (1996). Medial amygdaloid suppression of predatory attack behavior in the cat: II. Role of a GABAergic pathway from the medial to the lateral hypothalamus. *Brain Research, 716*, 72–83.
105. Kollack-Walker, S., & Newman, S. W. (1995). Mating and agonistic behavior produce different patterns of Fos immunolabeling in the male Syrian hamster brain. *Neuroscience, 66*, 721–736.
106. Pan, Y., Xu, L., Young, K. A., Wang, Z., & Zhang, Z. (2010). Agonistic encounters and brain activation in dominant and subordinate male greater long-tailed hamsters. *Hormones and Behavior, 58*, 478–484.
107. Halász, J., Liposits, Z., Kruk, M. R., & Haller, J. (2002). Neural background of glucocorticoid dysfunction-induced abnormal aggression in rats: Involvement of fear- and stress-related structures. *The European Journal of Neuroscience, 15*, 561–569.
108. Veening, J. G., et al. (2005). Do similar neural systems subserve aggressive and sexual behaviour in male rats? Insights from c-Fos and pharmacological studies. *European Journal of Pharmacology, 526*, 226–239.
109. Gobrogge, K. L., Liu, Y., Young, L. J., & Wang, Z. (2009). Anterior hypothalamic vasopressin regulates pair-bonding and drug-induced aggression in a monogamous rodent. *Proceedings of the National Academy of Sciences of the United States of America, 106*, 19144–19149.

110. Wang, Z., Hulihan, T. J., & Insel, T. R. (1997). Sexual and social experience is associated with different patterns of behavior and neural activation in male prairie voles. *Brain Research, 767*, 321–332.
111. Konoshenko, M. Y., Timoshenko, T. V., & Plyusnina, I. Z. (2013). c-Fos activation and intermale aggression in rats selected for behavior toward humans. *Behavioural Brain Research, 237*, 103–106.
112. Emery, N. J., et al. (2001). The effects of bilateral lesions of the amygdala on dyadic social interactions in rhesus monkeys (Macaca mulatta). *Behavioral Neuroscience, 115*, 515–544.
113. Takahashi, L. K., & Gladstone, C. D. (1988). Medial amygdaloid lesions and the regulation of sociosexual behavioral patterns across the estrous cycle in female golden hamsters. *Behavioral Neuroscience, 102*, 268–275.
114. Putkonen, P. T. (1966). Attack elicited by forebrain and hypothalamic stimulation in the chicken. *Experientia, 22*, 405–407.
115. Demski, L. S. (1973). Feeding and aggressive behavior evoked by hypothalamic stimulation in a cichlid fish. *Comparative Biochemistry and Physiology. A, Comparative Physiology, 44*, 685–692.
116. Martin, J. R. (1976). Motivated behaviors elicited from hypothalamus, midbrain, and pons of the Guinea pig (Cavia porcellus). *Journal of Comparative and Physiological Psychology, 90*, 1011–1034.
117. Sugerman, R. A., & Demski, L. S. (1978). Agonistic behavior elicited by electrical stimulation of the brain in western collared lizards. *Brain, Behavior and Evolution, 15*, 446–469.
118. Lipp, H. P. (1978). Aggression and flight behaviour of the marmoset monkey Callithrix jacchus: An ethogram for brain stimulation studies. *Brain, Behavior and Evolution, 15*, 241–259.
119. Roberts, W. W., Steinberg, M. L., & Means, L. W. (1967). Hypothalamic mechanisms for sexual, aggressive, and other motivational behaviors in the opossum. *Journal of Comparative and Physiological Psychology, 64*, 1–15.
120. Kruk, M. R., van der Poel, A. M., & de Vos-Frerichs, T. P. (1979). The induction of aggressive behaviour by electrical stimulation in the hypothalamus of male rats. *Behaviour, 70*, 292–322.
121. Woodworth, C. H. (1971). Attack elicited in rats by electrical stimulation of the lateral hypothalamus. *Physiology & Behavior, 6*, 345–353.
122. Smith, D. E., King, M. B., & Hoebel, B. G. (1970). Lateral hypothalamic control of killing: Evidence for a cholinoceptive mechanism. *Science, 167*, 900–901.
123. Bandler, R. J. (1970). Cholinergic synapses in the lateral hypothalamus for the control of predatory aggression in the rat. *Brain Research, 20*, 409–424.
124. Lammers, J. H., Kruk, M. R., Meelis, W., & van der Poel, A. M. (1988). Hypothalamic substrates for brain stimulation-induced patterns of locomotion and escape jumps in the rat. *Brain Research, 449*, 294–310.
125. Hoebel, B. G., & Teitelbaum, P. (1962). Hypothalamic control of feeding and self-stimulation. *Science, 135*, 375–377.
126. Herberg, L. J., & Blundell, J. E. (1967). Lateral hypothalamus: Hoarding behavior elicited by electrical stimulation. *Science, 155*, 349–350.
127. Lammers, J. H., Meelis, W., Kruk, M. R., & van der Poel, A. M. (1987). Hypothalamic substrates for brain stimulation-induced grooming, digging and circling in the rat. *Brain Research, 418*, 1–19.
128. Roeling, T. A., Kruk, M. R., Schuurmans, R., & Veening, J. G. (1993). Behavioural responses of bicucculline methiodide injections into the ventral hypothalamus of freely moving, socially interacting rats. *Brain Research, 615*, 121–127.
129. Adams, D. B., et al. (1993). Offense produced by chemical stimulation of the anterior hypothalamus of the rat. *Physiology & Behavior, 53*, 1127–1132.
130. Haller, J., et al. (1998). Aggressive experience affects the sensitivity of neurons towards pharmacological treatment in the hypothalamic attack area. *Behavioural Pharmacology, 9*, 469–475.

131. Hassanain, M., Bhatt, S., Zalcman, S., & Siegel, A. (2005). Potentiating role of interleukin-1β (IL-1β) and IL-1β type 1 receptors in the medial hypothalamus in defensive rage behavior in the cat. *Brain Research, 1048*, 1–11.
132. Xie, J., Kuenzel, W. J., Sharp, P. J., & Jurkevich, A. (2011). Appetitive and consummatory sexual and agonistic behaviour elicits FOS expression in aromatase and vasotocin neurons within the preoptic area and bed nucleus of the stria terminalis of male domestic chickens. *Journal of Neuroendocrinology, 23*, 232–243.
133. Wai, M. S. M., Lorke, D. E., Webb, S. E., & Yew, D. T. (2006). The pattern of c-fos activation in the CNS is related to behavior in the mudskipper. *Behavioural Brain Research, 167*, 318–327.
134. Delville, Y., De Vries, G. J., & Ferris, C. F. (2000). Neural connections of the anterior hypothalamus and agonistic behavior in golden hamsters. *Brain, Behavior and Evolution, 55*, 53–76.
135. Romero-Morales, L., et al. (2018). Neuronal activation associated with paternal and aversive interactions toward pups in the Mongolian gerbils (Meriones unguiculatus). *Hormones and Behavior, 105*, 47–57.
136. Li, Y., et al. (2018). Hypothalamic circuits for predation and evasion. *Neuron, 97*, 911–924.e5.
137. Park, S.-G., et al. (2018). Medial preoptic circuit induces hunting-like actions to target objects and prey. *Nature Neuroscience, 21*, 364–372.
138. Berridge, K. C., & Valenstein, E. S. (1991). What psychological process mediates feeding evoked by electrical stimulation of the lateral hypothalamus? *Behavioral Neuroscience, 105*, 3–14.
139. Falkner, A. L., Grosenick, L., Davidson, T. J., Deisseroth, K., & Lin, D. (2016). Hypothalamic control of male aggression-seeking behavior. *Nature Neuroscience, 19*, 596–604.
140. Falkner, A. L., Dollar, P., Perona, P., Anderson, D. J., & Lin, D. (2014). Decoding ventromedial hypothalamic neural activity during male mouse aggression. *Journal of Neuroscience: The Official Journal of the Society for Neuroscience, 34*, 5971–5984.
141. Chang, C.-H., & Gean, P.-W. (2019). The ventral hippocampus controls stress-provoked impulsive aggression through the ventromedial hypothalamus in post-weaning social isolation mice. *Cell Reports, 28*, 1195–1205.e3.
142. Roeling, T. A., et al. (1994). Efferent connections of the hypothalamic 'aggression area' in the rat. *Neuroscience, 59*, 1001–1024.
143. Toth, M., Fuzesi, T., Halasz, J., Tulogdi, A., & Haller, J. (2010). Neural inputs of the hypothalamic 'aggression area' in the rat. *Behavioural Brain Research, 215*, 7–20.
144. Bandler, R. (1982). Induction of 'rage' following microinjections of glutamate into midbrain but not hypothalamus of cats. *Neuroscience Letters, 30*, 183–188.
145. Mos, J., Kruk, M. R., Van der Poel, A. M., & Meelis, W. (1982). Aggressive behavior induced by electrical stimulation in the midbrain central gray of male rats. *Aggressive Behavior, 8*, 261–284.
146. Mos, J., et al. (1983). Effects of midbrain central gray lesions on spontaneous and electrically induced aggression in the rat. *Aggressive Behavior, 9*, 133–155.
147. Faber, C. L., et al. (2018). Distinct neuronal projections from the hypothalamic ventromedial nucleus mediate glycemic and behavioral effects. *Diabetes, 67*, 2518–2529.
148. Wang, L., et al. (2019). Hypothalamic control of conspecific self-defense. *Cell Reports, 26*, 1747–1758.e5.
149. Flak, J. N., et al. (2017). A leptin-regulated circuit controls glucose mobilization during noxious stimuli. *The Journal of Clinical Investigation, 127*, 3103–3113.
150. Zelena, D., Menant, O., Andersson, F., & Chaillou, E. (2018). Periaqueductal gray and emotions: The complexity of the problem and the light at the end of the tunnel, the magnetic resonance imaging. *Endocrine Regulations, 52*, 222–238.
151. Bandler, R., & Shipley, M. T. (1994). Columnar organization in the midbrain periaqueductal gray: Modules for emotional expression? *Trends in Neurosciences, 17*, 379–389.

152. Gil, M., Nguyen, N.-T., McDonald, M., & Albers, H. E. (2013). Social reward: Interactions with social status, social communication, aggression, and associated neural activation in the ventral tegmental area. *The European Journal of Neuroscience, 38*, 2308–2318.
153. Williamson, C. M., Klein, I. S., Lee, W., & Curley, J. P. (2019). Immediate early gene activation throughout the brain is associated with dynamic changes in social context. *Social Neuroscience, 14*, 253–265.
154. Golden, S. A., et al. (2016). Basal forebrain projections to the lateral habenula modulate aggression reward. *Nature, 534*, 688–692.
155. Mizumori, S. J., Cooper, B. G., Leutgeb, S., & Pratt, W. E. (2000). A neural systems analysis of adaptive navigation. *Molecular Neurobiology, 21*, 57–82.
156. Otis, J. M., et al. (2019). Paraventricular thalamus projection neurons integrate cortical and hypothalamic signals for cue-reward processing. *Neuron, 103*, 423–431.e4.
157. Kostowski, W., Cxlonkowski, A., Markowdka, L., & Markiewicz, L. (1975). Intraspecific aggressiveness after lesions of midbrain raphe nuclei in rats. *Pharmacology, 13*, 81–85.
158. Miczek, K. A., Altman, J. L., Appel, J. B., & Boggan, W. O. (1975). Para-chlorophenylalanine, serotonin and killing behavior. *Pharmacology, Biochemistry, and Behavior, 3*, 355–361.
159. Rosell, D. R., & Siever, L. J. (2015). The neurobiology of aggression and violence. *CNS Spectrums, 20*, 254–279.
160. Nelson, R. J., & Chiavegatto, S. (2001). Molecular basis of aggression. *Trends in Neurosciences, 24*, 713–719.
161. Olivier, B. (2015). Serotonin: A never-ending story. *European Journal of Pharmacology, 753*, 2–18.
162. de Boer, S. F., & Koolhaas, J. M. (2005). 5-HT1A and 5-HT1B receptor agonists and aggression: A pharmacological challenge of the serotonin deficiency hypothesis. *European Journal of Pharmacology, 526*, 125–139.
163. Faccidomo, S., Quadros, I. M. H., Takahashi, A., Fish, E. W., & Miczek, K. A. (2012). Infralimbic and dorsal raphé microinjection of the 5-HT(1B) receptor agonist CP-93,129: Attenuation of aggressive behavior in CFW male mice. *Psychopharmacology, 222*, 117–128.
164. Pytliak, M., Vargová, V., Mechírová, V., & Felšöci, M. (2011). Serotonin receptors – from molecular biology to clinical applications. *Physiological Research, 60*, 15–25.
165. Coccaro, E. F., Fanning, J. R., Phan, K. L., & Lee, R. (2015). Serotonin and impulsive aggression. *CNS Spectrums, 20*, 295–302.
166. Bielefeldt, A. Ø., Danborg, P. B., & Gøtzsche, P. C. (2016). Precursors to suicidality and violence on antidepressants: Systematic review of trials in adult healthy volunteers. *Journal of the Royal Society of Medicine, 109*, 381–392.
167. Glick, A. R. (2015). The role of serotonin in impulsive aggression, suicide, and homicide in adolescents and adults: A literature review. *International Journal of Adolescent Medicine and Health, 27*, 143–150.
168. Sharma, T., Guski, L. S., Freund, N., & Gøtzsche, P. C. (2016). Suicidality and aggression during antidepressant treatment: Systematic review and meta-analyses based on clinical study reports. *BMJ, 352*, i65.
169. Balázsfi, D., et al. (2018). Differential roles of the two raphe nuclei in amiable social behavior and aggression – An Optogenetic Study. *Frontiers in Behavioral Neuroscience, 12*, 163.
170. Hensler, J. G. (2006). Serotonergic modulation of the limbic system. *Neuroscience and Biobehavioral Reviews, 30*, 203–214.
171. Gamrani, H., Calas, A., Belin, M. F., Aguera, M., & Pujol, J. F. (1979). High resolution radioautographic identification of [3H]GABA labeled neurons in the rat nucleus raphe dorsalis. *Neuroscience Letters, 15*, 43–48.
172. Jackson, J., Bland, B. H., & Antle, M. C. (2009). Nonserotonergic projection neurons in the midbrain raphe nuclei contain the vesicular glutamate transporter VGLUT3. *Synapse (New York, N.Y.), 63*, 31–41.
173. Allers, K. A., & Sharp, T. (2003). Neurochemical and anatomical identification of fast- and slow-firing neurons in the rat dorsal raphe nucleus using juxtacellular labelling methods in vivo. *Neuroscience, 122*, 193–204.

174. Varga, V., et al. (2009). Fast synaptic subcortical control of hippocampal circuits. *Science, 326*, 449–453.
175. Sos, K. E., et al. (2017). Cellular architecture and transmitter phenotypes of neurons of the mouse median raphe region. *Brain Structure & Function, 222*, 287–299.
176. Shutoh, F., Ina, A., Yoshida, S., Konno, J., & Hisano, S. (2008). Two distinct subtypes of serotonergic fibers classified by co-expression with vesicular glutamate transporter 3 in rat forebrain. *Neuroscience Letters, 432*, 132–136.
177. Szőnyi, A., et al. (2019). Median raphe controls acquisition of negative experience in the mouse. *Science, 366*, eaay8746.
178. Binder, S., et al. (2019). Monosynaptic hippocampal-prefrontal projections contribute to spatial memory consolidation in mice. *Journal of Neuroscience: The Official Journal of the Society for Neuroscience, 39*, 6978–6991.
179. Sargin, D., Jeoung, H.-S., Goodfellow, N. M., & Lambe, E. K. (2019). Serotonin regulation of the prefrontal cortex: Cognitive relevance and the impact of developmental perturbation. *ACS Chemical Neuroscience, 10*, 3078–3093.
180. Fernandez, S. P., et al. (2016). Multiscale single-cell analysis reveals unique phenotypes of raphe 5-HT neurons projecting to the forebrain. *Brain Structure & Function, 221*, 4007–4025.
181. Van De Kar, L. D., & Lorens, S. A. (1979). Differential serotonergic innervation of individual hypothalamic nuclei and other forebrain regions by the dorsal and median midbrain raphe nuclei. *Brain Research, 162*, 45–54.
182. Niederkofler, V., et al. (2016). Identification of serotonergic neuronal modules that affect aggressive behavior. *Cell Reports, 17*, 1934–1949.
183. Soma, K. K. (2006). Testosterone and aggression: Berthold, birds and beyond. *Journal of Neuroendocrinology, 18*, 543–551.
184. Beeman, E. A. (1947). The effect of male hormone on aggressive behavior in mice. *Physiological Zoology, 20*, 373–405.
185. Albert, D. J., Walsh, M. L., & Jonik, R. H. (1993). Aggression in humans: What is its biological foundation? *Neuroscience and Biobehavioral Reviews, 17*, 405–425.
186. Archer, J. (1991). The influence of testosterone on human aggression. *British Journal of Psychology (London, England): 1953, 82*(Pt 1)), 1–28.
187. Book, A. S., Starzyk, K. B., & Quinsey, V. L. (2001). The relationship between testosterone and aggression: A meta-analysis. *Aggression and Violent Behavior, 6*, 579–599.
188. Soma, K. K., Scotti, M.-A. L., Newman, A. E. M., Charlier, T. D., & Demas, G. E. (2008). Novel mechanisms for neuroendocrine regulation of aggression. *Frontiers in Neuroendocrinology, 29*, 476–489.
189. Jasnow, A. M., Huhman, K. L., Bartness, T. J., & Demas, G. E. (2002). Short days and exogenous melatonin increase aggression of male Syrian hamsters (Mesocricetus auratus). *Hormones and Behavior, 42*, 13–20.
190. Wen, J. C., Hotchkiss, A. K., Demas, G. E., & Nelson, R. J. (2004). Photoperiod affects neuronal nitric oxide synthase and aggressive behaviour in male Siberian hamsters (Phodopus sungorus). *Journal of Neuroendocrinology, 16*, 916–921.
191. Kuriyama, K., & Ohkuma, S. (1995). Role of nitric oxide in central synaptic transmission: Effects on neurotransmitter release. *Japanese Journal of Pharmacology, 69*, 1–8.
192. Vincent, S. R. (2010). Nitric oxide neurons and neurotransmission. *Progress in Neurobiology, 90*, 246–255.
193. Moore, M. C., & Marler, C. A. (1987). Effects of testosterone manipulations on nonbreeding season territorial aggression in free-living male lizards, Sceloporus jarrovi. *General and Comparative Endocrinology, 65*, 225–232.
194. Trainor, B. C., & Marler, C. A. (2001). Testosterone, paternal behavior, and aggression in the monogamous California mouse (Peromyscus californicus). *Hormones and Behavior, 40*, 32–42.
195. He, F., Tai, F., Zhang, Y., & Zhang, X. (2012). Effects of castration on aggression and levels of serum sex hormones and their central receptors in mandarin voles (Microtus mandarinus). *Journal of Comparative Physiology. A, Neuroethology, Sensory, Neural, and Behavioral Physiology, 198*, 347–362.

196. Carré, J. M., et al. (2017). Exogenous testosterone rapidly increases aggressive behavior in dominant and impulsive men. *Biological Psychiatry, 82*, 249–256.
197. Tsai, L. W., & Sapolsky, R. M. (1996). Rapid stimulatory effects of testosterone upon myotubule metabolism and sugar transport, as assessed by silicon microphysiometry. *Aggressive Behavior, 22*, 357–364.
198. Foradori, C. D., Weiser, M. J., & Handa, R. J. (2008). Non-genomic actions of androgens. *Frontiers in Neuroendocrinology, 29*, 169–181.
199. Dixson, A. F. (1993). Sexual and aggressive behaviour of adult male marmosets (Callithrix jacchus) castrated neonatally, prepubertally, or in adulthood. *Physiology & Behavior, 54*, 301–307.
200. Klein, W. P., & Simon, N. G. (1991). Timing of neonatal testosterone exposure in the differentiation of estrogenic regulatory systems for aggression. *Physiology & Behavior, 50*, 91–93.
201. Motelica-Heino, I., Edwards, D. A., & Roffi, J. (1993). Intermale aggression in mice: Does hour of castration after birth influence adult behavior? *Physiology & Behavior, 53*, 1017–1019.
202. Butterfield, P. A., & Crook, J. H. (1968). The annual cycle of nest building and agonistic behaviour in captive Quelea quelea with reference to endocrine factors. *Animal Behaviour, 16*, 308–317.
203. Lucion, A. B., De-Almeida, R. M., & Da-Silva, R. S. (1996). Territorial aggression, body weight, carbohydrate metabolism and testosterone levels of wild rats maintained in laboratory colonies. *Brazilian Journal of Medical and Biological Research = Revista brasileira de pesquisas médicas e biológicas, 29*, 1657–1662.
204. Solomon, M. B., et al. (2009). Gonadal hormones modulate the display of conditioned defeat in male Syrian hamsters. *Hormones and Behavior, 56*, 423–428.
205. Trainor, B. C., Bird, I. M., & Marler, C. A. (2004). Opposing hormonal mechanisms of aggression revealed through short-lived testosterone manipulations and multiple winning experiences. *Hormones and Behavior, 45*, 115–121.
206. Terburg, D., Morgan, B., & van Honk, J. (2009). The testosterone–cortisol ratio: A hormonal marker for proneness to social aggression. *International Journal of Law and Psychiatry, 32*, 216–223.
207. Raisman, G., & Field, P. M. (1973). Sexual dimorphism in the neuropil of the preoptic area of the rat and its dependence on neonatal androgen. *Brain Research, 54*, 1–29. PubMed - NCBI. https://www.ncbi.nlm.nih.gov/pubmed/?term=raisman+Sexual+dimorphism+in+the+neuropil+of+the+preoptic+area+of+the+rat+and+its+dependence+on+neonatal+androgen.
208. Forger, N. G. (2018). Past, present and future of epigenetics in brain sexual differentiation. *Journal of Neuroendocrinology, 30*, e12492. 10.1111/jne.12492.
209. Ciofi, P., Lapirot, O. C., & Tramu, G. (2007). An androgen-dependent sexual dimorphism visible at puberty in the rat hypothalamus. *Neuroscience, 146*, 630–642.
210. Ghahramani, N. M., et al. (2014). The effects of perinatal testosterone exposure on the DNA methylome of the mouse brain are late-emerging. *Biology of Sex Differences, 5*, 8.
211. Murray, E. K., Hien, A., de Vries, G. J., & Forger, N. G. (2009). Epigenetic control of sexual differentiation of the bed nucleus of the stria terminalis. *Endocrinology, 150*, 4241–4247.
212. Cisternas, C. D., Cortes, L. R., Bruggeman, E. C., Yao, B., & Forger, N. G. (2020). Developmental changes and sex differences in DNA methylation and demethylation in hypothalamic regions of the mouse brain. *Epigenetics, 15*, 72–84.
213. Behzadi, G., Kalén, P., Parvopassu, F., & Wiklund, L. (1990). Afferents to the median raphe nucleus of the rat: Retrograde cholera toxin and wheat germ conjugated horseradish peroxidase tracing, and selective D-[3H]aspartate labelling of possible excitatory amino acid inputs. *Neuroscience, 37*, 77–100.
214. Hooks, B. M., et al. (2013). Organization of cortical and thalamic input to pyramidal neurons in mouse motor cortex. *Journal of Neuroscience: The Official Journal of the Society for Neuroscience, 33*, 748–760.
215. Lu, M. T., Preston, J. B., & Strick, P. L. (1994). Interconnections between the prefrontal cortex and the premotor areas in the frontal lobe. *The Journal of Comparative Neurology, 341*, 375–392.

Chapter 8
Distorted Circuitry in Violent Animals

Introduction

The mechanisms underlying aggression have long been considered unitary. This led to the belief that the behavioral methods crystallized in the first few decades of the twentieth century may not only clarify the mechanisms of aggression as a natural phenomenon but may also be relevant for understanding psychopathological and criminal aggression [1]. As a secondary consequence, novel treatments for aggression problems were preclinically tested by studying the classical methodologies: hypothalamic, resident–intruder, and maternal aggressions [2].

Over time, however, it became clear that brain structure and consequently function are more plastic than originally thought, which made it unlikely that the very same mechanisms operate in various disorders. Abnormal aggression models are endeavors that aim at mirroring this human diversity in the animal laboratory. Each model was developed with the clear purpose of modelling human etiological factors in animals and observing behavioral and neural consequences. The ultimate purpose of this research is the identification of distortions in brain mechanisms reflecting etiological factors and establishing their relationship with behavioral alterations, with the hope of identifying new leads for the treatment of aggression-related psychopathologies and ultimately crime.

Research with abnormal aggression models demonstrated that the distortions of aggressive behavior cannot be understood solely by the mechanisms of normal aggression. Different etiological factors induce specific brain alterations, which are associated with specific modifications of aggressive behavior. While natural manifestations of aggression are controlled essentially by one basic mechanism (with species-specific variants), each form of abnormal aggression appears to have its own mechanism, which is strongly influenced by its own etiological factor. As such, the use of plural words is justified: this is a discourse on the mechanisms of abnormal aggressions.

J. Haller, *Neurobiopsychosocial Perspectives on Aggression and Violence*,
Advances in Preventing and Treating Violence and Aggression,
https://doi.org/10.1007/978-3-030-46331-1_8

8.1 Background

In comparison with laboratory tests of animal aggression, models of abnormal aggression (animal violence) are rather new, which has a large impact on the current developmental stage of the area. Those studying the traditional models of normal aggression have used essentially the same few behavioral paradigms and historically had the time to explore the full spectrum of neuroscientific technologies. In contrast, those studying abnormal aggression have created models of their own, which they have studied mostly by methodologies that were available locally. In addition, other local conditions, e.g., the availability of funds and personnel, time allocable to research, personal scientific interests, etc., limit the pace of this research. Therefore, the development of the field is imbalanced in at least three ways. (1) Some models were investigated by a variety of methodologies and rather systematically. Other models were less well studied, which is shown by both the number of studies and the range of the technologies employed. (2) Each model has its own lead researcher who is reluctant to adopt the models of others. Consequently, models were seldom crosschecked, which questions the reliability of findings. The repeatability of findings is usually ensured, but those who replicate earlier findings often belong to the same research group. (3) Due to limitations by local conditions, a brain deficit observed in one model often remains uninvestigated in another. As such, an overlap of brain deficits may indicate similarities, but non-overlaps are sometimes due simply to chance.

Research into abnormal aggression models is currently in its heroic phase, when local teams attempt to explain everything based on their own models and methodologies, which results in an unintegrated collection of theories. All theories may be true, but all theories appear unilateral and incomplete, and the relationships between alternative theories remain unexplored. To give one single example, serotonin was shown to lose its aggression-controlling role in the glucocorticoid-deficit model of abnormal aggression, whereas in the early subjugation model, the serotonin–vasopressin imbalance hypothesis received a great emphasis (see below). The two phenomena may be interrelated, but their relationship was never investigated. Does vasopressin–serotonin imbalance play a role in abnormal aggression elicited by a chronic glucocorticoid deficit? In more general terms: Is the vasopressin–serotonin imbalance a general mechanism of abnormal aggression, or it is just a specific consequence of early subjugation? Dilemmas of this kind haunt the whole field. None can be addressed appropriately unless research groups start to study models other than their own and begin comparing mechanisms observed by one group with those observed by another group.

Below we present the findings obtained with the main models in a rather detailed way, because we consider these models as bridges between the mechanisms of normal aggression addressed in the previous chapter and the mechanisms of psychopathological and criminal aggressions addressed in the next. We will focus on those models that are directly relevant for this book, namely, those that are linked to genetic backgrounds and developmental stressors. Prenatal stressors will be omitted because these are better models of anxiety and depression than of abnormal aggression as shown above. Drug models, particularly those showing that anabolic–androgenic steroids [3], alcohol [4], and cocaine [5] result in abnormal aggression, will also be neglected together with those that investigate proximate brain mechanisms underlying abnormal forms of aggression [6]. These models are naturally important, but they are not directly relevant for the gene–life event–behavior trio.

8.2 Overview of the Main Findings

8.2.1 Genetic Models: Selection Lines for Aggression

8.2.1.1 Brief Description

The selection of mice for aggression was prompted by the high heritability of the trait in humans. As shown above, three such mouse line pairs exist of which two, the most studied, short and long attack latency [7] lines will be discussed here.

The aggressive short attack latency line shows strong signs of abnormality including excessive aggression and inappropriate targeting of attacks that results in harmful, potentially lethal bites [7–11]. They also attack pups, females, and anesthetized, nonthreatening males and are insensitive to appeasement signals from opponents. These attacks are performed against a background of reduced autonomic and glucocorticoid stress responses as compared to the timid line [12, 13].

8.2.1.2 Brain Alterations

The bulk of research on the aggressive line was done in the period when aggression research focused on neurochemical and pharmacological phenomena, and, for historical reasons, this approach was to some extent preserved later. (For the main epochs of aggression research, see previous section.) Most findings address issues related to the organizing and attuning systems of aggression control.

As opposed to long attack latency (timid) mice, the aggressive line does not require the neonatal surge of testosterone for the adult development of aggressiveness. This indirectly shows that the genetic component of aggression is very strong [14]. Nevertheless, the aggressive line shows higher testosterone blood levels and increased neural androgen receptor sensitivity in adulthood [15], suggesting that testosterone may still contribute to the increased aggression in this line. The aforementioned difference in glucocorticoid secretion in its turn may contribute to differences observed in the line-dependent functioning of the serotonergic system and hippocampus [12]. (See below for details regarding these differences.) Thus, hormonal-organizing systems may play a role in genetically determined abnormal aggression, a larger role being apparent for glucocorticoids.

Regarding attuning networks, an increased negative feedback by presynaptic 5-HT_{1A} serotonin receptors was suggested to result in decreased serotonergic neurotransmission in the aggressive line, which may support the serotonin deficiency hypothesis of aggression [16]. This was also supported by reduced serotonin content in the prefrontal cortex of the same line [17]. Nevertheless, other studies suggested that serotonin turnover is increased in the aggressive line; [18] moreover, the hippocampus of this line was more sensitive to serotonin than that of the timid line [19, 20]. This is reminiscent of controversies surrounding the role of serotonin in the control of normal aggression. (See previous chapter.) This awaits further studies as does the case of abnormal aggression. Findings on dopamine appear more congruent, although data are sparse: the aggressive line shows an upregulated dopamine system [7, 17].

In the accessory systems, structural brain alterations were reported. For instance, vasopressin neuron density in the bed nucleus of striae terminalis and vasopressinergic projections to the lateral septum are lower in the aggressive line [21], which potentially contributes to the lower activation of the lateral septum by fights [22]. Regarding the hippocampus, the aggressive line showed increased cell proliferation in the dentate gyrus [23] and decreased mossy fiber terminal fields [24], which is possibly explained by the differential expression of cytoskeleton and signal transduction genes and differential regulation of the raf/ERK pathway [25]. The relevance of these findings for aggression control remains to be elucidated.

Finally, both the rivalry and the predatory core circuitries were activated in the aggressive line by social conflicts. Under normal conditions, this pattern was only seen in maternal aggression, which is also violent and is also performed on the background of low glucocorticoid stress responses, suggesting that the coactivation of rivalry and predatory pathways is bound to this condition [26].

8.2.1.3 Overview and Conclusions

The selection of mice for aggression resulted in a series of brain alterations which range from functional changes, e.g., the altered activation of the aggression core circuitries, to structural ones, for instance, those seen in the bed nucleus striae terminalis, lateral septum, and hippocampus. It seems important that the core predatory and rivalry aggression circuits were co-activated in a model that is associated with reduced stress responses.

8.2.2 *Genetic Models: Selection Lines for Anxiety*

8.2.2.1 Brief Description

The rationale of including this model here is twofold: (i) anxiety and aggression are often associated in humans [27], and (ii) the rat line pair that was selected for extremes in anxiety showed abnormal forms of aggression in the resident–intruder test [8, 28]. Both high- and low-anxiety rats show excessive aggression although this was not as pronounced as with mice selected for aggression, and both attacked vulnerable targets of opponents (e.g., head, throat, and belly). The aggressiveness of the low-anxiety line appears to be more pronounced as the individuals belonging to it attack females and sedated opponents, which was not seen in the high-anxiety line [8, 28].

Autonomic and glucocorticoid stress responses to aggression were decreased in the high-anxiety rat line, whereas the low-anxiety rat line showed increased stress responses to fighting [8]. This is surprising for rats being characterized by low anxiety, but it occurs that responses to non-social and social stressors are different in this line; the former elicit increased glucocorticoid stress responses as expected, whereas the latter responded in an opposite way. These lines offer two forms of genetically determined abnormal aggressions as it regards stress responses.

8.2.2.2 Brain Alterations

In the lateral septum of the "more abnormal" low-anxiety line, vasopressin negatively associated with aggression as shown by release studies, and possibly as a consequence, the lateral septum was weakly activated by fights in this line. The opposite was observed in the high-anxiety line [29]. These findings were supported by experiments where vasopressin alone or vasopressin receptor antagonists were applied locally. Similar effects of vasopressin were observed when the maternal aggression of rats belonging to these strains was studied [30, 31].

An extensive immediate early gene activation study [28] suggested that the rivalry and predatory aggression core circuitries were co-activated in the low- but not in the high-anxiety line. In the latter, an increased activation of the core rivalry circuitry was observed. The same study also showed that dopamine release in the nucleus accumbens was increased in the low-anxiety but not in the high-anxiety line.

8.2.2.3 Overview and Conclusions

Although the model remains poorly investigated from the point of view of aggression research, it leads to several important conclusions as follows. (1) It draws attention to the role of vasopressinergic and dopaminergic systems in abnormal aggression, two neurotransmitter systems poorly studied in some other models. (2) It shows that the severity of abnormal aggression depends on the severity of brain alterations. (3) It suggests that male abnormal aggression and violent but still normal maternal aggression may have overlapping brain mechanisms.

8.2.3 The Post-weaning Social Isolation Model

8.2.3.1 Brief Description

Human evidence suggests that early neglect leads to a reactive emotional temperament [32] characterized by uncontrolled outbursts of anger and aggression [33, 34]. Post-weaning social isolation models this early social condition, and over six decades of research has significantly contributed to understanding the effects of social neglect on the aggressive behavior of different species [35–38]. Early studies, however, addressed aggression in quantitative terms as the concept of abnormal animal aggression was not developed yet.

The model discussed here involves the raising of rats in individual cages from weaning to early adulthood and their testing in the resident–intruder test as residents. They were also studied in social groups formed in adulthood. Although weaning and the placement of rats in individual cages elicit a transient stress response, glucocorticoid production is not altered in the subsequent weeks of isolation, and basal autonomic functions do not show changes either [39]. When rats were exposed to an intruder in their home cage, however, they showed a dramatic exacerbation of both glucocorticoid and autonomic stress responses, which was not ameliorated by repeated exposures to the resident–intruder test.

The behavior of rats underwent somewhat opposing changes in the resident–intruder test and during social cohabitation. In the former, rats isolated from weaning showed a marked behavioral arousal manifested in rapid switches from one behavior to another, increases in the number of bites delivered to opponents, and altered attack targeting and a decrease in social signals. Specifically, rats preferentially targeted their attacks on vulnerable body parts of opponents (head, throat, and belly) and failed to signal their attack intentions appropriately by offensive threats. In summary, they showed a behavioral pattern reminiscent of uncontrolled outbursts of aggression seen in some human psychopathologies.

When rats were introduced into social groups, they were timid and frequently showed unprovoked defensive behaviors and appeared "estranged" from companions, e.g., did not huddle with them during sleep. Their social behavior normalized approximately within 1 week; yet, abnormal behavior reoccurred when re-socialized rats were again studied in the resident–intruder test. Thus, social behavior was responsive to social experience, whereas aggressive behavior was not. This pattern of behavior was repeatedly observed in a number of studies [39–44].

8.2.3.2 Brain Alterations

Resident–intruder conflicts elicited an increased activation of the rivalry aggression circuitry at all its main levels from the prefrontal cortex (medial and lateral orbitofrontal cortices, anterior cingulate cortex), amygdala (bed nucleus of striae terminalis, medial and basolateral amygdala), hypothalamus (mediobasal hypothalamus, hypothalamic paraventricular nucleus) to the brainstem [41].

These functional changes were accompanied by significant changes in brain structure. Social isolation from weaning to early adulthood inhibited the development of the medial prefrontal cortex, as shown by its reduced thickness and the decreased dendritic arborization of its neurons and by reductions in the vascularization of, and glial density in, this area [43]. In addition, post-weaning social isolation induced a series of neural plasticity-related changes in the medial prefrontal cortex, particularly in its infralimbic region, in the medial amygdala, and ventral hippocampus, and reduced the projections of this hippocampal area to the prefrontal cortex [44]. Epigenetic changes likely contributed to the observed prefrontal alterations as shown by alterations in the methylation of the brain-derived neurotrophic factor gene in prefrontal regions. Note that brain-derived neurotrophic factor is an important engine of plasticity in general [45]. The factor was also closely associated with plasticity-related changes in the brain of the rats submitted to the model.

These findings were recently confirmed and complemented by an independent group, which also implicated the brain-derived neurotrophic factor in post-weaning social isolation-induced abnormal aggression. They showed that glutamatergic neurotransmission plays important roles in controlling the effects of this factor [46]. Another study by the same group showed that the ventral hippocampus beyond its connections to the prefrontal cortex (see above) affects abnormal aggression by its connections to the ventral hypothalamus [47]. This was evidenced by the specific optogenetic stimulation of those ventral hippocampal neurons that project to the ventral hypothalamus, a subregion of the rivalry aggression hypothalamic site.

Another recent study [44] addressed the strange finding mentioned above, specifically, that resocialization failed to abolish abnormal features of aggression despite that it eliminated social deficits observed at the beginning of resocialization. It was hypothesized that this was due to the reduced plasticity of the brain in adulthood which may be reinstated by fluoxetine administered concomitantly. Note that besides being an antidepressant, fluoxetine, when administered for several weeks, reactivates the neural plasticity in adults typical of younger ages [48]. This capacity of the compound was shown to be involved in its antidepressant effects; moreover, it was suggested that fluoxetine is promising for the treatment of amblyopia as it restores plasticity in the adult visual cortex [49]. Neither resocialization nor fluoxetine alone abolished abnormal aggression developed in response to post-weaning social isolation, but their combination did so, specifically by reactivating brain-derived neurotrophic factor-related neural plasticity. The causal involvement of this factor in the process was shown by the blockade of the TrkB receptor, which mediates the effects of brain-derived neurotrophic factor. This blockade abolished behavioral improvement induced by the combination of fluoxetine and resocialization, showing that epigenetic changes in the gene encoding for brain-derived neurotrophic factor is causally involved in behavioral disturbances.

8.2.3.3 Overview and Conclusions

Post-weaning social isolation massively alters the structure of major components of the core aggression circuitry, and, likely as a consequence, the circuitry was overactivated by social challenges. It is worth noting that this is one of the two abnormal aggression models where the role of epigenetic processes and alterations in neural plasticity were experimentally demonstrated.

Thus, the brain undergoes plastic changes under the effect of early isolation that cannot be redressed by resocialization in adulthood. When, however, neural plasticity was reactivated by fluoxetine, resocialization became effective. This suggests that fluoxetine may be used to enhance the efficacy of psychotherapies, because resocialization alone was poorly effective in reactive human aggression as well [50, 51].

8.2.4 The Peripubertal Stress Model

8.2.4.1 Brief Description

The model was based on human findings showing that the brain is highly susceptible to environmental perturbations during puberty, and mental disorders often emerge in this period [52, 53], including aggression-related psychopathologies. The model consists in exposing rats to predator odor, open field, and elevated open platform intermittently between 28 and 42 days of age. It was suggested that compared to social stress models, this excludes social learning, which may modify aggressive behavior by itself and as such may mask the pure effects of stress [54].

Peripubertal stressors increased aggression dramatically in adulthood [55]; rats readily attacked anaesthetized, nonthreatening opponents [56], and females [57]. In addition, attacks were damaging (targeted vulnerable body parts of opponents) and were poorly signaled socially [58]. Similar effects were observed in female rats [59]. Thus, non-social peripubertal stress elicited the full spectrum of abnormal aggression symptoms, and its consequences were gender-independent. It is noteworthy that the adult effects of peripubertal stressors were inhibited by glucocorticoid receptor blockers administered to juveniles concurrently with the stressor [60], demonstrating causal relationships between juvenile glucocorticoid stress and adult behavior. Abnormal aggressions developed on the background of normal baseline glucocorticoid production but blunted responses to social and non-social stressors [56, 58].

8.2.4.2 Brain Alterations

One array of changes emerging in this model concerns aggression-induced brain activation patterns [56]. This appears to be the only abnormal aggression model where activation was blunted in one subarea of the prefrontal cortex, particularly the medial orbitofrontal cortex. This is in line with some but not all human findings, as shown in the next section. Almost all subareas of the amygdala were over-activated by aggression, including the central amygdala, which plays multiple roles in predatory aggression (as shown in the previous chapter). Moreover, structural equation modelling suggested that aggression was triggered after peripubertal stress by a medial orbitofrontal cortex → medial amygdala → central amygdala pathway, which contains the main components of both the rivalry and predatory circuitry in an interesting connectivity sequence.

The second category of changes concerns neurotransmission. Specifically, abnormal aggression was associated with enhanced MAOA and 5-HTT gene expression in the prefrontal cortex [56] and enhanced CRHR1 gene expression in the hippocampus and central amygdala [61]. Note that the MAOA gene encodes the MAOA enzyme and 5-HTT encodes the serotonin transporter, whereas CRHR1 encodes the corticotropin-releasing hormone receptor type 1. All three were on the list of those genes that are associated aggression (see Chap. 3). Protein products of the former inhibit serotonin neurotransmission by breaking down or removing serotonin from the synapse, while the latter mediates the effects of the corticotropin-releasing hormone, which is involved in the control of the stress [62] and fear [63] responses in the paraventricular nucleus of the hypothalamus and central amygdala, respectively. Expression changes were accompanied by increased histone acetylation, a basic epigenetic phenomenon, and the consequences of peripubertal stressors were reversed by the administration of MAO_A enzyme inhibitors and CRHR1 receptor antagonists. This demonstrates the relevance of these epigenetic changes in abnormal aggression.

The third category of changes concern those observed in the expression of neuroligins, which are synaptic cell adhesion molecules that control the balance of neural excitation and inhibition [64]. Particularly, peripubertal stress reduced neuroligin-2 expression in the prefrontal cortex. In view of the roles played by neuroligins and other cell adhesion molecules in mediating the effects of stress on aggression [65, 66], this finding indicates that adhesion molecules are promising targets of investigations into the mechanisms that elicit the emergence of abnormal aggression.

Finally, recent studies involved other mechanisms in the control of peripubertal stress-induced abnormal aggression. These include changes in white matter integrity that predicted the subsequent development of the aggressive phenotype, [55] the modulation of glucocorticoid receptor expression in the central amygdala, which could be counteracted by treatment with the glucocorticoid receptor antagonist mifepristone [60], and disturbed excitation and inhibition balance in the lateral septum [67].

8.2.4.3 Overview and Conclusions

The exposure of rats to just three non-social stressors in the peripubertal period leads to unexpectedly strong behavioral and neural alterations in adulthood. The magnitude of changes appears exceptional when compared with the more modest effects of a larger number of social stressors (defeats) administered to juveniles in the same life period. (See next section.)

Peripubertal stressors altered the molecular connectivity of neurons and synapses, changed the functioning of various neurotransmitter systems by epigenetic processes, and modified the functioning of the aggression circuitry. These changes are likely interrelated although such relationships remain to be established. In the context of other discoveries, two mechanisms deserve emphasis. First, the role of serotonin is further complicated by this line of research. The concomitant augmentation of the MAO_A enzyme and the serotonin transporter suggests that abnormal aggression is associated with decreased serotonin in this model. This adjoins the controversies surrounding the roles of this neurotransmitter. Second, the activation of the central amygdala, moreover its key role in peripubertal stress-induced abnormal aggression, indicates the coactivation of the predatory aggression circuit with that of rivalry aggression. It is a pity that other key components of the predatory aggression circuitry particularly the lateral hypothalamus and periaqueductal gray were not investigated in this model so far.

8.2.5 The Early Subjugation Model

8.2.5.1 Brief Description

Early subjugation aims at modelling child abuse that is often followed by antisocial behavior in later stages of life [68]. This model was developed and extensively used in hamsters [69], but a rat variant of the model also exists [70]. Usually, juveniles are daily exposed to attacks by larger males between the age of 28–42 days (hamsters) and 26–40 days (rats), although the timing and the number of defeat experiences showed some variation over years in hamsters. Aggressive behavior was studied in the resident–intruder test. Signs of behavioral abnormality were not blatant in either species. In hamsters, subjugation increased aggression against smaller but decreased it against larger opponents, [69] accelerated the emergence of adult forms of aggression [71], and promoted attacks on juveniles [69, 72]. In rats, only increased attack counts were reported [70]. Abnormal features of attack were not studied expressly in either species. In both, behavioral consequences were highly persistent [70, 72]. Corticosterone was increased by subjugation alone (i.e., in the juvenile stage), but this effect disappeared within 2 weeks [73]. Subsequently, baseline glucocorticoid levels remained unaltered, but glucocorticoid stress responses were blunted [72]. Notably, subjugation in adulthood does not elicit similar effects, demonstrating that the responses discussed here are linked to a sensitive life period [72].

8.2.5.2 Brain Alterations

Brain alterations induced by early subjugation are poorly known. One study based its research scope on earlier findings by the same group, which showed that vasopressinergic and serotonergic neurotransmissions interactively control aggression at the level of hypothalamic attack sites [74–76]. Particularly, vasopressin stimulates aggression in this area, whereas serotonin inhibits it by its connections to vasopressinergic neurons. This led to the emergence of the vasopressin–serotonin balance hypothesis of aggression.

Early subjugation decreased the vasopressin content of hypothalamic attack sites and increased their serotonin innervation [69]. Similar changes were observed in the lateral septum. Subjugation also increased tyrosine hydroxylase activity in the medial amygdala [73]. This enzyme is the rate-limiting step of catecholamine synthesis and is usually expressed in the cell bodies of noradrenergic and dopaminergic neurons, which are located far away from the amygdala. Nevertheless, the enzyme is also expressed in the axon terminals of dopaminergic cells [77]. Thus, this finding indirectly shows that subjugation increased the dopaminergic innervation of the medial amygdala.

A more recent study showed that metabolic activity and the coordination of activity in brain areas related to motivation were altered by social subjugation [78]. Metabolic activity was evaluated based on cytochrome oxidase an enzyme crucially involved in energy metabolism. Although the study focused on sexual behavior, metabolic changes were observed in brain areas belonging to the accessory circuitry of aggression control, e.g., the bed nucleus striae terminalis, hypothalamic preoptic area, and ventral tegmental area. Unfortunately, the behavioral significance of such metabolic changes is unknown at present.

8.2.5.3 Overview and Conclusions

The neural mechanisms of early subjugation-induced abnormal aggression are poorly known, and the available findings are somewhat at variance with alterations expected based on earlier studies and seem to lead to opposing consequences. For instance, decreased vasopressinergic and increased serotonergic neurotransmission in hypothalamic attack sites should have decreased aggression based on studies by the same group in non-subjugated hamsters. At the same time, increased dopaminergic innervation is usually associated with increased aggression [79].

As child abuse rather reliably leads to aggression in adulthood, it is only a pity that its laboratory model is so poorly understood. Conflicting findings may be related to the complex behavioral outcome of early subjugation, which can increase or decrease aggression depending on the opponent and leads to few signs of behavioral abnormality. The merit of work performed with this model is that it drew attention to the importance of vasopressin–serotonin balance in hypothalamic attack sites.

8.2.6 *The Glucocorticoid-Deficit Model*

8.2.6.1 Brief Description

This model models hypo-glucocorticoid states observed in a variety of aggressive people. (See previous chapters.) The essence of the experimental manipulation is the removal of the adrenal glands (adrenalectomy) followed by low-level glucocorticoid replacement by subcutaneous tablets [80]. The former eliminates glucocorticoid production, whereas the latter ensures low and stable glucocorticoid blood levels, which are necessary for maintaining neuronal integrity [81]. Plasma glucocorticoid levels were unreactive to stressors and represented one-third of normal daytime glucocorticoid levels, similar to that seen in habitually violent offenders [82]. Rats were tested in the resident–intruder test, the experimental animal being the resident.

Glucocorticoid deficiency changed three important aspects of attack behavior: (i) Rats preferentially targeted their attacks at the head, throat, and belly of the opponent. Occasionally, bites were even aimed at the testes and the hind paws of intruders. Such attacks are damaging, moreover, potentially life-threatening, and are rarely delivered by controls. (ii) The intention of biting was poorly signaled socially, which made attacks unexpected to opponents. Quite often, the intruder was suddenly bitten while exploring the cage, i.e., without being in social contact with the resident. (iii) The delivery of attacks was associated with substantially reduced and shortened autonomic stress responses. Aggression-induced heart rate increases were halved as compared to controls and the response terminated while the rats were still fighting, whereas in controls, heart rates remained increased for about an hour *after* the termination of the conflict. This pattern was repeatedly observed [80, 83–86].

In summary, low and non-reactive glucocorticoid levels induced the emergence of vicious, unpredictable, and "cold-blooded" attacks – in blunt terms this pattern is reminiscent of psychopathic aggression. Changes were highly specific to the targeting and signaling of attacks as no other aspects of aggressive behavior were changed. Acutely decreased corticosterone production did not elicit this pattern, whereas repeated glucocorticoid injections abolished it in adrenalectomized rats, showing that behavioral–autonomic alterations were specific to the chronic glucocorticoid deficit.

8.2.6.2 Brain Alterations

Behavioral alterations were associated with major alterations in the aggression circuitry as follows. (1) The aggressive encounter activated the core pathway of predatory aggression together with that of rivalry aggression (i.e., the central amygdala–lateral hypothalamus–ventral periaqueductal gray pathways together with the medial amygdala–mediobasal hypothalamus–dorsal periaqueductal gray) [87]. The former was exclusively activated in controls, whereas the latter exclusively in mouse-killing rats [88]. The importance of the lateral hypothalamic ("predatory") activation was revealed by a subsequent study, showing that the optogenetic stimulation of this area elicited an attack pattern highly similar to that seen in adrenalectomized rats [89]. (2) The prefrontal control of aggression was altered. Specifically, the balance between local inhibitory (GABAergic) and excitatory (glutamatergic) neurotransmission was substantially altered by glucocorticoid deficiency in the agranular, infralimbic, lateral orbitofrontal, and medial orbitofrontal regions [90]. Importantly, the inhibition–excitation balance is believed to play important roles in information processing and decision-making in the prefrontal cortex [91], especially in conjunction with social behavior [92]. A multiple regression analysis revealed that the inhibition/excitation imbalance explained ~90% of behavioral variation, which assigns a large role to this specific prefrontal deficit. (3) Substance P communication between the medial amygdala and mediobasal hypothalamus, the importance of which was evidenced already by early brain stimulation studies [93, 94], was dramatically changed by glucocorticoid deficiency [95]. The expression of the neurokinin 1 receptor that mediates substance P neurotransmission was increased two- to threefold in the medial amygdala and six- to sevenfold in the mediobasal hypothalamus. Moreover, the blockade of these receptors in the hypothalamus specifically abolished violent forms of aggression [95, 96], which demonstrates the role of these receptors in abnormal aggression. (4) Serotonin lost its aggression-controlling role in adrenalectomized rats as shown by both the lack of correlation between aggression and the activation of the dorsal raphe [21] and non-responsiveness to the anti-aggressive agent buspirone, an 5-HT_{1A} serotonin receptor partial agonist [85, 86]. In controls, there was a tight negative correlation between aggression and dorsal raphe activation, whereas buspirone did reduce aggressiveness.

8.2.6.3 Overview and Conclusions

Glucocorticoid deficiency activated the predatory aggression core circuit in a social context, altered the functioning of prefrontal decision mechanisms, enhanced the communication between the medial amygdala and mediobasal hypothalamus via substance P neurotransmission, and suspended the role of serotonin in aggression control. All these changes were highly relevant for the emergence of abnormal aggression in this model as shown above. Note that the predatory circuit was not activated in the post-weaning social isolation (hyperarousal) model [41] but was activated in several other models associated with hypoarousal [26]. This suggests that the activation of the predatory circuit is typical to those etiological factors that decrease glucocorticoid secretion on the long run and which reduce arousal elicited by fights.

The several fold increase in Substance P (neurokinin 1) receptors in key areas of aggression control suggests that this receptor may serve as a lead for the treatment of certain aggression-related psychopathologies especially because antagonists of the receptor – which were developed as putative antidepressants [97] – abolished abnormal features of aggression (e.g., faulty attack targeting) without affecting normal, more mild forms of aggression.

8.3 Two Types of Core Pathways

The models briefly but as far as possible exhaustively reviewed above suggest the existence of two major core pathways that can lead to the development of aggression. (See Fig. 8.1.) One pathway operates in those models where aggression was associated with low basal glucocorticoid plasma levels and/or blunted stress responses, and aggression-induced autonomic activation is also low. This pathway was well characterized in the glucocorticoid deficiency model of abnormal aggression. In other models, less information is available, but the central amygdala was

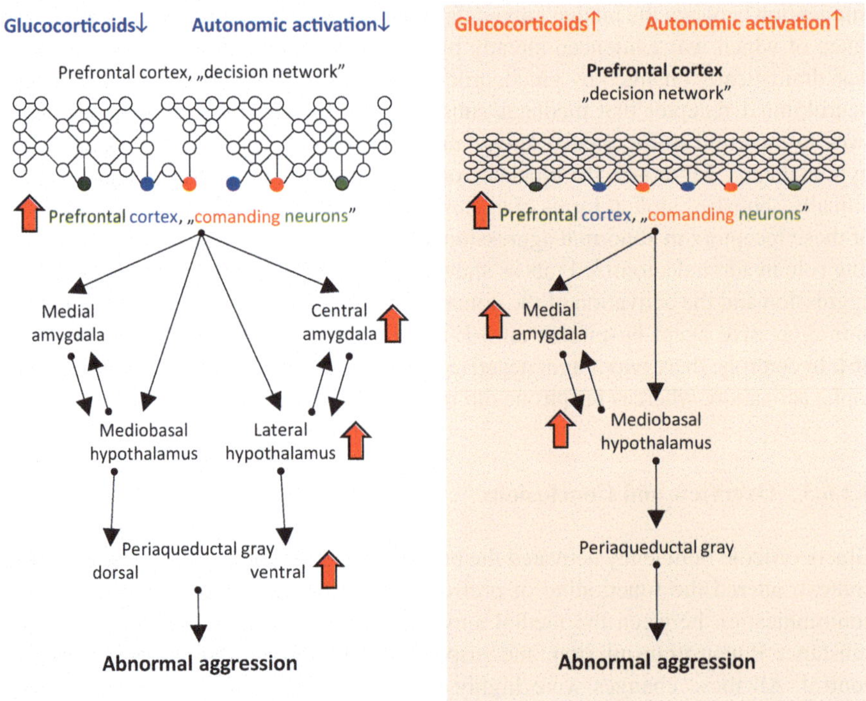

Fig. 8.1 The two basic types of abnormal aggression core circuitries. Red block arrows indicate those areas, which were activated more in abnormal than in normal aggression. The schematic was based on the template of normal aggression circuitries shown in the previous chapter. *Left-hand panel*. Abnormal aggression associated with blunted stress responses appears to be controlled by a combined rivalry–predatory circuitry. This is like that observed in maternal aggression, which is violent but still normal. The components of the circuitry undergo several other changes as shown in text. The upper part of the figure illustrates the imbalance between stimulation and inhibition within the prefrontal cortex. *Right-hand panel*. Abnormal aggression associated with increased stress responses appears to recruit the rivalry circuit only. Yet many components of the circuit are over-activated by aggression. Circuit components undergo many changes; the upper part of the schematic illustrates the developmental deficits observed in the prefrontal cortex. For other changes in the circuitries, see text

activated in each hypoarousal model. As this is one of the main areas where the rivalry and predatory core circuits diverge, moreover, from where predatory aggression can be elicited by electric stimulation [98], we believe that its activation indicates that the predatory circuit was involved in the control of this abnormal aggression type. The second core pathway was most extensively characterized in the post-weaning social isolation model, where aggression was displayed on the background of enhanced glucocorticoid and autonomic stress responses. In this model, an extensive restructuring of the aggression circuitry was observed; yet, aggression elicited the activation of the rivalry aggression circuitry without implicating the predatory circuitry. Noteworthy, the rivalry circuitry was over-activated as compared to controls. Additional deviations from the mechanisms that control aggression were described for each model separately.

8.4 What Do the Models Model? Theoretical Considerations

In principle, abnormal aggression models model aggression-related psychopathologies and indirectly criminal violence as psychopathological and criminal violence shows large overlaps as shown above. However, disorder modelling is often problematic because many clinical symptoms are human-specific. To circumvent such problems, one line of thought opts for symptom – rather than for disorder – modelling. For instance, decreased sucrose consumption in the chronic mild stress model of depression models the anhedonia symptom rather than depression as such [99], whereas the so-called alcohol deprivation effect models relapse rather than alcoholism [100].

Other modelling efforts, however, have taken on a more ambitious task and engaged in modelling whole disorders, e.g., posttraumatic stress disorder [101] or schizophrenia [102]. They also modelled subtypes of disorders, e.g., the predominantly inattentive subtype of attention-deficit/hyperactivity disorder [103] and its combined subtype [104]. Such approaches were sometimes considered misuses of the concept of modelling [105]. If feasible, however, disorder modelling may bring the animal model closer to the human condition and may unravel crucial insights into the mechanisms of disorders and the possibilities of treatment by being able to employ research technologies inapplicable in humans.

It was recently proposed that disorder modelling is possible with abnormal aggression models, based on a set of principles [106]. We reformulate these principles as follows. (1) The etiological factor of the human disorder must be analogous to the etiological factor used when the disorder was modelled in animals. Etiological factors may include genetic backgrounds, developmental exposures to chemicals, stressful life events, their interactions, or any other factor that can be perceived as being involved in the development of the disorder based on human studies. (2) There should be a similarity between the symptoms of the disorder as described in DSM5 [107] or ICD10 [108] and behavioral disturbances observed in the model. Note, however, that demands towards models should not exceed the exigency of diagnosis. Establishing diagnoses requires the presence of a limited number of symptoms, this number being specified for each disorder. No patient fulfills all the symptoms; that is sometimes even impossible. With animals, some symptoms cannot be fulfilled because they are rather human-specific, but if enough symptom-like behavioral deficits were observed, the disorder may be diagnosed within the model. The second restriction is that animals should not necessarily reproduce the symptoms literally. For instance, the DSM5 definition of conduct disorder lists under the heading "Serious Violations of Rules" symptoms like "Often stays out at night despite parental prohibitions…" and "Is often truant from school …." Such behaviors cannot be seen in rodents; however, the behavior of animals is governed by natural rules, which are obviously broken in models of abnormal aggression as shown above. These can serve as rodent equivalents of rule violations. In a similar vein, uncontrollable outbursts of aggression in intermittent explosive disorder may be modelled by excessive aggression associated with exaggerated behavioral and autonomic arousal in animals. (3) Animals should show behavioral disturbances that are not included among symptoms but are regularly observed in clinical research. For instance, decreased autonomic stress responses are regularly observed in antisocial personality disorder without this being listed among the symptoms in DSM5. The more associated features are present, the more specific the disorder model is. The presence of associated features should not replace the principle of showing a sufficient number of disorder-specific symptoms. (4) The brain mechanisms identified in the model should resemble brain deficits observed in the disorder, and there should be similarities in the effects of pharmacological agents.

These principles overlap with the criteria set forth by Willner 30 years ago for laboratory models of mental disorders [109]. He suggested that good models show predictive, face, and construct validity. Principle No. 1 on the list provided above is reminiscent of Willner's construct validity, i.e., theoretical rationale. On their turn, principles No. 2 and 3 are analogous with the concept of face validity (phenomenological similarity). The difference is that the principles outlined above make a distinction between diagnostic criteria and associated features and rely more on diagnostic manuals than the face validity criterion usually does. Finally, the predictive validity criterion was reproduced and extended by principle No. 4, requiring from the model predictive validity in pharmacological terms but also the existence of similarities in brain mechanisms. The application of the latter principle was made possible by the tremendous progress made by human brain imaging. Taken together, the principles proposed here are stricter than those proposed earlier, primarily because these principles were formulated for disorder models, whereas Willner's principles were expected to be fulfilled by more general symptom models.

Based on the principles listed above, it was suggested that abnormal aggression models developed in recent years may be, or may be developed into, disorder models. At present, two categories of models can be differentiated [106]: (i) Models associated with low arousal, which appear to model disorders like conduct and antisocial personality disorders, and (ii) models involving hyper-emotionality, which may model disorders associated with impulse control problems. Of particular interest are the pharmacologic arguments of the study, as a review of 14 pharmacological agents belonging to 5 substance classes showed that their effects depended to a great extent on the etiological factor of the models. Having two types of models suggests that abnormal aggression models are symptom-like rather than disorder-like models presently; however, more specific laboratory models of abnormal aggression are emerging. For instance, a model was built for intimate partner violence [110]. Transforming symptom-like models into true disorder models may need further studies, but the advantages of disorder modelling make the endeavor worthwhile. The possibilities of investigation are limited in humans by ethical constraints, which adds an extra value of appropriate disorder models.

8.5 General Overview

Although this line of research is still in its infancy as suggested above, abnormal aggression models led to some important conclusions.

1. Etiological factors of aggression-related psychopathologies elicited abnormal forms of aggression in animals. This suggests that the development of abnormal aggression follows shared rules, which justifies the use of animal abnormal aggression for modelling human conditions.
2. Changes in aggression were associated with a series of structural brain alterations in all the models. In the simplest case, e.g., in the early subjugation model, only changes in the connectivity of small brain regions were observed. In other cases, e.g., in the post-weaning social isolation model, both the thickness and the vascularization of the prefrontal cortex were altered with additional changes in neuronal architecture and glial density. The peripubertal stress model extends the area of structural changes to proteins that connect synapses and neurons. As shown in two of the models, the etiological factors of aggression-related psychopathologies activate epigenetic phenomena and plastic changes in the brain that are rather resistant to simple interventions.
3. Brain alterations can be considered mechanisms that alter aggressive behaviors as shown by a series of studies demonstrating that (i) the prevention of brain alterations prevent the development of behavioral alterations; (ii) counteracting brain alterations restore normal behavior; and (iii) etiologic factor-independent induction of brain alterations alter behavior in similar ways. The close relationship between brain alterations and behavior forecasts that the former may be used to envision novel treatment approaches for human aggression problems.
4. Novel treatment approaches were already proposed based on the findings with abnormal aggression models. Some of these proposals may address underlying causes and promise the "healing" of aggression. For example, reactivating the plasticity of the brain and inducing and directing new plastic changes in the right direction might disable the neural mechanisms of abnormal aggression. Other treatments, e.g., the antagonism of the neurokinin 1 receptors of Substance P, may be perceived as symptomatic treatments, which nevertheless may be useful.

5. The findings obtained so far reinforce the view that the role of serotonin in abnormal aggression is just as complex as its role in normal aggression. Serotonin may counteract but may also contribute to the emergence of abnormal aggression, depending on the brain area and the aspect of serotonin neurotransmission studied. On one hand, this may explain strange responses to serotonergic agents in some patients, whereas on the other suggests that more studies on serotonin are required. These should preferentially be done in abnormal aggression models as evidence suggests that serotonin is differentially involved in normal and abnormal aggression.
6. Recurrent findings indicate that vasopressin as a neurotransmitter and the hippocampus as a brain area play more important roles in the control of abnormal aggression than previously thought. This suggests that efforts to develop new treatment strategies should focus more than previously on vasopressin and the hippocampus.

These general conclusions were based on the shared etiological factors of aggression-related psychopathologies and abnormal animal aggression. Naturally, they are valid only if the two also share brain mechanisms. This will be investigated in the next section.

References

1. Siegel, A., & Victoroff, J. (2009). Understanding human aggression: New insights from neuroscience. *International Journal of Law and Psychiatry, 32*, 209–215.
2. Olivier, B. (2015). Serotonin: A never-ending story. *European Journal of Pharmacology, 753*, 2–18.
3. Melloni, R. H., & Ferris, C. F. (1996). Adolescent anabolic steroid use and aggressive behavior in golden hamsters. *Annals of the New York Academy of Sciences, 794*, 372–375.
4. Miczek, K. A., Weerts, E. M., Tornatzky, W., DeBold, J. F., & Vatne, T. M. (1992). Alcohol and 'bursts' of aggressive behavior: Ethological analysis of individual differences in rats. *Psychopharmacology, 107*, 551–563.
5. Ricci, L. A., Grimes, J. M., Knyshevski, I., & Melloni, R. H. (2005). Repeated cocaine exposure during adolescence alters glutamic acid decarboxylase-65 (GAD65) immunoreactivity in hamster brain: Correlation with offensive aggression. *Brain Research, 1035*, 131–138.
6. Fish, E. W., DeBold, J. F., & Miczek, K. A. (2005). Escalated aggression as a reward: Corticosterone and GABA(A) receptor positive modulators in mice. *Psychopharmacology, 182*, 116–127.
7. Benus, R. F., Bohus, B., Koolhaas, J. M., & van Oortmerssen, G. A. (1991). Behavioural differences between artificially selected aggressive and non-aggressive mice: Response to apomorphine. *Behavioural Brain Research, 43*, 203–208.
8. Neumann, I. D., Veenema, A. H., & Beiderbeck, D. I. (2010). Aggression and anxiety: Social context and neurobiological links. *Frontiers in Behavioral Neuroscience, 4*, 12.
9. Natarajan, D., de Vries, H., Saaltink, D.-J., de Boer, S. F., & Koolhaas, J. M. (2009). Delineation of violence from functional aggression in mice: An ethological approach. *Behavior Genetics, 39*, 73–90.
10. Natarajan, D., de Vries, H., de Boer, S. F., & Koolhaas, J. M. (2009). Violent phenotype in SAL mice is inflexible and fixed in adulthood. *Aggressive Behavior, 35*, 430–436.

11. Sluyter, F., et al. (2003). Toward an animal model for antisocial behavior: Parallels between mice and humans. *Behavior Genetics, 33*, 563–574.
12. Veenema, A. H., Koolhaas, J. M., & de Kloet, E. R. (2004). Basal and stress-induced differences in HPA axis, 5-HT responsiveness, and hippocampal cell proliferation in two mouse lines. *Annals of the New York Academy of Sciences, 1018*, 255–265.
13. Natarajan, D., & Caramaschi, D. (2010). Animal violence demystified. *Frontiers in Behavioral Neuroscience, 4*, 9.
14. Compaan, J. C., de Ruiter, A. J., Koolhaas, J. M., van Oortmerssen, G. A., & Bohus, B. (1992). Differential effects of neonatal testosterone treatment on aggression in two selection lines of mice. *Physiology & Behavior, 51*, 7–10.
15. Compaan, J. C., Wozniak, A., De Ruiter, A. J., Koolhaas, J. M., & Hutchison, J. B. (1994). Aromatase activity in the preoptic area differs between aggressive and nonaggressive male house mice. *Brain Research Bulletin, 35*, 1–7.
16. Caramaschi, D., de Boer, S. F., & Koolhaas, J. M. (2007). Differential role of the 5-HT1A receptor in aggressive and non-aggressive mice: An across-strain comparison. *Physiology & Behavior, 90*, 590–601.
17. Caramaschi, D., de Boer, S. F., de Vries, H., & Koolhaas, J. M. (2008). Development of violence in mice through repeated victory along with changes in prefrontal cortex neurochemistry. *Behavioural Brain Research, 189*, 263–272.
18. Veenema, A. H., et al. (2005). Differences in the effects of 5-HT(1A) receptor agonists on forced swimming behavior and brain 5-HT metabolism between low and high aggressive mice. *Psychopharmacology, 178*, 151–160.
19. Korte, S. M., et al. (1996). Enhanced 5-HT1A receptor expression in forebrain regions of aggressive house mice. *Brain Research, 736*, 338–343.
20. van Riel, E., Meijer, O. C., Veenema, A. H., & Joëls, M. (2002). Hippocampal serotonin responses in short and long attack latency mice. *Journal of Neuroendocrinology, 14*, 234–239.
21. Compaan, J. C., Buijs, R. M., Pool, C. W., De Ruiter, A. J., & Koolhaas, J. M. (1993). Differential lateral septal vasopressin innervation in aggressive and nonaggressive male mice. *Brain Research Bulletin, 30*, 1–6.
22. Veenema, A. H., & Neumann, I. D. (2007). Neurobiological mechanisms of aggression and stress coping: A comparative study in mouse and rat selection lines. *Brain, Behavior and Evolution, 70*, 274–285.
23. Veenema, A. H., et al. (2007). Differential effects of stress on adult hippocampal cell proliferation in low and high aggressive mice. *Journal of Neuroendocrinology, 19*, 489–498.
24. Hensbroek, R. A., Sluyter, F., Guillot, P. V., Van Oortmerssen, G. A., & Crusio, W. E. (1995). Y chromosomal effects on hippocampal mossy fiber distributions in mice selected for aggression. *Brain Research, 682*, 203–206.
25. Feldker, D. E. M., et al. (2003). Serial analysis of gene expression predicts structural differences in hippocampus of long attack latency and short attack latency mice. *The European Journal of Neuroscience, 17*, 379–387.
26. Haller, J., Tóth, M., Halasz, J., & De Boer, S. F. (2006). Patterns of violent aggression-induced brain c-fos expression in male mice selected for aggressiveness. *Physiology & Behavior, 88*, 173–182.
27. Chung, J. E., et al. (2019). Association between anxiety and aggression in adolescents: A cross-sectional study. *BMC Pediatrics, 19*, 115.
28. Beiderbeck, D. I., et al. (2012). High and abnormal forms of aggression in rats with extremes in trait anxiety--involvement of the dopamine system in the nucleus accumbens. *Psychoneuroendocrinology, 37*, 1969–1980.
29. Beiderbeck, D. I., Neumann, I. D., & Veenema, A. H. (2007). Differences in intermale aggression are accompanied by opposite vasopressin release patterns within the septum in rats bred for low and high anxiety. *The European Journal of Neuroscience, 26*, 3597–3605.
30. de Jong, T. R., Beiderbeck, D. I., & Neumann, I. D. (2014). Measuring virgin female aggression in the female intruder test (FIT): Effects of oxytocin, estrous cycle, and anxiety. *PLoS One, 9*, e91701.

31. Bosch, O. J., & Neumann, I. D. (2010). Vasopressin released within the central amygdala promotes maternal aggression. *The European Journal of Neuroscience, 31*, 883–891.
32. Tung, I., Noroña, A. N., Lee, S. S., Langley, A. K., & Waterman, J. M. (2018). Temperamental sensitivity to early maltreatment and later family cohesion for externalizing behaviors in youth adopted from foster care. *Child Abuse & Neglect, 76*, 149–159.
33. Chapple, C. L., Tyler, K. A., & Bersani, B. E. (2005). Child neglect and adolescent violence: Examining the effects of self-control and peer rejection. *Violence and Victims, 20*, 39–53.
34. Kotch, J. B., et al. (2008). Importance of early neglect for childhood aggression. *Pediatrics, 121*, 725–731.
35. Harlow, H. F., Dodsworth, R. O., & Harlow, M. K. (1965). Total social isolation in monkeys. *Proceedings of the National Academy of Sciences of the United States of America, 54*, 90–97.
36. Day, H. D., Seay, B. M., Hale, P., & Hendricks, D. (1982). Early social deprivation and the ontogeny of unrestricted social behavior in the laboratory rat. *Developmental Psychobiology, 15*, 47–59.
37. Potegal, M., & Einon, D. (1989). Aggressive behaviors in adult rats deprived of playfighting experience as juveniles. *Developmental Psychobiology, 22*, 159–172.
38. Kempes, M. M., Gulickx, M. M. C., van Daalen, H. J. C., Louwerse, A. L., & Sterck, E. H. M. (2008). Social competence is reduced in socially deprived rhesus monkeys (Macaca mulatta). *Journal of Comparative Psychology (Washington DC), 122*, 62–67.
39. Toth, M., Mikics, E., Tulogdi, A., Aliczki, M., & Haller, J. (2011). Post-weaning social isolation induces abnormal forms of aggression in conjunction with increased glucocorticoid and autonomic stress responses. *Hormones and Behavior, 60*, 28–36.
40. Tóth, M., Halász, J., Mikics, E., Barsy, B., & Haller, J. (2008). Early social deprivation induces disturbed social communication and violent aggression in adulthood. *Behavioral Neuroscience, 122*, 849–854.
41. Toth, M., et al. (2012). The neural background of hyper-emotional aggression induced by post-weaning social isolation. *Behavioural Brain Research, 233*, 120–129.
42. Tulogdi, A., et al. (2014). Effects of resocialization on post-weaning social isolation-induced abnormal aggression and social deficits in rats. *Developmental Psychobiology, 56*, 49–57.
43. Biro, L., et al. (2017). Structural and functional alterations in the prefrontal cortex after post-weaning social isolation: Relationship with species-typical and deviant aggression. *Brain Structure & Function, 222*, 1861–1875.
44. Mikics, É., et al. (2018). Social learning requires plasticity enhanced by fluoxetine through prefrontal Bdnf-TrkB signaling to limit aggression induced by post-weaning social isolation. *Neuropsychopharmacology, 43*, 235–245.
45. Andero, R., Choi, D. C., & Ressler, K. J. (2014). BDNF-TrkB receptor regulation of distributed adult neural plasticity, memory formation, and psychiatric disorders. *Progress in Molecular Biology and Translational Science, 122*, 169–192.
46. Chang, C.-H., Su, C.-L., & Gean, P.-W. (2018). Mechanism underlying NMDA blockade-induced inhibition of aggression in post-weaning socially isolated mice. *Neuropharmacology, 143*, 95–105.
47. Chang, C.-H., & Gean, P.-W. (2019). The ventral hippocampus controls stress-provoked impulsive aggression through the ventromedial hypothalamus in post-weaning social isolation mice. *Cell Reports, 28*, 1195–1205.e3.
48. Castrén, E., & Rantamäki, T. (2010). The role of BDNF and its receptors in depression and antidepressant drug action: Reactivation of developmental plasticity. *Developmental Neurobiology, 70*, 289–297.
49. Maya Vetencourt, J. F., et al. (2008). The antidepressant fluoxetine restores plasticity in the adult visual cortex. *Science, 320*, 385–388.
50. Currie, M., & Startup, M. (2012). Doing anger differently: Two controlled trials of percussion group psychotherapy for adolescent reactive aggression. *Journal of Adolescence, 35*, 843–853.
51. Weiss, B., et al. (2005). Iatrogenic effects of group treatment for antisocial youths. *Journal of Consulting and Clinical Psychology, 73*, 1036–1044.

52. Paus, T., Keshavan, M., & Giedd, J. N. (2008). Why do many psychiatric disorders emerge during adolescence? *Nature Reviews. Neuroscience, 9*, 947–957.
53. Kilford, E. J., Garrett, E., & Blakemore, S.-J. (2016). The development of social cognition in adolescence: An integrated perspective. *Neuroscience and Biobehavioral Reviews, 70*, 106–120.
54. Haller, J., Harold, G., Sandi, C., & Neumann, I. D. (2014). Effects of adverse early-life events on aggression and anti-social behaviours in animals and humans. *Journal of Neuroendocrinology, 26*, 724–738.
55. Walker, S. E., et al. (2018). Alterations in brain microstructure in rats that develop abnormal aggression following peripubertal stress. *The European Journal of Neuroscience, 48*, 1818–1832.
56. Márquez, C., et al. (2013). Peripuberty stress leads to abnormal aggression, altered amygdala and orbitofrontal reactivity and increased prefrontal MAOA gene expression. *Translational Psychiatry, 3*, e216.
57. Cordero, M. I., et al. (2012). Evidence for biological roots in the transgenerational transmission of intimate partner violence. *Translational Psychiatry, 2*, e106.
58. Papilloud, A., Guillot de Suduiraut, I., Zanoletti, O., Grosse, J., & Sandi, C. (2018). Peripubertal stress increases play fighting at adolescence and modulates nucleus accumbens CB1 receptor expression and mitochondrial function in the amygdala. *Translational Psychiatry, 8*, 156.
59. Cordero, M. I., Ansermet, F., & Sandi, C. (2013). Long-term programming of enhanced aggression by peripuberty stress in female rats. *Psychoneuroendocrinology, 38*, 2758–2769.
60. Papilloud, A., et al. (2019). Peripubertal stress-induced heightened aggression: Modulation of the glucocorticoid receptor in the central amygdala and normalization by mifepristone treatment. *Neuropsychopharmacology, 44*, 674–682.
61. Veenit, V., Riccio, O., & Sandi, C. (2014). CRHR1 links peripuberty stress with deficits in social and stress-coping behaviors. *Journal of Psychiatric Research, 53*, 1–7.
62. Makara, G. B., Stark, E., Kárteszi, M., Palkovits, M., & Rappay, G. (1981). Effects of paraventricular lesions on stimulated ACTH release and CRF in stalk-median eminence of the rat. *The American Journal of Physiology, 240*, E441–E446.
63. Liang, K. C., et al. (1992). Lesions of the central nucleus of the amygdala, but not the paraventricular nucleus of the hypothalamus, block the excitatory effects of corticotropin-releasing factor on the acoustic startle reflex. *Journal of Neuroscience: The Official Journal of the Society for Neuroscience, 12*, 2313–2320.
64. Südhof, T. C. (2008). Neuroligins and neurexins link synaptic function to cognitive disease. *Nature, 455*, 903–911.
65. Kohl, C., et al. (2013). The interplay of conditional NCAM-knockout and chronic unpredictable stress leads to increased aggression in mice. *Stress (Amsterdam, Netherlands), 16*, 647–654.
66. van der Kooij, M. A., et al. (2014). Impaired hippocampal neuroligin-2 function by chronic stress or synthetic peptide treatment is linked to social deficits and increased aggression. *Neuropsychopharmacology, 39*, 1148–1158.
67. Cordero, M. I., Just, N., Poirier, G. L., & Sandi, C. (2016). Effects of paternal and peripubertal stress on aggression, anxiety, and metabolic alterations in the lateral septum. *European Neuropsychopharmacology, 26*, 357–367.
68. Dodge, K. A., Bates, J. E., & Pettit, G. S. (1990). Mechanisms in the cycle of violence. *Science, 250*, 1678–1683.
69. Delville, Y., Melloni, R. H., & Ferris, C. F. (1998). Behavioral and neurobiological consequences of social subjugation during puberty in golden hamsters. *Journal of Neuroscience: The Official Journal of the Society for Neuroscience, 18*, 2667–2672.
70. Cunningham, R. L., & McGinnis, M. Y. (2008). Prepubertal social subjugation and anabolic androgenic steroid-induced aggression in male rats. *Journal of Neuroendocrinology, 20*, 997–1005.

71. Wommack, J. C., & Delville, Y. (2003). Repeated social stress and the development of agonistic behavior: Individual differences in coping responses in male golden hamsters. *Physiology & Behavior, 80*, 303–308.
72. Ferris, C. F., Messenger, T., & Sullivan, R. (2005). Behavioral and neuroendocrine consequences of social subjugation across adolescence and adulthood. *Frontiers in Zoology, 2*, 7.
73. Wommack, J. C., Salinas, A., Melloni, R. H., & Delville, Y. (2004). Behavioural and neuroendocrine adaptations to repeated stress during puberty in male golden hamsters. *Journal of Neuroendocrinology, 16*, 767–775.
74. Ferris, C. F., & Delville, Y. (1994). Vasopressin and serotonin interactions in the control of agonistic behavior. *Psychoneuroendocrinology, 19*, 593–601.
75. Ferris, C. F., et al. (1997). Vasopressin/serotonin interactions in the anterior hypothalamus control aggressive behavior in golden hamsters. *Journal of Neuroscience: The Official Journal of the Society for Neuroscience, 17*, 4331–4340.
76. Ferris, C. F., & Potegal, M. (1988). Vasopressin receptor blockade in the anterior hypothalamus suppresses aggression in hamsters. *Physiology & Behavior, 44*, 235–239.
77. Pickel, V. M., Joh, T. H., Field, P. M., Becker, C. G., & Reis, D. J. (1975). Cellular localization of tyrosine hydroxylase by immunohistochemistry. *The Journal of Histochemistry and Cytochemistry, 23*, 1–12.
78. Bastida, C. C., et al. (2014). Chronic social stress in puberty alters appetitive male sexual behavior and neural metabolic activity. *Hormones and Behavior, 66*, 220–227.
79. de Almeida, R. M. M., Ferrari, P. F., Parmigiani, S., & Miczek, K. A. (2005). Escalated aggressive behavior: Dopamine, serotonin and GABA. *European Journal of Pharmacology, 526*, 51–64.
80. Haller, J., van de Schraaf, J., & Kruk, M. R. (2001). Deviant forms of aggression in glucocorticoid hyporeactive rats: A model for 'pathological' aggression? *Journal of Neuroendocrinology, 13*, 102–107.
81. MacLennan, K. M., Smith, P. F., & Darlington, C. L. (1998). Adrenalectomy-induced neuronal degeneration. *Progress in Neurobiology, 54*, 481–498.
82. Virkkunen, M. (1985). Urinary free cortisol secretion in habitually violent offenders. *Acta Psychiatrica Scandinavica, 72*, 40–44.
83. Haller, J., Halász, J., Mikics, E., & Kruk, M. R. (2004). Chronic glucocorticoid deficiency-induced abnormal aggression, autonomic hypoarousal, and social deficit in rats. *Journal of Neuroendocrinology, 16*, 550–557.
84. Halász, J., Liposits, Z., Kruk, M. R., & Haller, J. (2002). Neural background of glucocorticoid dysfunction-induced abnormal aggression in rats: Involvement of fear- and stress-related structures. *The European Journal of Neuroscience, 15*, 561–569.
85. Haller, J., Tóth, M., & Halász, J. (2005). The activation of raphe serotonergic neurons in normal and hypoarousal-driven aggression: A double labeling study in rats. *Behavioural Brain Research, 161*, 88–94.
86. Haller, J., Horváth, Z., & Bakos, N. (2007). The effect of buspirone on normal and hypoarousal-driven abnormal aggression in rats. *Progress in Neuro-Psychopharmacology & Biological Psychiatry, 31*, 27–31.
87. Tulogdi, A., et al. (2010). Brain mechanisms involved in predatory aggression are activated in a laboratory model of violent intra-specific aggression. *The European Journal of Neuroscience, 32*, 1744–1753.
88. Tulogdi, A., et al. (2015). Neural mechanisms of predatory aggression in rats-implications for abnormal intraspecific aggression. *Behavioural Brain Research, 283*, 108–115.
89. Biro, L., et al. (2018). Task division within the prefrontal cortex: Distinct neuron populations selectively control different aspects of aggressive behavior via the hypothalamus. *Journal of Neuroscience: The Official Journal of the Society for Neuroscience, 38*, 4065–4075.
90. Halász, J., Tóth, M., Kalló, I., Liposits, Z., & Haller, J. (2006). The activation of prefrontal cortical neurons in aggression--a double labeling study. *Behavioural Brain Research, 175*, 166–175.

91. Ferguson, B. R., & Gao, W.-J. (2018). PV interneurons: Critical regulators of E/I balance for prefrontal cortex-dependent behavior and psychiatric disorders. *Frontiers in Neural Circuits, 12*, 37.
92. Selimbeyoglu, A., et al. (2017). Modulation of prefrontal cortex excitation/inhibition balance rescues social behavior in CNTNAP2-deficient mice. *Science Translational Medicine, 9*, eaah6733.
93. Yao, R., Rameshwar, P., Gregg, T., & Siegel, A. (2001). Co-localization of NK(1)-receptor mRNA with glutamate immunopositivity in cat hypothalamic neurons by the combination of in situ hybridization and immunohistochemistry. *Brain Research. Brain Research Protocols, 7*, 154–161.
94. Shaikh, M. B., Steinberg, A., & Siegel, A. (1993). Evidence that substance P is utilized in medial amygdaloid facilitation of defensive rage behavior in the cat. *Brain Research, 625*, 283–294.
95. Halasz, J., et al. (2008). The effect of neurokinin1 receptor blockade on territorial aggression and in a model of violent aggression. *Biological Psychiatry, 63*, 271–278.
96. Halasz, J., et al. (2009). Substance P neurotransmission and violent aggression: The role of tachykinin NK(1) receptors in the hypothalamic attack area. *European Journal of Pharmacology, 611*, 35–43.
97. Czéh, B., Fuchs, E., & Simon, M. (2006). NK1 receptor antagonists under investigation for the treatment of affective disorders. *Expert Opinion on Investigational Drugs, 15*, 479–486.
98. Han, W., et al. (2017). Integrated Control of Predatory Hunting by the Central Nucleus of the Amygdala. *Cell, 168*, 311–324.e18.
99. Willner, P., Muscat, R., & Papp, M. (1992). Chronic mild stress-induced anhedonia: A realistic animal model of depression. *Neuroscience and Biobehavioral Reviews, 16*, 525–534.
100. Vengeliene, V., Bilbao, A., & Spanagel, R. (2014). The alcohol deprivation effect model for studying relapse behavior: A comparison between rats and mice. *Alcohol, 48*, 313–320.
101. Zoladza, P. R., & Diamond, D. M. (2015). Psychosocial stress in rats: animal model ofPTSD based on clinically relevant risk factors. In C. Martin, V. Preedy, & V. B. Patel (Eds.), *Comprehensive guide to post-traumatic stress disorder*. Springer International Publishing.
102. Lipska, B. K., & Weinberger, D. R. (2000). To model a psychiatric disorder in animals: Schizophrenia as a reality test. *Neuropsychopharmacology, 23*, 223–239.
103. Sagvolden, T., Dasbanerjee, T., Zhang-James, Y., Middleton, F., & Faraone, S. (2008). Behavioral and genetic evidence for a novel animal model of attention-deficit/hyperactivity disorder predominantly inattentive subtype. *Behavioral and Brain Functions, 4*, 56.
104. Tomlinson, A., et al. (2015). Putative therapeutic targets for symptom subtypes of adult ADHD: D4 receptor agonism and COMT inhibition improve attention and response inhibition in a novel translational animal model. *European neuropsychopharmacology: The Journal of the European College of Neuropsychopharmacology, 25*, 454–467.
105. Wong, A. H. C., & Josselyn, S. A. (2016). Caution when diagnosing your mouse with schizophrenia: The use and misuse of model animals for understanding psychiatric disorders. *Biological Psychiatry, 79*, 32–38.
106. Haller, J. (2018). Preclinical models of conduct disorder - principles and pharmacologic perspectives. *Neuroscience and Biobehavioral Reviews, 91*, 112–120.
107. *American psychiatric association: Diagnostic and statistical manual of mental disorders, 5th edition*. American Psychiatric Association, Washington, 2013.
108. *The ICD-10 classification of mental and behavioral disorders*. World Health Organization, Geneva, 1999.
109. Willner, P. (1986). Validation criteria for animal models of human mental disorders: Learned helplessness as a paradigm case. *Progress in Neuro-Psychopharmacology & Biological Psychiatry, 10*, 677–690.
110. Poirier, G. L., Cordero, M. I., & Sandi, C. (2013). Female vulnerability to the development of depression-like behavior in a rat model of intimate partner violence is related to anxious temperament, coping responses, and amygdala vasopressin receptor 1a expression. *Frontiers in Behavioral Neuroscience, 7*, 35.

Chapter 9
The Neurobiology of Human Aggression and Violence

Introduction

For behavioral studies, the human brain was a black box for a long time, which was only occasionally illuminated by observations of the consequences of traumatic brain injuries and the findings of psychosurgery. Studies on neurotransmitters in the cerebrospinal fluid and blood and the effects of pharmacologic agents provided some information on brain functions, but these were unavoidably nonspecific from a functional anatomic point of view. This state of the art was radically changed by the advent of brain imaging techniques, which gradually evolved from purely anatomical to more functional observations and from studying resting-state functions to studying brain responses to various tasks. Aggression research, similar to all other fields of behavioral science, benefited greatly from these developments. Although brain imaging still has its limits, it allowed the dissection of the brain mechanisms of human aggression and violence in unprecedented detail.

This chapter overviews the main findings obtained so far with a focus on the brain areas that are generally believed to constitute the core circuitry of aggression control. Brain imaging studies were corroborated with findings on the consequences of brain injuries and of those obtained when brain areas were deliberately lesioned to limit pathological aggression.

9.1 Background

9.1.1 Brain Signatures and Brain Mechanisms

Aggression and psychopathologic and criminal violence are usually studied retrospectively, when participants are not engaged in aggressive behavior and are cooperative, as without their cooperation a psychological or brain imaging study

J. Haller, *Neurobiopsychosocial Perspectives on Aggression and Violence*,
Advances in Preventing and Treating Violence and Aggression,
https://doi.org/10.1007/978-3-030-46331-1_9

cannot be performed. These may be called aggression-history studies because their findings refer to previous rather than current behavior. The laboratory paradigms of aggression described in previous chapters study ongoing behavior and may be called manifest-aggression studies. Both are valid approaches but are basically different, which is often neglected when mechanisms of aggression are investigated. There are two important points here:

1. Aggression-history studies investigate the neural signatures of aggression-proneness. Aggression is evaluated by psychological and psychiatric inventories and criminal records. In their turn, brain mechanisms are investigated with a delay, by the methodologies that are briefly presented below. Such studies do reveal neural differences between aggressive and non-aggressive people but provide no information on the brain mechanisms that actually control fighting (Fig. 9.1).
2. Manifest-aggression studies investigate aggression by using the laboratory paradigms of aggression. Behavior is directly observed, and brain mechanisms are studied in parallel. Such studies are relevant for the brain mechanisms that elicit and maintain aggressive behavior. Naturally, the two types of studies can be combined, by studying both manifest-aggression and aggression histories.

Both types of studies provide important information, but these are essentially different. Aggression histories are associated with neural developmental trajectories and are embedded in the wider context of lifestyles [1, 2]. Aggressive personalities are associated with alterations in empathy, impulsivity, irritability, moral reasoning, punishment sensitivity, risk-taking proneness, etc. which all are important contributors of aggression; moreover, they have their own "brain signatures" [3–9]. Aggression-history studies may reveal structural and functional brain alterations associated with these traits. In contrast, manifest-aggression studies reveal mechanisms that are acutely activated by aggression, which may reveal the neural circuitries of its control.

Ostensibly, the two types of studies should be in line with each other: a deficit in a brain area should involve its poor functioning when recruited by aggression.

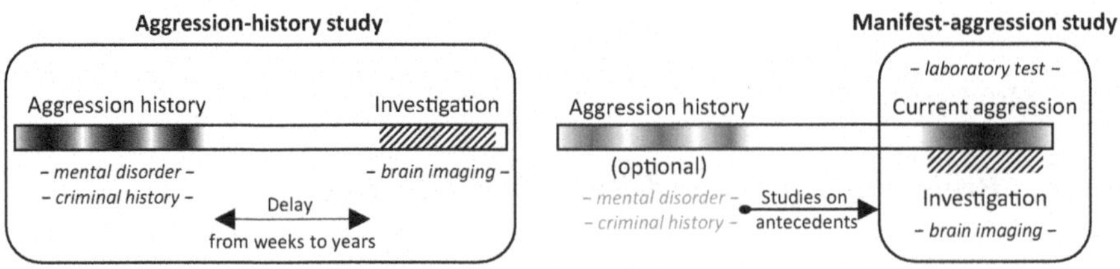

Fig. 9.1 *The two main types of human aggression studies. Left-hand panel.* The general schematic of studies that investigate the neural signature of aggressiveness based on inventories or records. Brain mechanisms are investigated when the participant is peaceful. *Right-hand panel.* The design of studies that investigate aggression while it unfolds in laboratory paradigms of human aggression. The two types of studies can be combined as shown in the schematic

Findings suggest, however, that this is not true, as shown in the post-weaning social isolation model of abnormal aggression in rats, where the prefrontal cortex was thinned by the procedure and had a poorer vascularization and dendritic branching, yet it was overactivated by fights as compared to controls. The same can and does happen in humans as shown below.

In general, the two phenomena are not clearly distinguished in the aggression literature. Comparing these two approaches will be the focus of this chapter.

9.1.2 Research Methods: A Brief History

The first methodology that provided information on the brain mechanisms of human aggression was surgical in nature. A Swedish language paper published in 1964 by the Japanese scientist and surgeon Sano [10], followed by an English one in 1966 [11], demonstrated that the electrolytic destruction of a relatively small region in the posteromedial human hypothalamus eliminates aggressiveness. The region is analogous with hypothalamic attack sites in animals [12].

Psychosurgery, however, is not a sustainable approach in human research although the method had a significant career in the clinic as shown later; however, traumatic brain injuries – accident versions of psychosurgery – provided important insights into the brain mechanisms of aggression control. This research line started with the famous case of Phineas Gage [13], who survived a severe traumatic brain injury in the nineteenth century. A significant portion of his prefrontal cortex was destroyed, following which, his personality changed without observable changes in his mental or physical faculties, to the amazement of contemporary physicians.

Modern research on the aggression-related consequences of brain injuries started from mid-twentieth century [14]. Novel approaches employ complex lesion–behavior mapping techniques [15] that allow inferences not only on the functional roles of various brain regions but also on their connectivity [16]. This approach already begun in aggression research [17]. Recently, stimulation techniques were also developed as counterparts of lesions [18].

Although brain injuries provided important information, pharmacology was the mainstream research technology before the advent of modern brain imaging techniques. Inspired by animal research and/or by the off-label effects of therapies of other psychopathologies, this research line clarified the role of dopamine, norepinephrine, and serotonin in controlling human aggression and developed pharmacotherapies that are still in use today [19–21].

The ultimate tools of modern aggression research are the brain imaging techniques. Current experimental technologies were introduced in the last quarter of the twentieth century by Mansfield [22] and Lauterbur [23] who developed magnetic resonance imaging for biological and medical research. Contemporary brain imaging techniques employ various techniques to study the structure and function of the brain in living humans. They are basically capable of four things: (i) revealing the 3D internal structure of the brain to allow for precise measurements; (ii) detecting the regional intensity of brain function by measuring blood flow or glucose consumption; (iii) visualizing fibers to investigate structural connectivity; and (iv) visualizing the distribution of certain neurotransmitter receptors to elucidate details of neural communication. These basic technological capacities were further exploited innovatively. For instance, the temporal correlation of activity was used to study the functional connectivity of spatially distributed brain regions [24]. 3D brain images were also used to study the surface of the cortex ("gyrification") or subcortical nuclei to investigate their integrity [25]. Thus, brain imaging is a collective term that covers a wide array of technologies.

The very same procedures can be employed while individuals rest and when they perform tasks. The former approach is typical to aggression-history studies; for instance, one can investigate the thickness of the prefrontal cortex in violent criminals compared to non-violent criminals and non-criminals. The second approach is typical to manifest-aggression studies. For instance, one can investigate prefrontal activations, e.g., regional changes in glucose consumption, while participants are engaged in the Taylor aggression paradigm to see contrasts between violent criminals and non-violent participants. In all cases, brain scans are compared, and differences are investigated. If, for instance, the cortex of violent criminals was thinner or it consumed less glucose in specific prefrontal cortical regions, it was assumed that that region was involved in aggression history or actual behavior. This assumption is strengthened by correlations between the level of aggressiveness and the magnitude of brain differences. Statistical calculations naturally need to be corrected for multiple comparisons, which make the obtaining of significant differences rather difficult. This means on one side that only highly reliable differences become statistically significant, whereas on the other it explains why roles are attributed to so small and patchily distributed areas.

Below we present the core circuitries of aggression to reveal their function in normal and abnormal states. As shown above, the psychological approach covers all forms of aggression; here it will be addressed as aggression by mentally healthy and non-criminal people. Psychopathologic and criminal violence will be presented in comparison with normal ("psychological") aggression; abnormal animal aggression will also be discussed.

9.2 Prefrontal Cortex

9.2.1 Extent, Subdivisions, and the Nature of Activation

The prefrontal cortex is the most frontal area of the brain that comprises about 30% of the total cortical area. It is conceptualized and divided into subareas in several ways. Figure 9.2 shows the three main approaches, together with examples of aggression-induced brain activation patterns.

It is often difficult to compare studies due to the variability in conceptualizations and terminologies, together with the patchy arrangement of aggression-related

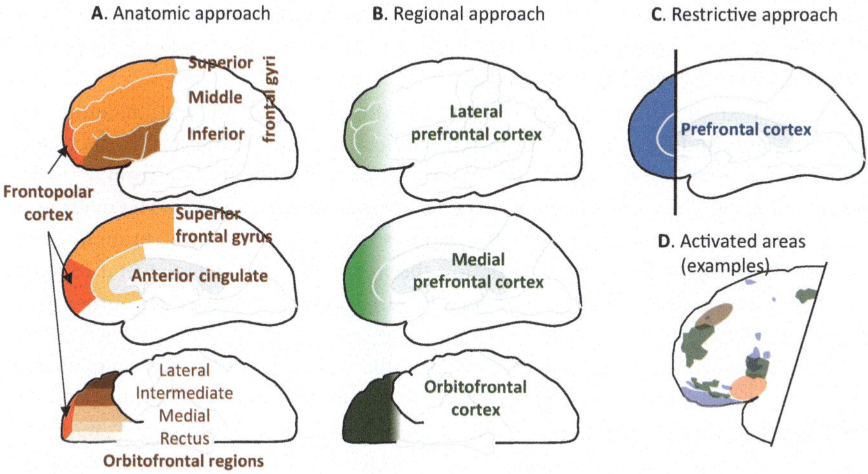

Fig. 9.2 *The prefrontal cortex: size, subdivisions, and activation patterns. Panel A.* The "anatomic approach" follows the gyrification of the area, by naming various parts based on the main gyri. *Panel B.* The "regional" approach divides the prefrontal cortex into an outer surface (lateral), an inner, inter-hemispheric surface (medial) and a ventral surface, which is called orbitofrontal. *Panel C.* The area is sometimes viewed as located rostrally to the corpus callosum, a thick nerve tract that connects the two hemispheres. This region contains little more than the frontopolar cortex. All three approaches are common, and brain areas are named according to the approach chosen by the author. *Panel D.* Alterations in the lateral prefrontal cortex of psychopathic murderers as shown by four different studies [26–29] (differentiated by color). Differences from non-murderers occur as small patches; several distinct patches were identified by some studies. Note these are not arranged along anatomical divisions, and even if named according to their general placement (e.g., dorsolateral prefrontal cortex), they usually do not overlap. The figure was compiled based on [30]

areas. This is likely due to the complex statistics related to repeated measures. In simple terms, the larger is the brain area that is studied, the more difficult it is to differentiate chance from true findings. Thus, the exact size and shape of the detected "patch" may not be as important as the prefrontal area where it belongs.

9.2.2 Findings

9.2.2.1 Theoretical Considerations, Lesions, and Stimulations

The prefrontal deficit theory is one of the most influential concepts of aggression control. The theory was originally based on the effects of brain lesions in animals and the consequences of traumatic brain injuries in humans [17, 31–35]. Injuries in the dorsolateral and ventromedial prefrontal cortex were consistently associated with a state called "acquired psychopathy." This is characterized by diminished moral reasoning, loss of empathy, liability to risk-taking, and aggressiveness. Lesions placed in other parts of the prefrontal region, e.g., in the orbitofrontal cortex or elsewhere in the brain, do not elicit psychopathy. Temporal lobe lesions, however, may also increase aggressiveness, but these may affect the amygdala; as such, their effects may not be specific to the cortex.

Recently, studies using anodal transcranial direct current stimulations indirectly supported the findings from brain lesion studies [36–38]. While lesions increased aggression, stimulation of the dorsolateral and ventromedial prefrontal cortex decreased it but not when directed to the inferior frontal gyrus [39]. The overlap of critical regions in lesion and stimulation studies is telling. In addition, brain imaging studies also support the prefrontal deficit theory. Raine [40] was the first to show that the metabolism of glucose is reduced in the prefrontal cortex of murderers, a finding that was replicated later by various other imaging techniques as shown below.

Despite this strong experimental evidence, the activation of the prefrontal cortex by aggression is a recurrent finding. As these findings ostensibly contradict one of the basic theories of aggression, their authors attribute activations to "emotional pain," "cognitive operations related to more intense social interaction," "compassion to the suffering opponent," "protection mechanism against experiencing negative emotions," etc. The following sections may be perceived as an attempt to reconcile these two types of findings.

Because the role of the prefrontal cortex in aggression may be a scientifically sensitive issue, we present the findings as exhaustively as possible. There was a cost to this broad approach: the large number of studies was referred to prevent their detailed discussion. In the tables presented below, we will not make distinction between various signs of the downregulation of prefrontal activity, e.g., diminished volume or thickness, decreased blood flow, glucose metabolism, etc., as all these symptoms are generally accepted signs of diminished function. Laterality and gender differences will also not be discussed. Although laterality may indeed be important, different authors found critical changes either on the left- or on the right-hand side of the brain, whereas other studies did not observe laterality effects. Similarly, gender differences are just as volatile as laterality. The question asked in the following sections is simple: Is there an association between aggressiveness and prefrontal cortex structure and function, and, if yes, what do these findings tell us about the role of this brain area?

9.2.2.2 Prefrontal Deficits: Aggression-History Studies

In these studies, people with a history of aggressive behavior were compared with people without a similar history (see Table 9.1). Participants fell into one of three categories:

1. Subjects labelled "healthy" who were devoid of psychopathologies and criminal histories. Typically, two groups were compared: one that had a life history of aggressive behavior and another that lacked that. Aggression histories were evaluated based on self and peer reports, e.g., based on psychological inventories. Past aggressions did not reach the level necessary for diagnosis or conviction.

Table 9.1 Prefrontal deficits associated with a history of aggression in healthy subjects ("psychological" aggression) and with psychopathologic and criminal aggression histories

General conditions	Aggression-related condition	Subregion	Association
"Psychological" aggression			
Healthy [41]	Aggression, proactive	CG a	↓
Healthy [42]	Aggressive, defiant	CG a	↓
Healthy [43]	Aggression	CG a	↓
Healthy [44]	Aggression, physical	OFC	↓
Healthy [41]	Aggression, reactive	OFC	↓
Healthy [41]	Aggression, proactive	OFC	↓
Healthy [43]	Aggression	OFC	↓
Healthy [45]	Aggression	PFC dl	↓
Healthy [45]	Aggression	PFC l	↓
Healthy [46]	Aggression, chronic	PFC l – WM	↓
Healthy [46]	Aggression, chronic	PFC m – WM	↓
Healthy [44]	Aggression, physical	PFC vm	↓
Healthy [41]	Aggression, reactive	CG a	→
Psychopathologies			
Antisocial personality disorder [47]		PFC	↓
Antisocial personality disorder [48]		PFC	↓
Antisocial personality disorder [49]		FP	↓
Antisocial personality disorder [49]		PFC vl	↓
Antisocial personality disorder [26]	Psychopathy	OFC	↓
Antisocial personality disorder [50]	Psychopathy	PFC – WM	↓Pb
Attention-deficit/hyperactivity [51]	Aggression	OFC	↓
Borderline personality disorder [52]		CG a	↓
Borderline personality disorder [53]	Act-out anger	PFC dl	↓
Borderline personality disorder [49]		FP	↓
Borderline personality disorder [54]		PFC – WM	↓
Borderline personality disorder [53]	Act-out anger	PFC al	↓
Borderline personality disorder [55]	Aggression	CG s	↓
Borderline personality disorder [49]		PFC vl	↓
Borderline personality disorder [56]	Impulsiveness	FP	↓**F**
Dementia [57]	Aggression	PFC d	↓
Disruptive behavior [58]	Aggression	CG a	↓
Disruptive behavior [59]	Aggression	FG m	↓
Disruptive behavior [58]	Aggression	PFC	↓
Disruptive behavior [59]	Aggression	FG s	↓
Epilepsy [60]	Aggression	PFC	↓
Personality disorder various [61]	Aggression	FG i	↓
Personality disorder various [61]	Aggression	FG s	↓
Borderline personality disorder [62]		CG a	↑

(continued)

Table 9.1 (continued)

General conditions	Aggression-related condition	Subregion	Association
Borderline personality disorder [62]		FG i	↑
Borderline personality disorder [62]		FG s	↑
Personality disorder various [63]	Intermittent explosive disorder	OFC	^5-HT2A
Personality disorder various [64]	Aggression, impulsive	OFC am	Ø SSRI
Posttraumatic stress disorder [65]	Aggression, impulsive	OFC	→
Various diagnoses [66]	Aggression	OFC	˅^Assym
Crime			
Offender [67]	Psychopathy	FG s – GA	↓
Offender [68]	Antisocial personality disorder	FG m	↓
Offender [28]	Psychopathy	OFC	↓
Offender [68]	Antisocial personality disorder	OFC	↓
Offender [69]	Psychopathy	PFC – WM	↓
Violent offender [70]		PFC dl	↓
Violent offender [70]	Psychopathy	PFC dm	↓
Violent offender [71]		PFC dm	↓
Violent offender [29]	Psychopathy	FP	↓
Violent offender [27]	Habitual	FP	↓
Violent offender [40]	Murder	PFC l	↓
Violent offender [40]	Murder	PFC m	↓
Violent offender [72]	Psychopathy	OFC	↓
Violent offender [27]	Habitual	OFC	↓
Violent offender [73]	"Affective" murder	PFC	↓
Violent offender [73]	"Predatory" murder	PFC	→
Violent offender [74]	Psychopathy, alcohol	PFC dl	˅^ALC
Violent offender [74]	Psychopathy, alcohol	OFC	˅^ALC
Violent offender [75]	Psychopathy	CG a	^5-HT1B
Violent offender [76]	Psychopathy	CG a	˅MAOA
Violent offender [76]	Psychopathy	PFC m	˅MAOA
Violent offender [76]	Psychopathy	OFC	˅MAOA
Violent offender [77]	Psychopathy	OFC	↑

Associations. ↓ negative association (PFC deficit – high aggression), ↓*Pb* participants were exposed to lead as children, ↓*F* only in females, → no association, ↑ positive association (PFC deficit – low aggression), ˅*MAOA* decreased MAO_A expression, ^$5\text{-}HT_{1B}$ increased serotonin 1B receptor binding, ^$5\text{-}HT_{2A}$ higher availability of the 5-HT2A serotonin receptor, ˅^*Assym* association with left/right asymmetry but not with volumes, ˅^*ALC* association with alcoholism but not with volumes, *Ø SSRI* a selective serotonin reuptake inhibitor lost its effect on PFC *prefrontal regions*, *a* anterior, *CG* cingulate cortex, *al* anterolateral, *am* anteromedial, *d* dorsal, *dl* dorsolateral, *FP* frontopolar cortex, *GA* gyral anomalies (low gyrification index), *iFG* inferior frontal gyrus, *il* inferolateral, *l* lateral, *m* medial, *mFG* middle frontal gyrus, *OFC* orbitofrontal cortex, *PFC* prefrontal cortex, *sFG* superior frontal gyrus, *vl* ventrolateral, *vm* ventromedial, *WM* white matter

2. Psychopathologic subjects were diagnosed with an aggression-related mental disorder, sometimes also having a comorbid disorder. In some studies, aggressive variants of the disorder were specifically studied; in others, aggression was not the focus. Such details were specified in the "Associated condition" column. Controls were labelled healthy and were rarely investigated for aggression histories. Thus, control groups may have included both categories mentioned above, i.e., they might have had a life history of aggression, which, however, did not fulfill diagnostic criteria.
3. Offenders with a criminal history. In many cases, they were incarcerated, while the study was performed. Two categories of studies were differentiated. "Offenders" were not selected based on the type of crime they committed, although, violent crime was common in this group. The term "violent crime" includes studies where offenders were selected for this type of behavior. Controls had no conviction record, which, however, did not exclude a life history of non-criminal aggression.

These findings show that a history of aggression is rather consistently associated with prefrontal deficits. The affected regions include those that led to "acquired psychopathy" when damaged and regions which, when stimulated, decreased aggression. These were the dorsolateral and ventromedial prefrontal cortex; however, dysfunctions were often also observed elsewhere. For instance, deficits were quite frequently located in the orbitofrontal and anterior cingulate cortex which may be explained by the complexity of the local networks. One can hypothesize that once one component of complex circuits is deficient, the whole network suffers.

These studies found that the level of aggressiveness did not differentiate participants. Prefrontal deficits were observed in people showing tolerable levels of aggression ("healthy"), as well as in those that showed psychopathologic or criminal aggression. Differences in the size and/or the location of deficits might exist, but statistical comparisons are difficult and complex even within studies, and cross-study comparisons cannot be performed. These findings suggest similar deficits in people displaying various forms of aggression. One can assume that while prefrontal deficits are associated with the general propensity to behave aggressively, aggression becomes psychopathological or criminal by other factors.

It is worth noting that the few conflicting findings were overwhelmingly observed in psychopathological and criminal aggression. While in healthy subjects, only one example of "non-association" was found, many more cases of non-association were observed in personality disorders and violent criminals. Moreover changes of the opposite nature – e.g., increased cortical thickness – were relatively frequently observed in borderline patients. In addition, counterintuitive findings were observed in psychopathologic and criminal aggression. For instance, increased 5-HT_{1B} serotonin receptor binding and 5-HT_{2A} serotonin receptor availability were found in psychopathic violent criminals, although serotonin should decrease aggression according to the serotonin deficit theory of aggression. In line with this observation, the typical impact of selective serotonin reuptake inhibitors on prefrontal functions – readily seen in controls – was not found in personality disorders (see, e.g., the study labelled by ØSSRI in the table). It seems that under certain conditions, psychopathologic and criminal aggression may deviate from the prefrontal deficit theory, and also they may become independent of the effects of serotonin.

9.2.2.3 Prefrontal Responses: Manifest-Aggression Studies

In these studies, participants were similar to those described above, with two notable differences:

(i) The studies evaluated changes in prefrontal functions that were elicited by the execution of various tasks. Usually, threat perception was investigated by pictures with different emotional valence. Frustration was induced by withdrawing an expected reward. Anger and aggression imagery were elicited by autobiographical memories, whereas aggression per se was studied by laboratory paradigms (e.g., Taylor aggression paradigm, ultimatum game, etc.). The behavioral domain the task referred to was indicated in the Table 9.2.
(ii) The controls of psychopathologic and criminal subjects were submitted to the same aggression tests. Thus, increased activation should be understood as increased responses compared to controls (see Table 9.2).

The general conclusion emerging from these studies is that aggressive behavior is associated with prefrontal activation in all its phases: when the threat was perceived, when anger was aroused, and when aggression was imagined or performed. There were few conflicting findings. Thus, the association of manifest aggression with prefrontal activation is typical, i.e., it is a not an unusual finding reported by a restricted number of studies. The activated areas are similar to those that showed deficits in aggression-history studies. It is noteworthy that there was a gradation in responses: participants diagnosed with an aggression-related psychopathology and those with criminal records displayed stronger prefrontal activations than healthy controls.

One possible explanation of these findings is that the prefrontal cortex was activated by factors other than aggression. This assumption is in line with some authors' explanations, who reported that their findings did not fit with the prefrontal deficit theory. In a way they were right, because such laboratory paradigms involve a variety of feelings. Participants may feel physical or psychological pain (e.g., in Taylor aggression paradigm or the ultimatum game, respectively), or they might also be concerned with the sufferings of the opponent. Yet, there are at least three arguments that weaken the assumption that aggressive responses were unrelated to prefrontal activations in these manifest-aggression studies:

1. Accepting this type of reasoning eliminates all theories on the role of the prefrontal cortex, because confounds attributed to manifest-aggression studies can just as well occur in aggression-history studies: aggression history may be confounded with the history of another feeling or behavior. In other words, if we adopt a defensive stance regarding manifest-aggression studies, the same stance should be adopted with aggression-history studies. This would question the role

Table 9.2 The impact of aggression on prefrontal functions in manifest-aggression studies

General conditions	Aggression-related condition	Behavioral domain	Subregion	Association
"Psychological" aggression				
Healthy [78]		Threat perception	Cg a	↑
Healthy [78]		Threat perception	Ofc	↑
Healthy [79]		Threat perception	Ofc	↑t
Healthy [80]		Threat perception	Ofc l	↑
Healthy [80]		Threat perception	Pcf m	↑
Healthy [81]		Social rejection	Pfc vl	↑
Healthy [82]		Frustration	Cg a	↑
Healthy [82]		Frustration	Pfc dl	↑
Healthy [82]		Frustration	Pcf m	↑
Healthy [83]		Frustration	Pfc vl	↑
Healthy [84]		Anger	Cg a	↑
Healthy [85]		Anger	Ofc	↑
Healthy [84]		Anger	Ofc	↑
Healthy [86]		Aggression imagery	Fp	↑
Healthy [87]		Aggression imagery	Pfc l	↑
Healthy [88]	Psychopathic traits	Aggression viewing	Fg m	↑
Healthy [89]		Aggression viewing	Pfc vm	↑
Healthy [90]		Aggression, virtual	Pfc l	↑$^{\vee}$ 5-ht
Healthy [90]		Aggression, virtual	Pcf m	↑$^{\vee}$ 5-ht
Healthy [91]		Aggression	Cg a	↑
Healthy [92]		Aggression	Cg a	↑
Healthy [93]		Aggression	Pfc dl	↑
Healthy [94]		Aggression	Pfc dl	↑
Healthy [95]		Aggression	Pfc dl	↑
Healthy [96]		Aggression	Pfc dm	↑
Healthy [92]		Aggression	Pfc d	↑
Healthy [97]		Aggression	Pfc d	↑
Healthy [96]		Aggression	Fg i	↑
Healthy [95]		Aggression	Pcf m	↑
Healthy [91]		Aggression	Pcf m	↑
Healthy [94]		Aggression	Pcf m	↑
Healthy [97]		Aggression	Pcf m	↑
Healthy [91]		Aggression	Ofc	↑
Healthy [92]		Aggression	Ofc	↑
Healthy [98]		Aggression	Ofc	↑
Healthy [97]		Aggression	Pfc vm	↑

(continued)

Table 9.2 (continued)

General conditions	Aggression-related condition	Behavioral domain	Subregion	Association
Healthy [99]		Aggression	Ofc	↓t
Healthy [86]		Aggression imagery	Pfc vm	↓
Psychopathologies				
Antisocial PD [100]		Threat conditioning	PFC dl	↑↑
Borderline PD [101]		Threat perception	PFC m	↑↑
Borderline PD [101]		Threat perception	PFC il	↑↑
Borderline PD [101]	Aggression	Anger imagery	OFC l	↑↑
Borderline PD [101]	Aggression	Anger imagery	PFC dl	↑↑
Borderline PD [95]	Intermittent explosive	Aggression	OFC	↑↑
Posttraumatic SD [102]	Aggression	Threat perception	CG a	↑↑
Posttraumatic SD [103]	Violence	Threat perception	CG a	↑↑
Posttraumatic SD [102]	Aggression	Threat perception	OFC	↑↑
Posttraumatic SD [103]	Violence	Threat perception	PFC m	↑↑
Crime				
Offender [104]	Psychopathy	Aggression	PFC d	↑↑
Offender [105]		Risk-taking	PFC dl	↑↑
Offender [106]	Aggressive	Threat perception	PFC dm	↑↑
Offender [104]	Psychopathic	Aggression	PFC l	↑↑
Offender [104]	Psychopathic	Aggression	PFC vm	↑↑
Violent offender [107]	Intimate partner v	Threat perception	CG a	↑↑
Violent offender [107]	Intimate partner v	Threat perception	FG m	↑↑
Violent offender [108]		Aggression	OFC	↑↑
Violent offender [109]		Anger	PFC vl	↑↑
Violent offender [108]		Aggression	PFC vm	↑↑
Offender [106]	Aggression	Threat perception	PFC dm	↓
Offender [104]	Psychopathy	Aggression	PFC m	↓
Violent offender [110]	Psychopathy	Threat perception	PFC a	↓T
Violent offender [109]		Anger	PFC dl	↓
Violent offender [107]	Intimate partner v	Threat perception	FG s	↓

Associations. ↓ negative (low PFC activity – high aggression), ↓*T* association depended on testosterone, → no association, ↑ positive association (high PFC activity – high aggression), ↑↑ positive association stronger than in controls submitted to the same test, ↑*T* association depended on testosterone, ↑*MAOA* in high-activity MAOA carriers, ↑*F* in females only, ˅*5-HT* inhibitory effect of PFC serotonin, ˅*MAOA* decreased MAO_A expression, ^*5-HT1B* stimulatory effect of serotonin 1B receptor binding, ^*5-HT2A* higher availability of receptor, ˅^*Assym* association with left/right asymmetry but not with volumes, ˅^*ALC* association with alcoholism but not with volumes, *ØMAOA* MAOA allele typically associated with aggression in controls did not show a similar association in the study group, *Ø5-HT* serotonin lost effect on PFC, *Prefrontal regions. a* anterior, *CG* cingulate cortex, *al* anterolateral, *am* anteromedial, *d* dorsal, *dl* dorsolateral, *FP* frontopolar cortex, *GA* gyral anomalies (gyrification), *FG* frontal gyrus, *i* inferior, *il* inferolateral, *l* lateral, *m* medial or middle, *OFC* orbitofrontal cortex, *PFC* prefrontal cortex, *s* superior, *vl* ventrolateral, *vm* ventromedial, *WM* white matter

of the prefrontal cortex in general. Eliminating prefrontal theories of aggression control is not in line with the totality of evidence because this stance implicates that associations with aggression were *always* secondary to other associations, which is very unlikely.

2. The degree of aggressiveness and the magnitude of prefrontal activations were positively correlated, and participants with a vicious aggression background showed stronger activations than those who were only occasionally aggressive in the past. Attributing such correlations to factors other than aggression would suggest that psychopathological and criminal aggression are associated with increased pain perception, higher sensitivity to the sufferings of others, and stronger cognitive efforts when faced with morally difficult decisions. Note that these were the "excuses" of those who tried to corroborate their own findings with the prefrontal deficit theory of aggression (see above). However, the symptoms of aggression-related psychopathologies and the characteristics of criminals suggest the opposite: people suffering from or committing these have reduced pain perception, decreased empathy, and diminished morality.
3. The stimulation of specific prefrontal neurons increased aggression in animals. Supporting assumptions on human aggression by arguments borrowed from animal research may not be an elegant choice, but this seems justified, as the implication of the prefrontal cortex in aggression control appears very similar in animals and humans. In both cases, prefrontal lesions increase aggression, whereas the indiscriminate stimulation of prefrontal neurons decreases aggression. Despite structural and functional deficits, the prefrontal cortex is activated by fights in both abnormal aggression models and excessive forms of human aggression. Moreover, the serotonergic system appears to lose its aggression-controlling role in animal models of abnormal aggression as in excessive, rule breaking human aggression. Recent technological advances have also made the stimulation of selected prefrontal neuron populations possible in animals. These studies showed that neurons called above "ruling" are intermingled with neurons having different roles, but their selective stimulation promotes aggression. Thus, they are not organized into aggression-promoting areas; rather, they are distinct functionally without being distinguishable spatially. One can hypothesize that such neurons exist in humans but have not yet been discovered due to the technical difficulty of stimulating intermingled neurons selectively.

9.2.3 Overview and Hypothesis

The available evidence shows rather clearly that aggressive personalities have prefrontal deficits but strongly recruit the prefrontal cortex when aggressive behavior is performed. We suggest that this apparent contradiction is quite acceptable from a theoretical point of view.

Prefrontal deficits are associated with increased anger and irritability, impulsivity, risk-taking, deficits in empathy and theory of mind, and indifference to rules and lack of moral reasoning [111–120]. Due to these features, people with prefrontal deficits are likely to lead risky lifestyles and have a "psychological landscape" which predisposes them to conflict.

On the other hand, the prefrontal cortex is essential for planning and executing complex behaviors [121, 122] by being involved in motor control [123–126] and the execution of goal-directed behaviors [127, 128]. Moreover, various subareas of the prefrontal cortex are preferentially involved in assigning value to external and internal sensations, the association of memories with current situations, the evaluation of the mental states of others, and in imagining future events [129]. Thus, one can hardly imagine how a behavior as complex as aggression could be performed without the active contribution of the prefrontal cortex.

Based on the above, the prefrontal deficit theory of aggression and the stimulatory control of aggressive behaviors by the prefrontal cortex do not contradict each other; rather they support each other. Prefrontal deficits appear to create "psychological landscapes" that lead to lifestyles that increase the likelihood of being involved in conflict. Moreover, the faulty "psychological landscape" alters judgment in such situations, which increases the likelihood of aggressive responding. Thus, chronic prefrontal deficits appear to affect personalities rather than to control behavior.

Once the conflict is initiated, the prefrontal cortex "takes the lead," and aggression ensues under its tight control. It is worthwhile to note that faulty judgment does not necessary mean decreased activity; wrong decisions may also need neural effort. In addition to such faulty activations of decision networks, "ruling networks," i.e., the neural populations that transmit commands to subcortical centers, are also activated, hence, the increased activation of prefrontal areas in aggression.

9.3 The Amygdala

9.3.1 *Size, Subdivisions, and Roles*

The amygdala is surprisingly small in humans; its size is almost negligible compared to the prefrontal cortex (see Fig. 9.3). Yet, this brain area plays wide ranging roles from controlling behaviors, e.g., aggressive and sexual behavior, to influencing emotions, storing emotional memory, and controlling the stress response. These functions are controlled interactively by several subunits, which have distinct input and output areas and a complex internal system of connections by which information is processed.

As Fig. 9.3 shows, the structure of the amygdala is less clear in humans than in animals. Authors divide the amygdala into subregions in different ways and also use a different nomenclature for the subunits such created. The main two approaches are shown in the Fig. 9.3. Note that even when authors use the same type of division of the amygdala, the size, shape, and location of subnuclei are often different.

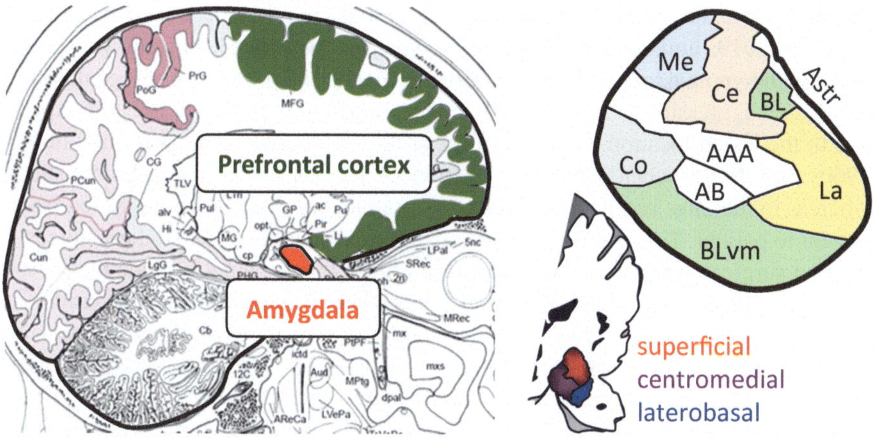

Fig. 9.3 *The amygdala: location in the brain and subdivisions. Left-hand panel.* A panel of the human brain atlas of Mai et al. [130], where the amygdala and the prefrontal cortex were highlighted in red and green, respectively. Other colors belong to the highlights of the atlas. *Right-hand panel.* The internal structure of the human amygdala according to two systems of classification [26, 131]. BL basolateral, Ce central, La lateral, Me medial, vm ventromedial

Consequently, the same term, e.g., "central," may identify different parts of the nucleus in different papers. Therefore, the roles of subdivisions which are so important in animals are poorly understood in humans.

9.3.2 Findings

9.3.2.1 Theoretical Considerations, Lesion, and Stimulations

The implicit consequence of the prefrontal deficit theory of aggression is that there must be a major drive for aggression which would be the target of the inhibitory influence of this area. This role is generally assigned to the amygdala. Enhanced amygdala functions, especially when associated with decreased prefrontal inhibition, are assumed to underlie both psychopathological aggression and violent crime. This hypothesis was formulated mostly based on lesion and stimulation studies, which support it. The next sections will deal with brain imaging studies.

Trials to limit otherwise intractable human aggression led the Japanese scientist Narabayashi and his colleagues to destroy parts of the amygdala with oil wax in 1963 [132]. The study was based on earlier surgical attempts to control epileptic seizures and was not prompted by aggression research on the roles played by the amygdala. Yet aggression was considerably inhibited by the surgery. This so-called amygdalotomy was rapidly adopted by a series of scientists, who confirmed initial observations. Lesions, mostly electrolytic in subsequent studies, were located bilaterally in the central [133], lateral [132], anteromedial [134], or medial [135] subdivisions of the amygdala. Occasionally the whole area was destroyed bilaterally [136]. In 2019, unilateral amygdalotomy was also performed, but this was combined with hypothalamic lesions to ascertain efficacy [137]. Overall, amygdalotomy eliminated aggression in 50–100% of patients depending on the study but irrespective to the lesion location. Note that most of these surgeries were performed in the 1960s and 1970s when the exact location of lesions could not be established, whereas in the most recent study, this was possible, but exact locations varied from patient to patient. This is telling for the spatial precision of earlier studies, suggesting that surgical errors may have decreased efficacy; one cannot exclude the possibility that efficacy was higher in those studies where surgery was more accurate.

Stimulation of the amygdala led to a variety of responses from fear to sadness and happiness, but uncontrollable outbursts of rage were also observed [138]. The variability of these outcomes was likely due the multiplicity of the roles of the amygdala but probably also to imprecise and poorly controlled stimulation sites, as these studies were performed decades ago. Note that the effects of stimulations were mirrored by the side effects of amygdalotomy.

Taken together, lesion studies clearly show that the amygdala plays a crucial role in human aggression. Stimulation studies also reveal that the unselected stimulation of the amygdala may lead to a variety of responses including but not limited to uncontrollable rage.

9.3.2.2 Amygdala Deficits: Aggression-History Studies

Table 9.3 presents the findings in a similar manner as for the prefrontal cortex. However, the findings are considerably less congruent than with the prefrontal cortex. Therefore, we considered more variables here. For instance, we considered the amygdala feature investigated by brain imaging. Most studies investigated the volume of the area; others investigated the volume or the density of gray matter; and a few investigated the surface deformations of the amygdala. Finally, others investigated resting-state functions, e.g., glucose consumption, oxygenation, etc.

In most studies (53%), the association was bilateral; in 40% of studies, it was seen on only the right-side amygdala, and in only 7% of the studies, it was seen on only the left-side amygdala. Laterality was considered, however, in fewer than half of the studies suggesting that, in most cases, significant differences were obtained only when the left- and right-side amygdala were considered together. As it regards genders, differences were sometimes observed, but this was not typical. For instance, findings by the same research group done in similar subjects lead to the same conclusions irrespective to gender [145, 146].

The totality of findings suggests that a history of aggressiveness and violence can be associated with both amygdala deficits and "amygdala gains" (e.g., increased volumes) the former being observed more frequently. This is less blatant in healthy subjects, where the only example of such a "gain" was relative: the volume of the amygdala was not larger in aggressive than non-aggressive participants; rather, only the amygdala/hippocampus ratio increased. With psychopathologies and crime,

Table 9.3 Amygdala deficits associated with a history of aggression in healthy subjects as well as with psychopathologic and criminal aggression histories

Control condition	Aggression-related condition	Subarea	Variable	Association
Healthy [139]	Aggression		Volume	↑H
Healthy [140]	Psychopathic traits		Gray matter	→
Healthy [141]	Psychopathic traits		Gray matter	→
Healthy [45]	Aggression		Volume	↓
Healthy [142]	Violence		Volume	↓
Alexithymia [143]	Reactive aggression		Volume	↑
Antisocial PD [26]	Psychopathy	Basolateral	Volume	↑
Antisocial PD [26]	Psychopathy	Central	Volume	↑
Antisocial PD [26]	Psychopathy	Lateral	Volume	↑
Alexithymia [143]	Proactive aggression		Volume	→
Various disorders [144]	Aggression		Volume	→
Various disorders [144]	Aggression	Dorsal	Volume	↓
Conduct disorder [145]			Volume	↓
Conduct disorder [146]			Gray matter	↓
Conduct disorder [8]			Gray matter	↓
Conduct disorder [147]			Function	↓
Antisocial PD [26]	Psychopathy	Basolateral	Volume	↓
Antisocial PD [147]	Psychopathy	Laterobasal	Function	↓
Borderline PD [55]	Aggression		Gray matter	↓
Borderline PD [148]	Intermittent explosive d.		Function	↓
Intermittent explosive [149]			Cell loss	↓
Violent offender [150]			Gray matter	↑
Violent offender [151]	Antisocial PD	Cortical	Surface	↑ MAO
Violent offender [152]	Antisocial PD		Volume	↑
Violent offender [153]	Psychopathy		Volume	→
Violent offender [154]	Domestic violence		Function	→
Violent offender [27]			Volume	→
Offender [155]	Psychopathy		Volume	↓
Offender [155]	Psychopathy	Cortical	Surface	↓
Offender [155]	Psychopathy	Central	Surface	↓
Offender [155]	Psychopathy	Basolateral	Surface	↓
Offender [155]	Psychopathy	Lateral	Surface	↓
Offender [72]	Psychopathy		Gray matter	↓

(continued)

Table 9.3 (continued)

Control condition	Aggression-related condition	Subarea	Variable	Association
Violent offender [156]			Gray matter	↓
Violent offender [151]	Antisocial PD	Basolateral	Surface	↓ MAO
Violent offender [28]	Psychopathy		Gray matter	↓
Violent offender [77]	Psychopathy		Gray matter	↓

The amygdala subarea was indicated only when this was specifically studied. Empty cells indicate that the whole area was considered together

Associations. ↑ positive association (e.g., high volume – high aggression), ↑*H* increased amygdala/hippocampus ratio without volume increase in the amygdala per se, ↑ *MAO* association valid for the MAO_A-low genotype, → no association, ↓ negative association (e.g., high volume – low aggression), ↓ MAO association valid for the MAO_A-low genotype. Not bolded arrow indicates marginally significant associations

however, the very same conditions may be associated with both deficits and increased amygdala volumes or increased functions. This did not seem to depend on the type of psychopathology or crime.

The association of aggression histories with both amygdala up- and downregulations cannot be easily explained, but a few studies suggest that this may be related to subregion-dependent changes. For instance, the dorsal part of the amygdala was smaller in aggressive than non-aggressive people, even though the amygdala as a whole showed no volumetric changes [144]. In psychopathic subjects, the central and lateral amygdala were larger than in controls, but the basolateral region was smaller [26]. In the same vein, the cortical amygdala was larger, but the basolateral amygdala was smaller in violent offenders than controls [151]. Regional differences were observed in other two studies. Whereas some areas such as the laterobasal complex [147] and the cortical–central–basolateral–lateral subnuclei [155] showed differences, other amygdala regions did not show differences. In animals, amygdala subnuclei played differential roles in aggression, and the same may be true for human studies; however, only a few studies investigated the amygdala in such detail.

9.3.2.3 Amygdala Responses: Manifest-Aggression Studies

The studies reviewed here investigated functional changes in the amygdala related to tasks performed in parallel (see Fig. 9.4.). These tasks and other details of such studies were described in the similar section on the prefrontal cortex (Table 9.4).

The share of studies where the changes were observed on the right-hand side amygdala (44%) was approximately equal to the share of those where differences were on the left-side amygdala (40%). Bilateral changes were observed in a minority of studies (16%). Note that laterality was not an issue in about one-third of studies. As with gender, such differences were observed in only a minority of studies.

Table 9.4 *Actual aggression and amygdala activation*

Control condition	Aggression-related condition	Area	Behavioral domain	Association
Healthy [157]			Frustration	↑
Healthy [79]			Threat perception	↑
Healthy [158]	Antisocial tendencies		Threat perception	↑ OX
Healthy [159]			Threat perception	↑Ph
Healthy [160]			Anger	↑
Healthy [161]	High provocation		Anger	↑
Healthy [93]			Anger	↑
Healthy [162]	Prize fighters		Aggression viewing	↑
Healthy [163]			Aggression viewing	↑
Healthy [164]		Centromedial	Aggression viewing	↑
Healthy [165]			Aggression imagery	↑
Healthy [166]			Aggression	↑
Healthy [167]			Aggression	↑
Healthy [92]			Aggression	↑
Healthy [168]			Aggression	↑
Healthy [161]	High provocation		Aggression	↑
Healthy [169]	Aggression		Frustration	↓
Healthy [170]			Aggression viewing	↓
Healthy [171]	Psychopathic traits		Aggression imagery	↓
Healthy [98]		Basolateral	Aggression	↓
Borderline PD [172]			Threat perception	↑
Borderline PD [101]			Threat perception	↑↑
Borderline PD [173]			Threat perception	↑↑
Borderline PD [174]			Threat perception	↑↑
Conduct disorder [175]			Threat perception	↑↑
Conduct disorder [176]	Severe		Threat perception	↑↑
Intermittent explosive d [177]			Threat perception	↑↑

(continued)

Table 9.4 (continued)

Control condition	Aggression-related condition	Area	Behavioral domain	Association
Intermittent explosive d [178]			Threat perception	↑↑
Intermittent explosive d [179]			Threat perception	↑↑
Intermittent explosive d [180]			Threat perception	↑↑
Posttraumatic SD [103]		Basolateral	Threat perception	↑↑
Conduct disorder [181]			Aggression viewing	↑↑
Antisocial PD [182]	Psychopathy		Aggression viewing	↑↑
Borderline PD [95]	Aggression		Aggression	↑↑
Antisocial PD [175]			Threat perception	→
Disruptive behavior [183]	Psychopathic traits		Threat perception	→
Intermittent explosive d [180]			Threat perception	ˇSSRI
Conduct disorder [184]	Psychopathic traits		Threat perception	↓
Conduct disorder [185]	Psychopathic traits		Aggression attitude	↓
Offender [186]	Psychopathy		Threat perception	↑↑
Violent offender [187]	Antisocial PD or Intermittent explosive		Anger	↑↑
Violent offender [105]			Risk-taking	↑↑
Violent offender [188]	Intimate partner v		Aggression, verbal	↑↑
Violent offender [108]			Aggression	↑↑
Offender [189]	Psychopathy		Threat perception	→

The amygdala subarea was indicated only when this was specifically studied. Empty cells indicate that the whole area was considered together

Associations. ↑ positive associations (e.g., higher activity associates with higher aggression), ↑*OX* association valid for certain oxytocin polymorphisms, ↑ *Ph* association valid for certain physical features of participants, ↑↑ activation larger than seen in healthy controls, → no association, ↓ negative association (e.g., higher activity associates with lower aggression), ˇ*SSRI* selective serotonin reuptake inhibition (serotonin upregulation) loses its effects

This time the findings were in full agreement with the theory, as frustration, threat perception, anger, viewing aggressive scenes, and aggression all increased amygdala activity. In addition, the amygdala was more strongly activated when the subject had a history of violence. Conflicting findings were few and were mostly observed in healthy subjects. In one instance, the upregulation of serotonergic neurotransmission failed to induce changes in intermittent explosive disorder although such changes were observed in controls. Notably, such serotonin insensitivities were also observed in the prefrontal cortex and models of abnormal animal aggression.

Importantly, participants showed subnucleus-related changes. It was observed that aggression increased the activation of the whole amygdala bilaterally [168] but decreased the activation of the basolateral amygdala unilaterally [98]. Although the findings were reported in two different studies, these were performed by the same research group in similar subjects. Subarea-related differences were reported by two other groups [103, 164], the most interesting being the one that indicates a task division between amygdala subareas. In this study, healthy participants watched videos displaying a violent conflict between two people [164]. The centromedial amygdala was activated in those who focused on the aggressor, whereas the basolateral amygdala was activated in those who focused on the victim. Although there are few studies, these disparate findings suggest that the role of various amygdala subareas in aggression may be as differential as in animals.

9.3.2.4 Prefrontal–Amygdala Connectivity

One important assumption of the prefrontal deficit theory of aggression is that aggression becomes violence when the pro-aggressive effects of the amygdala are liberated from the inhibitory control of the prefrontal cortex. The findings reviewed so far offer partial support for this hypothesis. The aggression-promoting role of the amygdala seems to hold true albeit only acutely, i.e., while aggression is initiated and performed. In contrast, the aggression-related activation of the prefrontal cortex, as shown by the manifest-aggression studies reviewed in the previous section, does not support the inhibition of the amygdala by the prefrontal cortex. Yet, one can still assume that if the prefrontal cortex–amygdala connectivity diminished, the influence of the prefrontal cortex on the amygdala weakened even if the prefrontal cortex was activated. In other words, enhanced prefrontal activation had little chance to affect the amygdala if the connectivity between the two areas was compromised. Unsurprisingly, the connectivity of the prefrontal cortex and amygdala was intensely studied. We will not discuss this issue in detail here but emphasize that this connectivity can be either stronger or weaker in aggressive people.

As expected based on the prefrontal deficit hypothesis, the prefrontal cortex–amygdala connectivity was decreased in aggressive borderline personality disordered subjects [190], violent offenders [108], and affective murderers [73]. Thus, one might assume that in these cases the amygdala was released from prefrontal control and enhanced aggression; however, connectivity was *increased* in healthy people showing psychopathic traits [88], borderline patients [191], violent posttraumatic patients [103], and in aggressive patients who had various psychiatric diagnoses [102]. In addition, connectivity remained unchanged in "predatory" murderers [73], i.e., those who kill for gain as opposed to "affective" murderers who kill due to uncontrolled emotions. These findings suggest that in some aggressive people at least, the prefrontal cortex controls the amygdala more strongly than usual.

Recent findings, however, show that the prefrontal–amygdala coupling is more complex than generally thought. For instance, the three main facets of psychopathy, e.g., fearless dominance, self-centered impulsivity, and coldheartedness, were associated with connectivities that were segmented along prefrontal cortical and amygdalar subnuclei; some of these were weakened, whereas others were strengthened [88]. For instance, weak basolateral amygdala–ventrolateral prefrontal cortex coupling was seen in egotistically impulsive psychopathic individuals, whereas stronger basolateral amygdala–anterior cingulate coupling was seen in those showing coldheartedness. The existence of multiple, differentially affected prefrontal–amygdala connectivities was evidenced in several other aggression types [192, 193]. Other findings on their turn suggest that the strength of functional connectivity may change dynamically over a social conflict depending on social signals [168, 194].

Studying connectivity is crucial because the efficacy of information transfer depends to a great extent on its strength. One area may become activated in vain if it can only weakly affect other areas because of decreased connectivities; however, the phenomenon is poorly understood at present. Opposite changes in connectivity may underlie similar behaviors, and various aspects of the same psychopathology may be explained by distinct sub-connectivities between subareas belonging to the same major areas. Finally, functional connectivity may be different at the beginning and the end of the very same social conflict.

9.3.3 Overview and Comparisons with Animal Findings

Aggressive behavior is carried out under the strong positive influence of the amygdala, as shown by both lesion and manifest-aggression studies. Stronger activations were observed in psychopathologies and violent crime, suggesting that normal and abnormal forms of aggression are differentiated by the degree of amygdala activation. No differences, however, were observed in various types of psychopathologic and criminal aggression as all appear to be supported by the amygdala irrespective to the associated feelings and behaviors.

The amygdala also supported aggression in animals, but the activation of certain amygdala subareas was preferentially associated with hypoarousal- and hyperarousal-driven aggression. The former appeared to be governed by the predation-linked central amygdala, whereas hyperarousal-driven aggression by a host of other subnuclei out of which the role of the medial amygdala was the most prominent. Such a dissociation of roles is not evident in humans because the division of its subdivisions is poorly established and because subnuclei were rarely studied separately. A few findings do show, however, that the subnuclei of the human amygdala are differentially involved in various aggression-related processes, as shown by both their differential activation patterns and their preferential coupling to prefrontal areas. Although the relationship between amygdala subdivisions and types of human aggression remains to be established, the findings obtained so far are encouraging for this type of work.

Regarding the relationship between a durable association of amygdala structure and aggressiveness, findings are mixed. A role for subnuclei can be assumed here as well. However, independent of different amygdala structure and resting-state functions, people appear to prepare for and to perform aggression under the stimulatory influence of enhanced amygdala activation.

9.4 The Hypothalamus and the Periaqueductal Gray

Both structures are located deep in the brain, near to small aqueous cavities, which makes their study by brain imaging difficult. Their activation can be detected, but the chances of differentiating subregions are low, at least with the usual techniques. Therefore, we will discuss these brain areas only briefly, focusing on surgical procedures in the case of the hypothalamus.

9.4.1 The Hypothalamus

The hypothalamus is a diencephalic area located close to the third brain ventricle (see Fig. 9.4). The earliest evidence of its involvement in aggression came from Sano [11] who – based on animal work, particularly on that performed by Hess [195] – mapped the area electrophysiologically by recording autonomic responses while stimulating various regions of the hypothalamus and, after identifying a small circumscribed region that elicited strong autonomic responses, electrolytically destroyed it and observed that patients' aggressiveness was practically eliminated. The surgery was done in intractably violent patients who were kept isolated in high-security facilities.

The aggression-related region was soon named the "triangle of Sano," and thousands possibly tens of thousands of similar surgeries were performed primarily in Japan and the USA [197]. The number of surgeries has decreased over time, but did not disappear; reports from 1988 [197, 198], 2003 [199], and 2019 [137] demonstrate that these are performed till today.

The conclusion of these studies was that after bilateral hypothalamotomy, about 70% of patients refrained from aggression even when provoked, about an additional 25% did not initiate aggression themselves but responded to provocation, whereas the aggressiveness of the remaining 5% was either unchanged or even increased. Given the difficulties of targeting such a small target, this success rate clearly shows

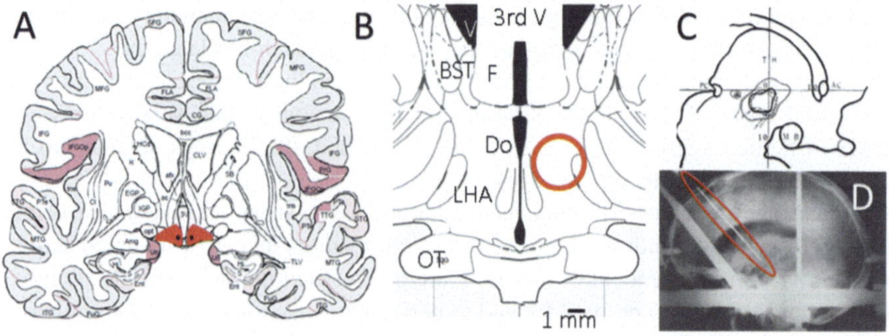

Fig. 9.4 *The hypothalamus and the triangle of Sano.* (**a**) The hypothalamus labelled by red on a panel of the brain atlas of Mai et al. [130] The black dot shows the approximate location and size of the triangle of Sano. (**b**) Modern reconstruction [12] of the area where lesions eliminated pathological human aggression (based on the same brain atlas). The lesions were likely placed within the red circle. (**c**) Schematic of the lesioned area in an early study by Sano [11]. (**d**) An early radiograph depicting the location of the electrode by which electrolytic lesions were administered to a patient [196]. The electrode was outlined by the red ellipse. The apparatus keeping the head in place is also visible. *Key abbreviations.* third V third brain ventricle, BST bed nucleus of striae terminalis, Do dorsal hypothalamic nucleus, F fornix, LHA lateral hypothalamus

that the destruction of a hypothalamic area that is analogous to animal hypothalamic attack sites eliminates aggression (see dot on Fig. 9.4a).

In one study, an accidental intraoperative stimulation of the "triangle of Sano" elicited uncontrollable outbursts of anger in a patient [200], further supporting the notion that this brain area is tightly involved in the control of aggression. Relatively recently, hypothalamic deep brain stimulation was employed to limit human aggression, with a remarkable success [201]. These and subsequent studies demonstrated that the long-term high-frequency stimulation of the "triangle of Sano" reliably reduced aggression, the effect lasting at least years [201–204], although in some cases, the co-stimulation of the nucleus accumbens was required to maintain the effect over time [205]. This methodology has the prospect of becoming over time an established treatment for limiting pathological aggression. Yet, it is in sharp contrast with lesion findings, which is often overlooked when the two methodologies are comparatively discussed [206, 207]. Specifically, it is difficult to understand how aggression could be inhibited by both the elimination and the stimulation of the very same area. The explanation may lie in observations showing that chronic deep brain stimulation inhibits the stimulated area by increasing inhibitory GABA release in the axons of afferent connections [208]. This is in line with the beneficial effects of hypothalamic deep brain stimulation on epileptic seizures and hypersexuality [207, 209], because these should be aggravated, rather than improved, if such stimulations activated the hypothalamus. Consequently, the high-frequency deep brain simulation of the "triangle of Sano" is in fact a functional "lesion," and findings with the two methods support rather than contradict each other.

Brain imaging studies focusing on manifest aggression are also in line with the assumption that the hypothalamus is involved in controlling aggression. Witnessing a violent conflict [164], sensing the danger of aggression [210], angry faces (threat perception) [79], and aggression [97] are all associated by hypothalamic activation. Importantly, the hypothalamus was activated in a laboratory paradigm of human aggression, activation being stronger in criminal psychopaths [104].

Taken together, these findings demonstrate that in humans the hypothalamus plays roles comparable to that seen in non-human animals; particularly, this brain area appears indispensable for the execution of aggressive behavior. Due to the technical reasons mentioned above, the anatomical subtleties of hypothalamic involvement remained hidden so far. The findings suggest, however, that this brain area is not only involved in aggression but also in its abnormal forms, e.g., psychopathic violence.

9.4.2 The Periaqueductal Gray

This brain area surrounds the aqueduct, which connects the third and fourth brain ventricles (see Fig. 9.5). Novel brain imaging techniques allowed its detailed study despite the vicinity of an aqueous cavity [211, 212] and showed that the animal and human periaqueductal gray play comparable roles in the homeostatic regulation of salient functions such as pain, anxiety, and autonomic control [213]. Unfortunately, similar methods have not been employed so far by those interested in aggression control.

All knowledge regarding the role of the periaqueductal gray in human aggression comes from a restricted number of brain imaging studies because lesion and stimulation studies are lacking with this brain structure. The available studies, however,

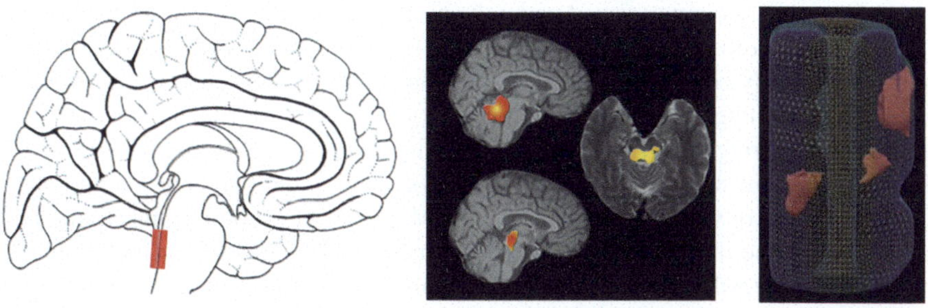

Fig. 9.5 *The location of the periaqueductal gray and activation patterns. Left-hand panel.* The approximate position and size of the human periaqueductal gray (red square). *Middle panel.* Activations enhanced by aggression-related tasks (compiled based on three studies) [157, 214, 215]. Note that the brain imaging signal does not differentiate finer structures in the area. *Right-hand panel.* High resolution 3D representation of PAG activations by high-field strength functional magnetic resonance technique [216]. Unfortunately, this was not employed in aggression research so far

cover essential information, by showing that frustration and [157] viewing [181] and performing aggression within the framework of a modified ultimatum game [214] increased periaqueductal gray activation. This effect was stronger in conduct disorder [181, 216] and was also influenced by testosterone [215]. In aggressive combat veterans, the periaqueductal gray showed a marginally stronger resting-state functional connectivity with the centromedial amygdala [65], which is reminiscent of a pathway that controls predatory attacks in animals. Note that the difference from non-violent veterans was nominally significant; it became marginal after correcting for multiple comparisons.

Obviously, the role of the periaqueductal gray in human aggression is far from being elucidated; yet the available findings are consistent with roles seen in animals.

9.5 Overview and Conclusions

9.5.1 The Human Circuitry of Abnormal Aggression

The quantity and quality of information on the key components of the aggression circuitry are highly variable. There are many studies on the prefrontal cortex which show that a history of aggression, particularly psychopathologic and criminal aggression, is associated with dysfunctions in this area. Manifest-aggression studies also consistently show that the prefrontal cortex is activated under the influence of aggression-provoking external influences and internal feelings and remains activated when aggression is performed. Moreover, such activations are stronger in abnormal forms of human aggression.

Consequently, the prefrontal deficit theory of aggression should be rethought. Based on the available information, prefrontal deficits are more likely related to risky lifestyles than to the brain control of aggression. Preparations to fight and the fights per se are likely performed under the positive control of the prefrontal cortex.

Amygdala–prefrontal connectivity also needs rethinking as the issue is not as simple as usually considered. First, aggression cannot be attributed to the disconnection of the amygdala from the inhibitory control of the prefrontal cortex as both are activated during aggression. Therefore, neither appears able to inhibit the other. Second, there are several connecting pathways between the two areas, which may be strengthened or weakened independently. Moreover, functional connectivity can change over time in line with incoming information. This line of research is in its beginning phase, when simple answers are sought for complex interactions.

Findings on the amygdala and hypothalamus are in line with expectations, but the spatial resolution of mechanistic explanations is poor. Both areas appear indispensable for the execution of aggressive behavior, and both appear to contribute to the emergence of abnormal human aggression. Yet, the differential involvement of subareas which is so important in animals is poorly understood. Finally, information on the periaqueductal gray is limited but is compatible with, rather than proves, its importance in aggression control. For a graphical summary, see Fig. 9.6.

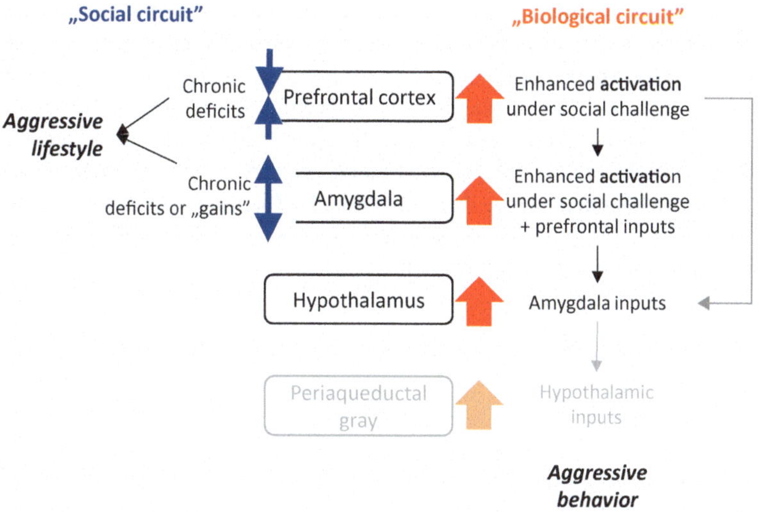

Fig. 9.6 The social and biological circuits of abnormal human aggression. The findings of aggression-history studies suggest that resting-state structural and functional alterations in the prefrontal cortex and amygdala "create" personalities that frequently engage in aggression due to their chosen lifestyle. This was called above the "social circuit." Manifest-aggression studies, however, show that the core circuitry of aggression is activated at its entire length while the individual performs aggression. This "biological circuit" is proposed to drive actual manifestations of aggression. *Gray*, based mostly on animal studies; *blue arrows*, volume and gray matter changes. Note that the prefrontal cortex is usually deficient, whereas the amygdala may either increase or decrease in size. *Block red arrows*, increased activation while the individual is aggressive

9.5.2 Arousal and Aggression Types

The mechanisms of abnormal animal aggression and those controlling psychopathologic and criminal violence are surprisingly similar. In both cases, abnormal aggression is associated with prefrontal deficits, which do not prevent the area to be overactivated by actual aggression. The overactivation of the amygdala and hypothalamus appears to play roles in both, and serotonin also appears to lose its aggression-controlling role. Both the animal and human circuits appear to be controlled directly by local neuronal effects via MAO_A enzyme polymorphisms and the hormone testosterone.

Despite similarities, however, there is a major difference between the two circuitries. In animals, two major circuitries were discovered. One controlled aggression that emerged on the background of decreased arousal and was controlled by a circuit that underlies predatory aggression under normal circumstances. The other was observed in models of hyperarousal, where the "traditional" rivalry circuit was activated with major changes in the structure of the core circuit and in associated and attuning systems. No such differential pathways were revealed in humans despite the fact that some forms of psychopathologic aggression are associated with hypoarousal whereas others with hyperarousal. Despite differential emotional backgrounds, human forms of abnormal aggression appeared rather similar regarding their neural background as far as the core circuitry of aggression is concerned. Importantly, however, the mechanisms of abnormal animal aggression diverge at levels where information are deficient in humans, particularly at the level of the amygdala, hypothalamus, and periaqueductal gray. As such, the lack of arousal-specific pathways appears to be due to technical difficulties and lack of knowledge rather than to a true similarity of pathways that control behaviorally and emotionally distinct forms of human aggression.

References

1. Hare, R. D., & Neumann, C. S. (2009). Psychopathy: Assessment and forensic implications. *Canadian Journal of Psychiatry, 54*, 791–802.
2. Provençal, N., Booij, L., & Tremblay, R. E. (2015). The developmental origins of chronic physical aggression: Biological pathways triggered by early life adversity. *The Journal of Experimental Biology, 218*, 123–133.
3. Baskin-Sommers, A. R., Wallace, J. F., MacCoon, D. G., Curtin, J. J., & Newman, J. P. (2010). Clarifying the factors that undermine behavioral inhibition system functioning in psychopathy. *Personality Disorders, 1*, 203–217.
4. Coccaro, E. F., Bergeman, C. S., Kavoussi, R. J., & Seroczynski, A. D. (1997). Heritability of aggression and irritability: A twin study of the Buss-Durkee aggression scales in adult male subjects. *Biological Psychiatry, 41*, 273–284.
5. Dolan, M., Anderson, I. M., & Deakin, J. F. (2001). Relationship between 5-HT function and impulsivity and aggression in male offenders with personality disorders. *The British Journal of Psychiatry: the Journal of Mental Science, 178*, 352–359.
6. Pujara, M., Motzkin, J. C., Newman, J. P., Kiehl, K. A., & Koenigs, M. (2014). Neural correlates of reward and loss sensitivity in psychopathy. *Social Cognitive and Affective Neuroscience, 9*, 794–801.
7. Raine, A., & Yang, Y. (2006). Neural foundations to moral reasoning and antisocial behavior. *Social Cognitive and Affective Neuroscience, 1*, 203–213.
8. Sterzer, P., Stadler, C., Poustka, F., & Kleinschmidt, A. (2007). A structural neural deficit in adolescents with conduct disorder and its association with lack of empathy. *NeuroImage, 37*, 335–342.
9. Wilson, M., & Daly, M. (1985). Competitiveness, risk taking, and violence: The young male syndrome. *Ethology and Sociobiology, 6*, 59–73.
10. Sano, K. (1964). Neurosurgical considerations of the hypothalamic mechanisms of emotion. *Nō to Shinkei, 16*, 815–824.
11. Sano, K., Yoshioka, M., Ogashiwa, M., Ishijima, B., & Ohye, C. (1966). Postero-medial hypothalamotomy in the treatment of aggressive behaviors. *Confinia Neurologica, 27*, 164–167.
12. Haller, J. (2013). The neurobiology of abnormal manifestations of aggression–A review of hypothalamic mechanisms in cats, rodents, and humans. *Brain Research Bulletin, 93*, 97–109.
13. Damasio, H., Grabowski, T., Frank, R., Galaburda, A. M., & Damasio, A. R. (1994). The return of Phineas Gage: Clues about the brain from the skull of a famous patient. *Science, 264*, 1102–1105.
14. Vondracek, V., Horvai, I., & Student, V. (1964). Aggression following cephalic trauma. *Psychiatrie, Neurologie und medizinische Psychologie (Leipz.), 16*, 104–107.

15. de Haan, B., & Karnath, H.-O. (2018). A hitchhiker's guide to lesion-behaviour mapping. *Neuropsychologia, 115*, 5–16.
16. Gleichgerrcht, E., Fridriksson, J., Rorden, C., & Bonilha, L. (2017). Connectome-based lesion-symptom mapping (CLSM): A novel approach to map neurological function. *NeuroImage: Clinical, 16*, 461–467.
17. Cristofori, I., et al. (2016). Brain regions influencing implicit violent attitudes: A lesion-mapping study. *Journal of Neuroscience, 36*, 2757–2768.
18. Fregni, F., et al. (2005). Anodal transcranial direct current stimulation of prefrontal cortex enhances working memory. *Experimental Brain Research, 166*, 23–30.
19. Swann, A. C. (2003). Neuroreceptor mechanisms of aggression and its treatment. *The Journal of Clinical Psychiatry, 64*(Suppl 4), 26–35.
20. Insel, T. R., Zohar, J., Benkelfat, C., & Murphy, D. L. (1990). Serotonin in obsessions, compulsions, and the control of aggressive impulses. *Annals of the New York Academy of Sciences, 600*, 574–585; discussion 585–586.
21. Eichelman, B. (1988). Toward a rational pharmacotherapy for aggressive and violent behavior. *Hospital & Community Psychiatry, 39*, 31–39.
22. Mansfield, P., & Maudsley, A. A. (1976). Line scan proton spin imaging in biological structures by NMR. *Physics in Medicine and Biology, 21*, 847–852.
23. Lauterbur, P. C. (1980). Progress in n.m.r. zeugmatography imaging. *Philosophical Transactions of the Royal Society of London. Series B, Biological Sciences, 289*, 483–487.
24. Biswal, B. B., Van Kylen, J., & Hyde, J. S. (1997). Simultaneous assessment of flow and BOLD signals in resting-state functional connectivity maps. *NMR in Biomedicine, 10*, 165–170.
25. Magnotta, V. A., et al. (1999). Quantitative in vivo measurement of gyrification in the human brain: Changes associated with aging. *Cerebral Cortex, 1991*(9), 151–160.
26. Boccardi, M., et al. (2011). Cortex and amygdala morphology in psychopathy. *Psychiatry Research, 193*, 85–92.
27. Tiihonen, J., et al. (2008). Brain anatomy of persistent violent offenders: More rather than less. *Psychiatry Research, 163*, 201–212.
28. Ermer, E., Cope, L. M., Nyalakanti, P. K., Calhoun, V. D., & Kiehl, K. A. (2012). Aberrant paralimbic gray matter in criminal psychopathy. *Journal of Abnormal Psychology, 121*, 649–658.
29. Gregory, S., et al. (2012). The antisocial brain: Psychopathy matters. *Archives of General Psychiatry, 69*, 962–972.
30. Haller, J. (2014). *Neurobiological bases of abnormal aggression and violent behaviour*. Vienna: Springer.
31. Max, J. E., et al. (2006). Predictors of personality change due to traumatic brain injury in children and adolescents six to twenty-four months after injury. *The Journal of Neuropsychiatry and Clinical Neurosciences, 18*, 21–32.
32. Pardini, M., et al. (2011). Prefrontal cortex lesions and MAO-A modulate aggression in penetrating traumatic brain injury. *Neurology, 76*, 1038–1045.
33. Barrash, J., Tranel, D., & Anderson, S. W. (2000). Acquired personality disturbances associated with bilateral damage to the ventromedial prefrontal region. *Developmental Neuropsychology, 18*, 355–381.
34. Barrash, J., et al. (2011). Dimensions of personality disturbance after focal brain damage: Investigation with the Iowa scales of personality change. *Journal of Clinical and Experimental Neuropsychology, 33*, 833–852.
35. Tranel, D., Bechara, A., & Denburg, N. L. (2002). Asymmetric functional roles of right and left ventromedial prefrontal cortices in social conduct, decision-making, and emotional processing. *Cortex: A Journal Devoted to the Study of the Nervous System and Behavior, 38*, 589–612.

36. Choy, O., Raine, A., & Hamilton, R. H. (2018). Stimulation of the prefrontal cortex reduces intentions to commit aggression: A randomized, double-blind, placebo-controlled, stratified, Parallel-Group Trial. *Journal of Neuroscience, 38*, 6505–6512.
37. Gilam, G., et al. (2018). Attenuating anger and aggression with neuromodulation of the vmPFC: A simultaneous tDCS-fMRI study. *Cortex: A Journal Devoted to the Study of the Nervous System and Behavior, 109*, 156–170.
38. Dambacher, F., et al. (2015). Reducing proactive aggression through non-invasive brain stimulation. *Social Cognitive and Affective Neuroscience, 10*, 1303–1309.
39. Dambacher, F., et al. (2015). No effects of bilateral tDCS over inferior frontal gyrus on response inhibition and aggression. *PLoS One, 10*, e0132170.
40. Raine, A., et al. (1994). Selective reductions in prefrontal glucose metabolism in murderers. *Biological Psychiatry, 36*, 365–373.
41. Yang, Y., Joshi, S. H., Jahanshad, N., Thompson, P. M., & Baker, L. A. (2017). Neural correlates of proactive and reactive aggression in adolescent twins. *Aggressive Behavior, 43*, 230–240.
42. Boes, A. D., Tranel, D., Anderson, S. W., & Nopoulos, P. (2008). Right anterior cingulate: A neuroanatomical correlate of aggression and defiance in boys. *Behavioral Neuroscience, 122*, 677–684.
43. Ducharme, S., et al. (2011). Right anterior cingulate cortical thickness and bilateral striatal volume correlate with child behavior checklist aggressive behavior scores in healthy children. *Biological Psychiatry, 70*, 283–290.
44. Chester, D. S., Lynam, D. R., Milich, R., & DeWall, C. N. (2017). Physical aggressiveness and gray matter deficits in ventromedial prefrontal cortex. *Cortex: A Journal Devoted to the Study of the Nervous System and Behavior, 97*, 17–22.
45. Thijssen, S., et al. (2015). Brain morphology of childhood aggressive behavior: A multi-informant study in school-age children. *Cognitive, Affective, & Behavioral Neuroscience, 15*, 564–577.
46. Coccaro, E. F., et al. (2018). Reduced frontal grey matter, life history of aggression, and underlying genetic influence. *Psychiatry Research: Neuroimaging, 271*, 126–134.
47. Raine, A., Lencz, T., Bihrle, S., LaCasse, L., & Colletti, P. (2000). Reduced prefrontal gray matter volume and reduced autonomic activity in antisocial personality disorder. *Archives of General Psychiatry, 57*, 119–127; discussion 128–129.
48. Yang, Y., et al. (2005). Volume reduction in prefrontal gray matter in unsuccessful criminal psychopaths. *Biological Psychiatry, 57*, 1103–1108.
49. Goethals, I., et al. (2005). Brain perfusion SPECT in impulsivity-related personality disorders. *Behavioural Brain Research, 157*, 187–192.
50. Beckwith, T. J., Dietrich, K. N., Wright, J. P., Altaye, M., & Cecil, K. M. (2018). Reduced regional volumes associated with total psychopathy scores in an adult population with childhood lead exposure. *Neurotoxicology, 67*, 1–26.
51. Cha, J., et al. (2015). Neural correlates of aggression in medication-naive children with ADHD: Multivariate analysis of morphometry and Tractography. *Neuropsychopharmacology, 40*, 1717–1725.
52. Hazlett, E. A., et al. (2005). Reduced anterior and posterior cingulate gray matter in borderline personality disorder. *Biological Psychiatry, 58*, 614–623.
53. Bertsch, K., et al. (2018). Neural correlates of emotional action control in anger-prone women with borderline personality disorder. *Journal of Psychiatry & Neuroscience, 43*, 161–170.
54. Carrasco, J. L., et al. (2012). Microstructural white matter damage at orbitofrontal areas in borderline personality disorder. *Journal of Affective Disorders, 139*, 149–153.
55. Soloff, P., Nutche, J., Goradia, D., & Diwadkar, V. (2008). Structural brain abnormalities in borderline personality disorder: A voxel-based morphometry study. *Psychiatry Research, 164*, 223–236.
56. Soloff, P. H., Meltzer, C. C., Becker, C., Greer, P. J., & Constantine, D. (2005). Gender differences in a fenfluramine-activated FDG PET study of borderline personality disorder. *Psychiatry Research, 138*, 183–195.

57. Hirono, N., Mega, M. S., Dinov, I. D., Mishkin, F., & Cummings, J. L. (2000). Left fronto-temporal hypoperfusion is associated with aggression in patients with dementia. *Archives of Neurology, 57*, 861–866.
58. Fahim, C., et al. (2011). Neuroanatomy of childhood disruptive behavior disorders. *Aggressive Behavior, 37*, 326–337.
59. Raschle, N. M., Menks, W. M., Fehlbaum, L. V., Tshomba, E., & Stadler, C. (2015). Structural and functional alterations in right dorsomedial prefrontal and left insular cortex co-localize in adolescents with aggressive behaviour: An ALE meta-analysis. *PLoS One, 10*, e0136553.
60. Juhász, C., Behen, M. E., Muzik, O., Chugani, D. C., & Chugani, H. T. (2001). Bilateral medial prefrontal and temporal neocortical hypometabolism in children with epilepsy and aggression. *Epilepsia, 42*, 991–1001.
61. Goyer, P. F., et al. (1994). Positron-emission tomography and personality disorders. *Neuropsychopharmacology, 10*, 21–28.
62. Juengling, F. D., et al. (2003). Positron emission tomography in female patients with borderline personality disorder. *Journal of Psychiatric Research, 37*, 109–115.
63. Rosell, D. R., et al. (2010). Increased serotonin 2A receptor availability in the orbitofrontal cortex of physically aggressive personality disordered patients. *Biological Psychiatry, 67*, 1154–1162.
64. New, A. S., et al. (2002). Blunted prefrontal cortical 18fluorodeoxyglucose positron emission tomography response to meta-chlorophenylpiperazine in impulsive aggression. *Archives of General Psychiatry, 59*, 621–629.
65. Varkevisser, T., Gladwin, T. E., Heesink, L., van Honk, J., & Geuze, E. (2017). Resting-state functional connectivity in combat veterans suffering from impulsive aggression. *Social Cognitive and Affective Neuroscience, 12*, 1881–1889.
66. Antonucci, A. S., et al. (2006). Orbitofrontal correlates of aggression and impulsivity in psychiatric patients. *Psychiatry Research, 147*, 213–220.
67. Miskovich, T. A., et al. (2018). Abnormal cortical gyrification in criminal psychopathy. *NeuroImage: Clinical, 19*, 876–882.
68. Raine, A., Yang, Y., Narr, K. L., & Toga, A. W. (2011). Sex differences in orbitofrontal gray as a partial explanation for sex differences in antisocial personality. *Molecular Psychiatry, 16*, 227–236.
69. Sethi, A., et al. (2015). Emotional detachment in psychopathy: Involvement of dorsal default-mode connections. *Cortex: A Journal Devoted to the Study of the Nervous System and Behavior, 62*, 11–19.
70. Leutgeb, V., et al. (2016). Altered cerebellar-amygdala connectivity in violent offenders: A resting-state fMRI study. *Neuroscience Letters, 610*, 160–164.
71. Amen, D. G., Stubblefield, M., Carmicheal, B., & Thisted, R. (1996). Brain SPECT findings and aggressiveness. *Annals of Clinical Psychiatry, 8*, 129–137.
72. Ermer, E., Cope, L. M., Nyalakanti, P. K., Calhoun, V. D., & Kiehl, K. A. (2013). Aberrant paralimbic gray matter in incarcerated male adolescents with psychopathic traits. *Journal of the American Academy of Child and Adolescent Psychiatry, 52*, 94–103.e3.
73. Raine, A., et al. (1998). Reduced prefrontal and increased subcortical brain functioning assessed using positron emission tomography in predatory and affective murderers. *Behavioral Sciences & the Law, 16*, 319–332.
74. Laakso, M. P., et al. (2002). Prefrontal volumes in habitually violent subjects with antisocial personality disorder and type 2 alcoholism. *Psychiatry Research, 114*, 95–102.
75. da Cunha-Bang, S., et al. (2017). Serotonin 1B receptor binding is associated with trait anger and level of psychopathy in violent offenders. *Biological Psychiatry, 82*, 267–274.
76. Kolla, N. J., et al. (2015). Lower monoamine oxidase-a total distribution volume in impulsive and violent male offenders with antisocial personality disorder and high psychopathic traits: An [(11)C] Harmine Positron Emission Tomography Study. *Neuropsychopharmacology, 40*, 2596–2603.
77. Leutgeb, V., et al. (2015). Brain abnormalities in high-risk violent offenders and their association with psychopathic traits and criminal recidivism. *Neuroscience, 308*, 194–201.

78. Blair, R. J., Morris, J. S., Frith, C. D., Perrett, D. I., & Dolan, R. J. (1999). Dissociable neural responses to facial expressions of sadness and anger. *Brain: A Journal of Neurology, 122*(Pt 5), 883–893.
79. Hermans, E. J., Ramsey, N. F., & van Honk, J. (2008). Exogenous testosterone enhances responsiveness to social threat in the neural circuitry of social aggression in humans. *Biological Psychiatry, 63*, 263–270.
80. Sugiura, M., et al. (2009). Extraction of situational meaning by integrating multiple meanings in a complex environment: A functional MRI study. *Human Brain Mapping, 30*, 2676–2688.
81. Chester, D. S., Lynam, D. R., Milich, R., & DeWall, C. N. (2018). Neural mechanisms of the rejection-aggression link. *Social Cognitive and Affective Neuroscience, 13*, 501–512.
82. Siegrist, J., et al. (2005). Differential brain activation according to chronic social reward frustration. *Neuroreport, 16*, 1899–1903.
83. Abler, B., Walter, H., & Erk, S. (2005). Neural correlates of frustration. *Neuroreport, 16*, 669–672.
84. Dougherty, D. D., et al. (1999). Anger in healthy men: A PET study using script-driven imagery. *Biological Psychiatry, 46*, 466–472.
85. Kimbrell, T. A., et al. (1999). Regional brain activity during transient self-induced anxiety and anger in healthy adults. *Biological Psychiatry, 46*, 454–465.
86. Strenziok, M., et al. (2011). Developmental effects of aggressive behavior in male adolescents assessed with structural and functional brain imaging. *Social Cognitive and Affective Neuroscience, 6*, 2–11.
87. Montag, C., et al. (2012). Does excessive play of violent first-person-shooter-video-games dampen brain activity in response to emotional stimuli? *Biological Psychology, 89*, 107–111.
88. Yoder, K. J., Porges, E. C., & Decety, J. (2015). Amygdala subnuclei connectivity in response to violence reveals unique influences of individual differences in psychopathic traits in a nonforensic sample. *Human Brain Mapping, 36*, 1417–1428.
89. King, J. A., Blair, R. J. R., Mitchell, D. G. V., Dolan, R. J., & Burgess, N. (2006). Doing the right thing: A common neural circuit for appropriate violent or compassionate behavior. *NeuroImage, 30*, 1069–1076.
90. Wolf, D., et al. (2018). Central serotonin modulates neural responses to virtual violent actions in emotion regulation networks. *Brain Structure & Function, 223*, 3327–3345.
91. Repple, J., et al. (2017). From provocation to aggression: The neural network. *BMC Neuroscience, 18*, 73.
92. Skibsted, A. P., et al. (2017). Aggression-related brain function assessed with the point subtraction aggression paradigm in fMRI. *Aggressive Behavior, 43*, 601–610.
93. Klimecki, O. M., Sander, D., & Vuilleumier, P. (2018). Distinct brain areas involved in anger versus punishment during social interactions. *Scientific Reports, 8*, 10556.
94. Achterberg, M., van Duijvenvoorde, A. C. K., Bakermans-Kranenburg, M. J., & Crone, E. A. (2016). Control your anger! The neural basis of aggression regulation in response to negative social feedback. *Social Cognitive and Affective Neuroscience, 11*, 712–720.
95. New, A. S., et al. (2009). Laboratory induced aggression: A positron emission tomography study of aggressive individuals with borderline personality disorder. *Biological Psychiatry, 66*, 1107–1114.
96. Chester, D. S., & DeWall, C. N. (2016). The pleasure of revenge: Retaliatory aggression arises from a neural imbalance toward reward. *Social Cognitive and Affective Neuroscience, 11*, 1173–1182.
97. Lotze, M., Veit, R., Anders, S., & Birbaumer, N. (2007). Evidence for a different role of the ventral and dorsal medial prefrontal cortex for social reactive aggression: An interactive fMRI study. *NeuroImage, 34*, 470–478.
98. Buades-Rotger, M., Beyer, F., & Krämer, U. M. (2017). Avoidant responses to interpersonal provocation are associated with increased amygdala and decreased mentalizing network activity. *eNeuro, 4*, ENEURO.0337-16.2017.

99. Mehta, P. H., & Beer, J. (2010). Neural mechanisms of the testosterone-aggression relation: The role of orbitofrontal cortex. *Journal of Cognitive Neuroscience, 22*, 2357–2368.
100. Schneider, F., et al. (2000). Functional imaging of conditioned aversive emotional responses in antisocial personality disorder. *Neuropsychobiology, 42*, 192–201.
101. Herpertz, S. C., et al. (2001). Evidence of abnormal amygdala functioning in borderline personality disorder: A functional MRI study. *Biological Psychiatry, 50*, 292–298.
102. Heesink, L., et al. (2018). Neural activity during the viewing of emotional pictures in veterans with pathological anger and aggression. *European Psychiatry, 47*, 1–8.
103. Neumeister, P., et al. (2017). Interpersonal violence in posttraumatic women: Brain networks triggered by trauma-related pictures. *Social Cognitive and Affective Neuroscience, 12*, 555–568.
104. Veit, R., et al. (2010). Aberrant social and cerebral responding in a competitive reaction time paradigm in criminal psychopaths. *NeuroImage, 49*, 3365–3372.
105. Reyna, V. F., et al. (2018). Brain activation covaries with reported criminal behaviors when making risky choices: A fuzzy-trace theory approach. *Journal of Experimental Psychology. General, 147*, 1094–1109.
106. Pardini, D. A., & Phillips, M. (2010). Neural responses to emotional and neutral facial expressions in chronically violent men. *Journal of Psychiatry & Neuroscience, 35*, 390–398.
107. Bueso-Izquierdo, N., et al. (2016). Are batterers different from other criminals? An fMRI study. *Social Cognitive and Affective Neuroscience, 11*, 852–862.
108. da Cunha-Bang, S., et al. (2017). Violent offenders respond to provocations with high amygdala and striatal reactivity. *Social Cognitive and Affective Neuroscience, 12*, 802–810.
109. Tonnaer, F., Siep, N., van Zutphen, L., Arntz, A., & Cima, M. (2017). Anger provocation in violent offenders leads to emotion dysregulation. *Scientific Reports, 7*, 3583.
110. Volman, I., et al. (2016). Testosterone modulates altered prefrontal control of emotional actions in psychopathic offenders(1,2,3). *eNeuro, 3*, ENEURO.0107-15.2016.
111. Birbaumer, N., et al. (2005). Deficient fear conditioning in psychopathy: A functional magnetic resonance imaging study. *Archives of General Psychiatry, 62*, 799–805.
112. Berlin, H. A., Rolls, E. T., & Kischka, U. (2004). Impulsivity, time perception, emotion and reinforcement sensitivity in patients with orbitofrontal cortex lesions. *Brain: A Journal of Neurology, 127*, 1108–1126.
113. Blumer, D., & Benson, D. F. (1975). Personality changes with frontal and temporal lobe lesions. In D. Blumer & D. F. Benson (Eds.), *Psychiatric aspects of neurological disease* (pp. 151–169). New York: Grune & Stratton.
114. Shamay-Tsoory, S. G., Harari, H., Aharon-Peretz, J., & Levkovitz, Y. (2010). The role of the orbitofrontal cortex in affective theory of mind deficits in criminal offenders with psychopathic tendencies. *Cortex: A Journal Devoted to the Study of the Nervous System and Behavior, 46*, 668–677.
115. Deckel, A. W., Hesselbrock, V., & Bauer, L. (1996). Antisocial personality disorder, childhood delinquency, and frontal brain functioning: EEG and neuropsychological findings. *Journal of Clinical Psychology, 52*, 639–650.
116. Dinn, W. M., & Harris, C. L. (2000). Neurocognitive function in antisocial personality disorder. *Psychiatry Research, 97*, 173–190.
117. Gansler, D. A., et al. (2011). Prefrontal regional correlates of self-control in male psychiatric patients: Impulsivity facets and aggression. *Psychiatry Research, 191*, 16–23.
118. Matsuo, K., et al. (2009). A voxel-based morphometry study of frontal gray matter correlates of impulsivity. *Human Brain Mapping, 30*, 1188–1195.
119. Spitzer, M., Fischbacher, U., Herrnberger, B., Grön, G., & Fehr, E. (2007). The neural signature of social norm compliance. *Neuron, 56*, 185–196.
120. Herzberg, M. P., et al. (2018). Risk taking, decision-making, and brain volume in youth adopted internationally from institutional care. *Neuropsychologia, 119*, 262–270.
121. Koechlin, E. (2016). Prefrontal executive function and adaptive behavior in complex environments. *Current Opinion in Neurobiology, 37*, 1–6.

122. Romanski, L. M. (2012). Chapter 33: Convergence of auditory, visual, and somatosensory information in ventral prefrontal cortex. In M. M. Murray & M. T. Wallace (Eds.), *The neural bases of multisensory processes*. Boca Raton: CRC Press/Taylor & Francis.
123. Petrides, M. (2005). Lateral prefrontal cortex: Architectonic and functional organization. *Philosophical Transactions of the Royal Society of London. Series B, Biological Sciences, 360*, 781–795.
124. Hoshi, E., & Tanji, J. (2007). Distinctions between dorsal and ventral premotor areas: Anatomical connectivity and functional properties. *Current Opinion in Neurobiology, 17*, 234–242.
125. Miyachi, S., et al. (2005). Organization of multisynaptic inputs from prefrontal cortex to primary motor cortex as revealed by retrograde transneuronal transport of rabies virus. *Journal of Neuroscience, 25*, 2547–2556.
126. Abe, M., & Hanakawa, T. (2009). Functional coupling underlying motor and cognitive functions of the dorsal premotor cortex. *Behavioural Brain Research, 198*, 13–23.
127. Bie, B., Brown, D. L., & Naguib, M. (2011). Synaptic plasticity and pain aversion. *European Journal of Pharmacology, 667*, 26–31.
128. Shackman, A. J., et al. (2011). The integration of negative affect, pain and cognitive control in the cingulate cortex. *Nature Reviews. Neuroscience, 12*, 154–167.
129. Dixon, M. L., Thiruchselvam, R., Todd, R., & Christoff, K. (2017). Emotion and the prefrontal cortex: An integrative review. *Psychological Bulletin, 143*, 1033–1081.
130. Mai, J. K., Assheuer, J., & Paxinos, G. (1998). *Atlas of the human brain*. Amsterdam: Academic.
131. Bzdok, D., Laird, A. R., Zilles, K., Fox, P. T., & Eickhoff, S. B. (2013). An investigation of the structural, connectional, and functional subspecialization in the human amygdala. *Human Brain Mapping, 34*, 3247–3266.
132. Narabayashi, H., Nagao, T., Saito, Y., Yoshida, M., & Nagahata, M. (1963). Stereotaxic amygdalotomy for behavior disorders. *Archives of Neurology, 9*, 1–16.
133. Balasubramaniam, V., & Kanaka, T. S. (1975). Amygdalotomy and hypothalamotomy – A comparative study. *Confinia Neurologica, 37*, 195–201.
134. Heimburger, R. F., Whitlock, C. C., & Kalsbeck, J. E. (1966). Stereotaxic amygdalotomy for epilepsy with aggressive behavior. *JAMA, 198*, 741–745.
135. Hitchcock, E., & Cairns, V. (1973). Amygdalotomy. *Postgraduate Medical Journal, 49*, 894–904.
136. Lee, G. P., et al. (1998). Clinical and physiological effects of stereotaxic bilateral amygdalotomy for intractable aggression. *The Journal of Neuropsychiatry and Clinical Neurosciences, 10*, 413–420.
137. García-Muñoz, L., et al. (2019). Effect of unilateral amygdalotomy and hypothalamotomy in patients with refractory aggressiveness. *Gaceta Médica de México, 155*, S49–S55.
138. Faria, M. A. (2013). Violence, mental illness, and the brain – A brief history of psychosurgery: Part 3 – from deep brain stimulation to amygdalotomy for violent behavior, seizures, and pathological aggression in humans. *Surgical Neurology International, 4*, 91.
139. Gilliam, M., et al. (2015). Maternal depression in childhood and aggression in young adulthood: Evidence for mediation by offspring amygdala-hippocampal volume ratio. *Journal of Child Psychology and Psychiatry, 56*, 1083–1091.
140. De Brito, S. A., et al. (2009). Size matters: Increased grey matter in boys with conduct problems and callous-unemotional traits. *Brain: A Journal of Neurology, 132*, 843–852.
141. de Oliveira-Souza, R., et al. (2008). Psychopathy as a disorder of the moral brain: Fronto-temporo-limbic grey matter reductions demonstrated by voxel-based morphometry. *NeuroImage, 40*, 1202–1213.
142. Pardini, D. A., Raine, A., Erickson, K., & Loeber, R. (2014). Lower amygdala volume in men is associated with childhood aggression, early psychopathic traits, and future violence. *Biological Psychiatry, 75*, 73–80.

143. Farah, T., Ling, S., Raine, A., Yang, Y., & Schug, R. (2018). Alexithymia and reactive aggression: The role of the amygdala. *Psychiatry Research: Neuroimaging, 281*, 85–91.
144. Gopal, A., et al. (2013). Dorsal/ventral parcellation of the amygdala: Relevance to impulsivity and aggression. *Psychiatry Research, 211*, 24–30.
145. Fairchild, G., et al. (2013). Brain structure abnormalities in adolescent girls with conduct disorder. *Journal of Child Psychology and Psychiatry, 54*, 86–95.
146. Fairchild, G., et al. (2011). Brain structure abnormalities in early-onset and adolescent-onset conduct disorder. *The American Journal of Psychiatry, 168*, 624–633.
147. Poeppl, T. B., et al. (2019). A view behind the mask of sanity: Meta-analysis of aberrant brain activity in psychopaths. *Molecular Psychiatry, 24*, 463–470.
148. New, A. S., et al. (2007). Amygdala-prefrontal disconnection in borderline personality disorder. *Neuropsychopharmacology, 32*, 1629–1640.
149. Coccaro, E. F., Lee, R., McCloskey, M., Csernansky, J. G., & Wang, L. (2015). Morphometric analysis of amygdala and hippocampus shape in impulsively aggressive and healthy control subjects. *Journal of Psychiatric Research, 69*, 80–86.
150. Schiffer, B., et al. (2011). Disentangling structural brain alterations associated with violent behavior from those associated with substance use disorders. *Archives of General Psychiatry, 68*, 1039–1049.
151. Klasen, M., et al. (2018). Neural networks underlying trait aggression depend on MAOA gene alleles. *Brain Structure & Function, 223*, 873–881.
152. Barkataki, I., Kumari, V., Das, M., Taylor, P., & Sharma, T. (2006). Volumetric structural brain abnormalities in men with schizophrenia or antisocial personality disorder. *Behavioural Brain Research, 169*, 239–247.
153. Bertsch, K., et al. (2013). Brain volumes differ between diagnostic groups of violent criminal offenders. *European Archives of Psychiatry and Clinical Neuroscience, 263*, 593–606.
154. George, D. T., et al. (2004). A select group of perpetrators of domestic violence: Evidence of decreased metabolism in the right hypothalamus and reduced relationships between cortical/subcortical brain structures in position emission tomography. *Psychiatry Research, 130*, 11–25.
155. Yang, Y., Raine, A., Narr, K. L., Colletti, P., & Toga, A. W. (2009). Localization of deformations within the amygdala in individuals with psychopathy. *Archives of General Psychiatry, 66*, 986–994.
156. Kiehl, K. A., et al. (2018). Age of gray matters: Neuroprediction of recidivism. *NeuroImage: Clinical, 19*, 813–823.
157. Yu, R., Mobbs, D., Seymour, B., Rowe, J. B., & Calder, A. J. (2014). The neural signature of escalating frustration in humans. *Cortex: A Journal Devoted to the Study of the Nervous System and Behavior, 54*, 165–178.
158. Waller, R., et al. (2016). An oxytocin receptor polymorphism predicts amygdala reactivity and antisocial behavior in men. *Social Cognitive and Affective Neuroscience, 11*, 1218–1226.
159. Carré, J. M., Murphy, K. R., & Hariri, A. R. (2013). What lies beneath the face of aggression? *Social Cognitive and Affective Neuroscience, 8*, 224–229.
160. Fabiansson, E. C., Denson, T. F., Moulds, M. L., Grisham, J. R., & Schira, M. M. (2012). Don't look back in anger: Neural correlates of reappraisal, analytical rumination, and angry rumination during recall of an anger-inducing autobiographical memory. *NeuroImage, 59*, 2974–2981.
161. Repple, J., et al. (2018). Sex differences in the neural correlates of aggression. *Brain Structure & Function, 223*, 4115–4124.
162. Schöne, M., et al. (2019). Neurobiological correlates of violence perception in martial artists. *Brain and Behavior: A Cognitive Neuroscience Perspective, 9*, e01276.
163. Beaver, J. D., Lawrence, A. D., Passamonti, L., & Calder, A. J. (2008). Appetitive motivation predicts the neural response to facial signals of aggression. *Journal of Neuroscience, 28*, 2719–2725.

164. Van den Stock, J., Hortensius, R., Sinke, C., Goebel, R., & de Gelder, B. (2015). Personality traits predict brain activation and connectivity when witnessing a violent conflict. *Scientific Reports, 5*, 13779.
165. Decety, J., & Porges, E. C. (2011). Imagining being the agent of actions that carry different moral consequences: An fMRI study. *Neuropsychologia, 49*, 2994–3001.
166. Buades-Rotger, M., & Krämer, U. M. (2018). From words to action: Implicit attention to antisocial semantic cues predicts aggression and amygdala reactivity to angry faces in healthy young women. *Aggressive Behavior, 44*, 624–637.
167. da Cunha-Bang, S., et al. (2018). Men with high serotonin 1B receptor binding respond to provocations with heightened amygdala reactivity. *NeuroImage, 166*, 79–85.
168. Buades-Rotger, M., et al. (2016). Endogenous testosterone is associated with lower amygdala reactivity to angry faces and reduced aggressive behavior in healthy young women. *Scientific Reports, 6*, 38538.
169. Pawliczek, C. M., et al. (2013). Anger under control: Neural correlates of frustration as a function of trait aggression. *PLoS One, 8*, e78503.
170. Mathiak, K., & Weber, R. (2006). Toward brain correlates of natural behavior: fMRI during violent video games. *Human Brain Mapping, 27*, 948–956.
171. Glenn, A. L., Raine, A., & Schug, R. A. (2009). The neural correlates of moral decision-making in psychopathy. *Molecular Psychiatry, 14*, 5–6.
172. Minzenberg, M. J., Fan, J., New, A. S., Tang, C. Y., & Siever, L. J. (2007). Fronto-limbic dysfunction in response to facial emotion in borderline personality disorder: An event-related fMRI study. *Psychiatry Research, 155*, 231–243.
173. Koenigsberg, H. W., et al. (2009). Neural correlates of emotion processing in borderline personality disorder. *Psychiatry Research, 172*, 192–199.
174. Donegan, N. H., et al. (2003). Amygdala hyperreactivity in borderline personality disorder: Implications for emotional dysregulation. *Biological Psychiatry, 54*, 1284–1293.
175. Herpertz, S. C., et al. (2008). Emotional processing in male adolescents with childhood-onset conduct disorder. *Journal of Child Psychology and Psychiatry, 49*, 781–791.
176. Sterzer, P., Stadler, C., Krebs, A., Kleinschmidt, A., & Poustka, F. (2005). Abnormal neural responses to emotional visual stimuli in adolescents with conduct disorder. *Biological Psychiatry, 57*, 7–15.
177. Coccaro, E. F., McCloskey, M. S., Fitzgerald, D. A., & Phan, K. L. (2007). Amygdala and orbitofrontal reactivity to social threat in individuals with impulsive aggression. *Biological Psychiatry, 62*, 168–178.
178. Coccaro, E. F., et al. (2016). Differential fMRI BOLD responses in amygdala in intermittent explosive disorder as a function of past alcohol use disorder. *Psychiatry Research: Neuroimaging, 257*, 5–10.
179. McCloskey, M. S., et al. (2016). Amygdala hyperactivation to angry faces in intermittent explosive disorder. *Journal of Psychiatric Research, 79*, 34–41.
180. Cremers, H., Lee, R., Keedy, S., Phan, K. L., & Coccaro, E. (2016). Effects of escitalopram administration on face processing in intermittent explosive disorder: An fMRI study. *Neuropsychopharmacology, 41*, 590–597.
181. Michalska, K. J., Zeffiro, T. A., & Decety, J. (2016). Brain response to viewing others being harmed in children with conduct disorder symptoms. *Journal of Child Psychology and Psychiatry, 57*, 510–519.
182. Decety, J., Chen, C., Harenski, C. L., & Kiehl, K. A. (2015). Socioemotional processing of morally-laden behavior and their consequences on others in forensic psychopaths. *Human Brain Mapping, 36*, 2015–2026.
183. Marsh, A. A., et al. (2008). Reduced amygdala response to fearful expressions in children and adolescents with callous-unemotional traits and disruptive behavior disorders. *The American Journal of Psychiatry, 165*, 712–720.
184. Jones, A. P., Laurens, K. R., Herba, C. M., Barker, G. J., & Viding, E. (2009). Amygdala hypoactivity to fearful faces in boys with conduct problems and callous-unemotional traits. *The American Journal of Psychiatry, 166*, 95–102.

185. Cardinale, E. M., et al. (2018). Externalizing behavior severity in youths with callous-unemotional traits corresponds to patterns of amygdala activity and connectivity during judgments of causing fear. *Development and Psychopathology, 30*, 191–201.
186. Müller, J. L., et al. (2003). Abnormalities in emotion processing within cortical and subcortical regions in criminal psychopaths: Evidence from a functional magnetic resonance imaging study using pictures with emotional content. *Biological Psychiatry, 54*, 152–162.
187. Spoont, M. R., Kuskowski, M., & Pardo, J. V. (2010). Autobiographical memories of anger in violent and non-violent individuals: A script-driven imagery study. *Psychiatry Research, 183*, 225–229.
188. Lee, T. M. C., Chan, S. C., & Raine, A. (2008). Strong limbic and weak frontal activation to aggressive stimuli in spouse abusers. *Molecular Psychiatry, 13*, 655–656.
189. Larson, C. L., et al. (2013). The interplay of attention and emotion: Top-down attention modulates amygdala activation in psychopathy. *Cognitive, Affective, & Behavioral Neuroscience, 13*, 757–770.
190. Herpertz, S. C., et al. (2017). Brain mechanisms underlying reactive aggression in borderline personality disorder-sex matters. *Biological Psychiatry, 82*, 257–266.
191. Soloff, P. H., Abraham, K., Ramaseshan, K., Burgess, A., & Diwadkar, V. A. (2017). Hypermodulation of brain networks by the amygdala among women with Borderline Personality Disorder: Network signatures of affective interference during cognitive processing. *Journal of Psychiatric Research, 88*, 56–63.
192. Aghajani, M., et al. (2017). Disorganized amygdala networks in conduct-disordered juvenile offenders with callous-unemotional traits. *Biological Psychiatry, 82*, 283–293.
193. Aghajani, M., et al. (2016). Dissociable relations between amygdala subregional networks and psychopathy trait dimensions in conduct-disordered juvenile offenders. *Human Brain Mapping, 37*, 4017–4033.
194. Brinkmann, L., et al. (2017). Dissociation between amygdala and bed nucleus of the stria terminalis during threat anticipation in female post-traumatic stress disorder patients. *Human Brain Mapping, 38*, 2190–2205.
195. Hess, W. R. (1928). Stammganglien-Reizversuche. *Berichte Gesamt Physiol, 42*, 554–555.
196. Schvarcz, J. R., Driollet, R., Rios, E., & Betti, O. (1972). Stereotactic hypothalamotomy for behaviour disorders. *Journal of Neurology, Neurosurgery, and Psychiatry, 35*, 356–359.
197. Dieckmann, G., Schneider-Jonietz, B., & Schneider, H. (1988). Psychiatric and neuropsychological findings after stereotactic hypothalamotomy, in cases of extreme sexual aggressivity. *Acta Neurochirurgica. Supplementum (Wien), 44*, 163–166.
198. Ramamurthi, B. (1988). Stereotactic operation in behaviour disorders. Amygdalotomy and hypothalamotomy. *Acta Neurochirurgica. Supplementum (Wien), 44*, 152–157.
199. Pedrosa-Sánchez, M., & Sola, R. G. (2003). Modern day psychosurgery: A new approach to neurosurgery in psychiatric disease. *Revue Neurologique, 36*, 887–897.
200. Bejjani, B. P., et al. (2002). Aggressive behavior induced by intraoperative stimulation in the triangle of Sano. *Neurology, 59*, 1425–1427.
201. Franzini, A., Marras, C., Ferroli, P., Bugiani, O., & Broggi, G. (2005). Stimulation of the posterior hypothalamus for medically intractable impulsive and violent behavior. *Stereotactic and Functional Neurosurgery, 83*, 63–66.
202. Franzini, A., Messina, G., Cordella, R., Marras, C., & Broggi, G. (2010). Deep brain stimulation of the posteromedial hypothalamus: Indications, long-term results, and neurophysiological considerations. *Neurosurgical Focus, 29*, E13.
203. Hernando, V., Pastor, J., Pedrosa, M., Peña, E., & Sola, R. G. (2008). Low-frequency bilateral hypothalamic stimulation for treatment of drug-resistant aggressiveness in a young man with mental retardation. *Stereotactic and Functional Neurosurgery, 86*, 219–223.
204. Benedetti-Isaac, J. C., et al. (2015). Seizure frequency reduction after posteromedial hypothalamus deep brain stimulation in drug-resistant epilepsy associated with intractable aggressive behavior. *Epilepsia, 56*, 1152–1161.

205. Harat, M., Rudaś, M., Zieliński, P., Birska, J., & Sokal, P. (2015). Deep brain stimulation in pathological aggression. *Stereotactic and Functional Neurosurgery, 93*, 310–315.
206. Gouveia, F. V., et al. (2019). Amygdala and hypothalamus: Historical overview with focus on aggression. *Neurosurgery, 85*, 11–30.
207. Barbosa, D. A. N., et al. (2017). The hypothalamus at the crossroads of psychopathology and neurosurgery. *Neurosurgical Focus, 43*, E15.
208. Benazzouz, A., & Hallett, M. (2000). Mechanism of action of deep brain stimulation. *Neurology, 55*, S13–S16.
209. Rizzi, M., et al. (2017). Exploring the brain through posterior hypothalamus surgery for aggressive behavior. *Neurosurgical Focus, 43*, E14.
210. Mutic, S., Brünner, Y. F., Rodriguez-Raecke, R., Wiesmann, M., & Freiherr, J. (2017). Chemosensory danger detection in the human brain: Body odor communicating aggression modulates limbic system activation. *Neuropsychologia, 99*, 187–198.
211. Cacciola, A., et al. (2019). Mapping the structural connectivity between the periaqueductal gray and the cerebellum in humans. *Brain Structure & Function, 224*, 2153–2165.
212. Menant, O., Andersson, F., Zelena, D., & Chaillou, E. (2016). The benefits of magnetic resonance imaging methods to extend the knowledge of the anatomical organisation of the periaqueductal gray in mammals. *Journal of Chemical Neuroanatomy, 77*, 110–120.
213. Linnman, C., Moulton, E. A., Barmettler, G., Becerra, L., & Borsook, D. (2012). Neuroimaging of the periaqueductal gray: State of the field. *NeuroImage, 60*, 505–522.
214. White, S. F., Brislin, S. J., Sinclair, S., & Blair, J. R. (2014). Punishing unfairness: Rewarding or the organization of a reactively aggressive response? *Human Brain Mapping, 35*, 2137–2147.
215. Goetz, S. M. M., et al. (2014). Testosterone rapidly increases neural reactivity to threat in healthy men: A novel two-step pharmacological challenge paradigm. *Biological Psychiatry, 76*, 324–331.
216. Satpute, A. B., et al. (2013). Identification of discrete functional subregions of the human periaqueductal gray. *Proceedings of the National Academy of Sciences of the United States of America, 110*, 17101–17106.

Chapter 10
Biological Factors of Psychological Change

Introduction

One of the basic concepts of this book was that the various factors that control aggression and violence are hierarchically stratified. The earlier chapters investigated the system from genes to neurobiological mechanisms, which were interactively shaped by heredity and environmental influences mediated by glucocorticoids. Here we briefly overview the last level of the hierarchical system: the level where neurobiological mechanisms translate into psychological features.

Naturally, each mechanism addressed so far is important; nevertheless, the ultimate integration level is psychological. For example, we have very specific ideas about the genetic, endocrine, and neural mechanisms that control anger [1, 2] yet all these mechanisms converge into a feeling, which is a psychological concept.

Given the complexity of the psychology of aggression and violence, one cannot strive at its exhaustive presentation in a single chapter. Instead, we address here the basic mechanisms that mediate the translation of biological processes into risk factors of psychological malfunction and the impact of these on psychopathological and criminal violence.

10.1 From Biology to Psychology: Opponents and Historical Backgrounds

Not everybody shares the idea that social and biological processes are crucial for understanding psychopathological and criminal violence. A passionate criticism of the findings and concepts discussed throughout this book reads as follows. "People

J. Haller, *Neurobiopsychosocial Perspectives on Aggression and Violence*, Advances in Preventing and Treating Violence and Aggression,
https://doi.org/10.1007/978-3-030-46331-1_10

do not commit crime because, for example, they are male, teenagers or belong to an ethnic minority. [...] Neither do people commit crime because, for example, they are unemployed, have many siblings, a slow resting heart rate, a poor educational record, a particular gene, a mother who smoked during pregnancy, or grew up in public housing. [...] People commit acts of crime because they perceive and choose (habitually or after some deliberation) a particular kind of act of crime as an action alternative in response to a specific motivation [...]" (page 71 in [3]). Although the quotation refers to crime in general, violent crime is in the focus of the cited study, and its main idea can easily be generalized. Briefly, violent crime and, in more general terms, aggression are explained by the psychology of the moment not by ultimate causes of various sorts including social and biological antecedents.

Such "anti-sociological" and "anti-biological" viewpoints may be rooted in age-old concepts on the functioning of the mind and can be attributed indirectly to Aristotle, who divided the human mind (soul) into three major components [4]: a distinctive "vegetative soul," which operates the body and is present already in plants and therefore vegetative; an "animal soul" that controls basic needs (e.g., hunger); and a "thinking soul" that is specifically human. Possibly influenced by this age-old concept, many today still believe that our consciousness, thinking, personality, etc. (i.e., Aristotle's "thinking soul") are separate from other psychic functions and are to a great extent independent of the brain. The "vegetative" and "animal" souls may be the product of the brain, but the "thinking soul" may not. However, this is a philosophical position. In practice, we have seen in the earlier chapters that disturbed mental functioning is closely linked to disturbed brain function, which may be lesser or greater, but is always detectable. Of course, there is the possibility that, in addition to the psychological factors that are biologically based, there also are psychological functions that have no biological basis. This cannot be challenged or proved at this time and is therefore ignored.

In a way, we agree with the author of the quotation, because we also think that risk factors are not causes. Violence in many cases but not always can be explained as resulting from proximate choices rather than remote conditions and events (see below). Life-long inclinations towards certain types of decisions such as the seeking of situations and environments where violence can be expressed cannot, however, be understood in terms of momentary choices. In addition, it is difficult to imagine how can people deliberately chose to be mentally ill, because violent crime and psychopathologic aggression are often comorbid and share overlapping genetic, endocrine, and neural backgrounds.

Risk factors naturally do not replace proximate causes – this is where we agree with the quotation. Rather, they explain them and as such are crucially important. This last chapter is dedicated to this issue. We attempt to interpret the primarily biological approach adopted so far from a wider perspective. We begin the chapter with a simple diagram that summarizes our view, although we will explain this in much more detail later (see Fig. 10.1).

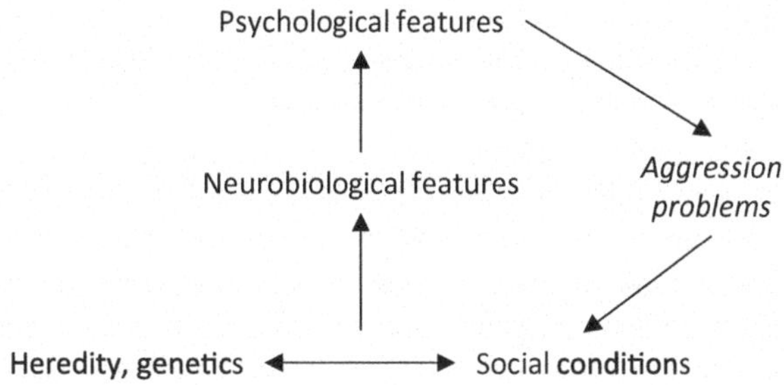

Fig. 10.1 Global relationships between risk factors for crime

10.2 Risks and Determinisms

10.2.1 Biology as a Risk Factor for Altered Psychology

A detailed presentation of the psychological factors of aggression and violence and of the way they derive from social and biological processes would require another book. Therefore, we will merely illustrate with examples how different types of risks emerge from each other and eventually become psychological risks.

The work selected as the first example [5] examined the relationship between genetic and social conditions as interacting risk factors for aggression. This relationship corresponds to that shown at the bottom of Fig. 10.1. The genetic predisposing factors chosen for the cited study were MAOA and COMT gene polymorphisms. Both were discussed above in the chapter on genetic factors. As a social factor, parenting style was studied. The study, based on data obtained from about 1400 adolescents, found that the two genetic predisposing factors promoted aggressiveness when combined with a negative (harsh) parenting style. The interplay of genetic and social risk factors was associated with a tendency to reactive aggression such as overreaction to both imaginary and real provocations, whereas proactive aggression did not depend on this specific gene–environment interaction, i.e., the interaction was specific to one aggression type.

The second example is a study on marginalized populations of the United States [6]. Most parents in the surveyed population belonged to the lowest income category and lived in sub-letted accommodation, and few had a college or university degree. Children who grew up in this environment were exposed to physical violence, early neglect, and trauma and were often raised in a criminal environment. Thus, their early childhood aggregated all the sociological risk factors described above. As adults, these individuals had lower than average plasma cortisol levels, identified above as a risk of crime, and proinflammatory responses to stress, which also constitutes a risk factor for lifetime aggression [7]. In addition, the study also identified an epigenetic risk, specifically the increased methylation of the gene encoding interleukin-6 which is a proinflammatory cytokine present in the brain. In short, this study is an example for the first upward arrow of Fig. 10.1, by showing how social factors affect neurobehavioral development by inducing epigenetic alterations and modifying cortisol secretion.

For a third example, we selected a study [1], which examined the relationships between brain function (a biological factor), two psychological phenomena, e.g., anger and rumination, and an aggression-related variable, e.g., the tendency to deliver punishment to an innocent third party. Participants were exposed to abusive remarks while in the functional magnetic resonance imaging device and were asked to reflect or ruminate on what they had heard. The intensities of anger and rumination, as investigated by psychological tests, were separately associated with the activation of two prefrontal regions, the anterior cingulate and medial prefrontal cortex, respectively. In addition, the latter was also associated with the subjects' tendency to punish people uninvolved in insulting by bursts of verbal aggression. This highlights the relationship between brain function, emotions, and violence, being in fact an experimental evidence for the second upward arrow of Fig. 10.1.

As stated above, it was not our intention here to describe such complex phenomena in detail. Our main goal was to highlight that the main assumption of this section, i.e., that risk factors are organized into a stratified system of interactions, is supported by empirical evidence and, within this system, biological change induces psychological change.

None of the interactions evidenced by these studies appear deterministic as all were statistical in nature. Social marginalization, low cortisol and inflammatory responses to stress, and the activation of the medial prefrontal cortex increased the likelihood of aggression but did not inevitably result in an aggressive response. Social and biological antecedents resulted in psychological features, e.g., impulsiveness and irritability that made aggressive outbursts only more likely. There are, however, biological phenomena that are more causally linked to aggression, e.g., those that are responsible for the technical execution of the behavior.

10.2.2 Biology as a Causal Factor

Aggression and violence depend on emotions, which may or may not be under control, and on cognitive decisions, which may or may not be well founded (see below). Beyond this level of integration, however, there are in addition brain mechanisms that ultimately control fixed action patterns collectively called aggression or violence based on their aim (biological approach), form (psychological approach), conformity with circumstances and normal functioning (psychiatric approach), or rules and law (law enforcement approach). Brain mechanisms directly controlling movements that organize into behavioral patterns, such as hypothalamic attack sites, motor brain areas, etc., are innate and are present in all individuals; moreover, all species studied so far and their ontogenetic emergence are part of the natural developmental program of the organism. Indeed, such innate neural mechanisms are indispensable for the execution of aggression as demonstrated by the findings of psychosurgery in humans and stimulation/lesion studies in animals.

One may consider such mechanisms as mere tools that are used by the organism to physically implement commands resulting from higher-order decision-making processes. Ostensibly, the carrying out of commands, as opposed to decision-making, has no psychological dimension. Yet, tools, even simpler ones such as knives, have properties that make them appropriate for a given purpose or which impede their proper use and, moreover, may have properties that make them dangerous. This holds true for the brain mechanisms that are responsible for the execution of movements that go to make up behavior.

To choose examples from the mechanisms discussed earlier, those that directly control the execution of attacks may lose their ability to be controlled by serotonin in abnormal models of animal aggression and in human psychopathologic and criminal aggression. In these cases, one of the main limiting factors of aggression was eliminated. Similarly, structural changes in the prefrontal cortex may shift the balance between inhibition and excitation such that executory commands sent to hypothalamic attack sites may overpower inhibitory commands sent to other brain areas. In more general terms, the set point of the system may be shifted due to genetic and/or developmental factors, which may make executory mechanisms more responsive to impulses.

These phenomena can be considered more deterministic than the ones discussed previously from two points of view. First, psychological functions need executory mechanisms, because decision cannot be implemented without them. For instance, flying needs both wings and neural mechanisms that control wings. Without these, one must invent devices to be able to fly. Similarly, the decision to fight needs brain mechanisms that can coordinate movements into a fight; if these mechanisms were lacking, anger never led to aggression. Note that while cases of "missing" aggression mechanisms were not reported so far, the neural mechanisms of aggression can be interrupted by surgery, and this eliminates aggressiveness, which demonstrates that the existence of innate aggression circuits are deterministically involved in the execution of aggression. Second, the innate or acquired properties of aggression circuitries, e.g., their sensitivity to stimulation, determine the way the organism will respond to a social challenge. Upregulated inhibitory mechanisms promote peacefulness, whereas the increased excitability of the circuitry promotes aggressiveness. These intrinsic properties of the system seem to determine inclinations which are manifested under all circumstances and define momentary decisions related to particular situations.

The existence of deterministic biological mechanisms raises a question that is metaphorically represented in the title of the next section.

10.2.3 Who Is Flying the Plane?

We deliberately reuse the metaphor by Siegel [8] for the second time in a book [9]: The metaphoric question nicely summarizes the essence of the problem. Are people freely choosing to be aggressive or violent as certain criminological theories suggest or are their choices determined by social conditions, as other criminological theories assume, or by their biological constitution as most studies referred to in this book suggest? In brief, is the metaphorical plane flown by free will – psychology – or biology?

Conceptualizing free will as the unimpeded ability to choose between possible options is compatible with the idea that most people are endowed with this capacity most of the time. Yet, there are at least two conditions which deprive them from this liberty, and both have repercussions for aggression. The first condition is related to emotions whereas the second to the ability to recognize the possible options.

The choices of those who are overcome with emotions, for instance, are not unimpeded as it is strongly limited by their own emotions as seen in reactive aggression. This is the first example for the dominating role of biology over free will: the deliberate cognitive choice between options is overshadowed by the physiological and psychological effects of emotions, which make the individual biased towards aggressive responses. If such emotional outbursts are frequent, the individual may be diagnosed with intermittent explosive disorder; moreover, s/he may be convicted for crime if anger outbursts inflict significant pain and damage on the victim.

The second example for the dominant role of biologic traits is based on findings showing that in certain psychopathologies, such as psychopathy, the prefrontal cortex is underdeveloped and, conversely, prefrontal injuries lead to a similar condition called acquired psychopathy. In this case, free will is not hampered by a stronger factor, such as emotion, but by the inability of recognizing all possibilities that are applicable in a situation. Such cognitive deficits were shown, among others, in antisocial personality disorder and violent crime, where the major aim of cognitive behavioral therapy is to make individuals aware of formerly unrecognized alternative possibilities of responding a challenge [10, 11]. We stress that these conditions are not equivalent with intellectual disability, which naturally can also limit the recognition of alternative behavioral options. Individuals with antisocial personality disorders, just like violent criminals, however, do not show generalized intellectual deficits, yet they still fail to consider options that are easily recognized by healthy and non-violent individuals. Deficits in recognizing non-aggressive options – whatever the reason was – limit the choices of individuals, which is in fact a limitation of free will.

We stress that the purpose of this argument was not to question the existence of free will; however, there are highly emotional situations when will becomes biased, and mental states that prevent the recognition of all alternative possibilities. In such specific cases, altered brain structure and/or function results in an altered psychology, which limits free will. This also weakens the position of those who exclusively attribute violent crime to deliberate momentary choices.

10.3 The Dual Mechanism of Aggression Control: A Hypothesis

As a general conclusion of this and previous chapters, we suggest that the mechanisms that lead to aggression-related psychopathologies and violent crime have two important sub-mechanisms (see Fig. 10.2).

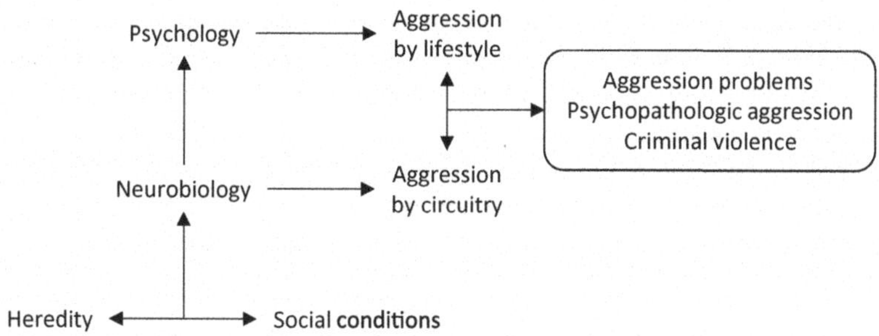

Fig. 10.2 The proposed dual mechanism of the emergence of aggression problems

Structural and functional alterations in the prefrontal cortex and amygdala disturb information processing, which leads to psychological deficits such as impulsiveness and irritability, lack of empathy and foresight, stress resilience or stress hyper-responsiveness, etc. These cognitive and emotional deficits lead to lifestyles and strategic decisions that make violence likely in general, especially when the unfavorable social conditions that contributed to the emergence of this psychological state persist. This was called "aggression by lifestyle" in Fig. 10.2 and predicts a long history of aggression and violence.

Diminished inhibitory and enhanced stimulatory control at neural level makes the aggression circuitry highly responsive to stimuli that activate it. Consequently, aggression is easily released from inhibition either by provocation or by the prospect of gain. This was called "aggression by circuitry" in Fig. 10.2 and predicts that aggression is easily triggered under various circumstances. Although this is a state-like feature, its persistence over time transforms it into a trait.

We suggest that aggression-related psychopathologies and violent crime emerge when the two mechanisms co-occur. If the circuitry can adequately be controlled, aggression-prone lifestyles may still allow the adaptation of behavior to circumstances, and avoiding of penalties. If living conditions are normal, the upregulation of the circuitry will only occasionally lead to aggression, which may be perceived less unfavorably by the social environment. The presence of one type of dysfunction may result in psychopathic traits but not psychopathy, in aggression histories but not criminal records. If, however, the two sub-mechanisms co-occur, aggression may reach levels that are abnormal from the point of view of both psychiatry and law.

10.4 Risks and Liability

As discussed in detail above, the proximate cause of crime in general and of violent crime in particular is a decision, yet such decisions are influenced by a series of risk factors, which can have a crucial impact on them. This unavoidably raises the question of legal responsibility, especially in the case of those who were exposed to multiple risk factors during their life and who also suffer from an aggression-related psychopathology. The question is extremely complex, and the answers given so far sometimes become philosophical. We believe, however, that addressing the issue is appropriate in a chapter already involved in discussing the relationship between free will and risk factors and by the end of a book that overviewed research findings and concepts that are highly relevant in this respect.

At present, there are four concurring positions on liability as follows:

1. The traditional view considers that those who are aware of their deeds and can differentiate rightful from wrong are responsible for all crimes they commit. Only intellectual disability or impaired cognition, such as psychosis, exempts someone from liability. This position is reluctant to consider risk factors due to limitations of judgment.
2. The representatives of the utilitarian position consider that all citizens have the right to live undisturbed by crime. In this regard, it does not matter whether the offender acted voluntarily or under the compelling effect of risk factors. S/he should be separated from the society for the sake of the potential victims. In this respect, the technique of separation, e.g., mental clinic or jail, is not particularly relevant.
3. According to the biomedical approach, the ability to make good decisions is often only apparent because the perpetrator acted under covert constraints. People who adopt this position would reduce the number of those sentenced to prison and increase the number of those referred to mental hospitals; however, perpetrators of crime would not be referred for separation but for medical treatment and healing.
4. According to the social reformer position, society, with very few exceptions, is guilty of crime, and the problem can be solved by transforming society, and criminals must not be punished but educated. It is expected that this long-term project would eliminate the very causes of crime as these are understood by criminological theories.

Each of the four positions, presented in a polarized manner, is logical and acceptable within its own terms; however, all four also have weaknesses. The traditional view does not tell us where to draw the line between the altered states of mind and the strength of the influence of risk factors. If the former is interpreted in a somewhat broader sense, this and the "biologizing" position become identical. The utilitarian position assumes that punishment discourages the perpetrator from repeating the crime, which seldom happens as shown by the high rates of recidivism worldwide. The biomedical approach is partly fueled by the belief that the propensity to commit a violent crime is curable, for which there is very little evidence. Finally, social welfare movements will probably need a very long time before reforms succeed, which lowers their chance of solving current problems.

The central problem with all four approaches, however, remains the elusive border between risk factors that can be overcome by personal effort and/or social reforms, those which have consequences that require medical treatment, and those that can be addressed by legal punishment only. To answer dilemmas of this kind, a new scientific field emerged, e.g., "neurolaw [12], which aims at integrating law and neuroscientific discoveries, e.g., those that were addressed in this book. The postscript will be devoted to the question of which this new science is the embodiment.

References

1. Denson, T. F., Pedersen, W. C., Ronquillo, J., & Nandy, A. S. (2009). The angry brain: Neural correlates of anger, angry rumination, and aggressive personality. *Journal of Cognitive Neuroscience, 21*, 734–744.
2. Wagels, L., et al. (2019). Exogenous testosterone and the monoamine-oxidase A polymorphism influence anger, aggression and neural responses to provocation in males. *Neuropharmacology, 156*, 107491.
3. Wikström, P.-O. H. (2014). Why crime happens: A situational action theory. In *Analytical sociology* (pp. 71–94). Wiley. https://doi.org/10.1002/9781118762707.ch03.
4. Aristotle. (2020). *De Anima (On the soul)*. Oxford: Oxford University Press.
5. Zhang, W., Cao, C., Wang, M., Ji, L., & Cao, Y. (2016). Monoamine Oxidase A (MAOA) and Catechol-OMethyltransferase (COMT) gene polymorphisms interact with maternal parenting in association with adolescent reactive aggression but not proactive aggression: Evidence of differential susceptibility. *Journal of Youth and Adolescence, 45*, 812–829.
6. Janusek, L. W., Tell, D., Gaylord-Harden, N., & Mathews, H. L. (2017). Relationship of childhood adversity and neighborhood violence to a proinflammatory phenotype in emerging adult African American men: An epigenetic link. *Brain, Behavior, and Immunity, 60*, 126–135.
7. Coccaro, E. F., et al. (2016). Tryptophan, kynurenine, and kynurenine metabolites: Relationship to lifetime aggression and inflammatory markers in human subjects. *Psychoneuroendocrinology, 71*, 189–196.
8. Siegel, A., & Douard, J. (2011). Who's flying the plane: Serotonin levels, aggression and free will. *International Journal of Law and Psychiatry, 34*, 20–29.
9. Haller, J. (2014). *Neurobiological bases of abnormal aggression and violent behaviour*. Vienna: Springer.
10. Davidson, K., Halford, J., Kirkwood, L., & Newton-Howes, G. (2010). CBT for violent men with antisocial personality disorder. Reflections on the experience of carrying out therapy in MASCOT, a pilot randomised controlled trial. *Personality and Mental Health, 4*, 86–95.
11. Vaske, J., Galyean, K., & Cullen, T. (2011). Toward a biosocial theory of offender rehabilitation: Why does cognitive-behavioral therapy work? *Journal of Criminal Justice, 39*, 90–102.
12. Jones, O. D., & Shen, F. X. (2012). Law and neuroscience in the United States. In M. T. Spranger (Ed.), *International neurolaw. A comparative analysis*. Berlin: Springer.

Postscript

Before closing this book, we invite the reader to a thought experiment. Suppose you are a judge who has to deal with a cocaine addict. The person provoked a mass fight in a public place, and that's why he came before you. During the procedure, the defender presents you with the photograph shown in Fig. A.1. Referring to the obvious differences between the two brains, the lawyer asks you to acquit the defendant because his liability is questionable: Cocaine altered his brain such that he is no longer able to assess the consequences of his actions. How will you decide?

Supposing that as a judge you are a layperson in neurosciences; as such, you may rightly wonder how to capture the brains of living people on a photograph? Furthermore, you might ask what is "brain metabolism," what is "brain disease," how does it relate to criminal behavior, etc. Now change roles and suppose the judge turns to you because you are an expert in the field. What would be your advice?

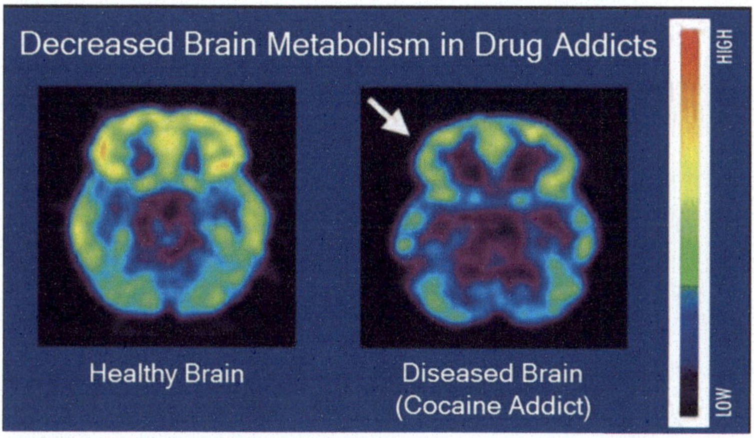

Fig. A.1 The photograph to be judged by the thought experiment

J. Haller, *Neurobiopsychosocial Perspectives on Aggression and Violence*, Advances in Preventing and Treating Violence and Aggression,
https://doi.org/10.1007/978-3-030-46331-1

This thought experiment is not entirely imaginary. Judges, lawyers, and policemen are faced with the advancement of neurobiology more and more frequently and are challenged with similar dilemmas as documented earlier in this book.

The importance of understanding the neurobiology of aggression cannot be better demonstrated than by the emergence of a science that specifically addresses similar questions. This science is called "neurolaw." To our best knowledge, the term is only about 25 years old, and at its beginnings aimed at addressing primarily legal issues, for instance, ensuring the best medical care and health insurance for those who suffered brain injuries. Later, around 2008–2009, the discipline began to make significant progress, and it was at that time that it formulated much more exciting questions by using neuroscience to investigate legal issues and providing expert neuroscientific opinion on legal responsibility.

Integrating law and neuroscience is naturally not easy because most legal experts have rather superficial and often false neuroscientific information, whereas most neuroscientists have even more superficial knowledge of law. As a result, training programs were initiated to teach neuroscience to legal experts, initially at the University of California and later at Vanderbilt University. Similar programs have already appeared in Europe.

One may wonder, however, whether neuroscience can adequately respond to this emerging public demand. Undoubtedly, the field evolved a great deal in recent decades. There have been major advances in animal research and brain imaging techniques related to aggression and violence. Looking objectively at the field, however, one must acknowledge that there is still much to do. The problem is not so much the scientific technology, although methods should and actually are continuously improved. Beyond technology, however, gaps can be attributed to a significant degree to the deficient integration of existing knowledge. The crosschecking of various fields of aggression research shows that communication between them is possible because in the case of behaviors as ancient as aggression, the four fields biology, psychology, psychiatry, and law enforcement address phenomena that derive one from another and are explained by similar and interconnected mechanisms. Second, integration is worthwhile, because each field has technologies, concepts, and findings that are useful for the other.

This book was a test to evaluate the prospects of, and to contribute modestly to future endeavors of a better integration.

Index

J. Haller, *Neurobiopsychosocial Perspectives on Aggression and Violence*, Advances in Preventing and Treating Violence and Aggression, https://doi.org/10.1007/978-3-030-46331-1

H

The manufacturer's authorised representative in the EU is Springer Nature Customer Service Centre GmbH, Europaplatz 3, 69115 Heidelberg, Germany. If you have any concerns regarding our products, please contact ProductSafety@springernature.com

Printed and bound by CPI Group (UK) Ltd, Croydon, CR0 4YY
30/09/2026
02225504-0013